MW01674436

Renal Replacement Therapy: An Issue of Nephrology Clinics

Renal Replacement Therapy: An Issue of Nephrology Clinics

Editor: Penny Summers

AMERICAN
MEDICAL PUBLISHERS
www.americanmedicalpublishers.com

AMERICAN
MEDICAL PUBLISHERS
www.americanmedicalpublishers.com

Cataloging-in-Publication Data

Renal replacement therapy : an issue of nephrology clinics / edited by Penny Summers.
p. cm.
Includes bibliographical references and index.
ISBN 978-1-63927-275-4
1. Hemodialysis. 2. Therapeutics. 3. Kidneys--Diseases--Treatment. 4. Nephrology. I. Summers, Penny.
RC901.7.H45 R46 2021
617.461 059--dc23

© American Medical Publishers, 2021

American Medical Publishers,
41 Flatbush Avenue,
1st Floor, New York,
NY 11217, USA

ISBN 978-1-63927-275-4 (Hardback)

This book contains information obtained from authentic and highly regarded sources. Copyright for all individual chapters remain with the respective authors as indicated. All chapters are published with permission under the Creative Commons Attribution License or equivalent. A wide variety of references are listed. Permission and sources are indicated; for detailed attributions, please refer to the permissions page and list of contributors. Reasonable efforts have been made to publish reliable data and information, but the authors, editors and publisher cannot assume any responsibility for the validity of all materials or the consequences of their use.

Trademark Notice: Registered trademark of products or corporate names are used only for explanation and identification without intent to infringe.

Contents

Preface

Over the recent decade, advancements and applications have progressed exponentially. This has led to the increased interest in this field and projects are being conducted to enhance knowledge. The main objective of this book is to present some of the critical challenges and provide insights into possible solutions. This book will answer the varied questions that arise in the field and also provide an increased scope for furthering studies.

Renal replacement therapy is a therapy in which normal blood-filtering function of the kidneys is replaced. It is primarily used during renal failure when the kidneys are not functioning properly and involves acute and chronic kidney diseases. Hemodiafiltration, dialysis and hemofiltration are the therapies used in this domain. These therapies help in the filtration of blood with or without machines. The process of hemodialysis, hemofiltration and hemodiafiltration can be continuous or intermittent. It uses either an arteriovenous route or a venovenous route. Kidney transplantation also falls under the umbrella of renal replacement therapy. This book unravels the recent studies in the field of renal replacement therapy. It strives to provide a fair idea about this discipline and to help develop a better understanding of the latest advances within this field. This book will serve as a valuable source of reference for graduate and post graduate students.

I hope that this book, with its visionary approach, will be a valuable addition and will promote interest among readers. Each of the authors has provided their extraordinary competence in their specific fields by providing different perspectives as they come from diverse nations and regions. I thank them for their contributions.

Editor

1

Kocuria kristinae septic arthritis associated with infectious endocarditis in a hemodialysis patient with diabetes mellitus

Taro Horino*, Yoshiko Shimamura, Koji Ogata, Kosuke Inoue and Yoshio Terada

Abstract

Background: *Kocuria kristinae* is an aerobic Gram-positive coccus that is considered ubiquitous and non-pathogenic in healthy individuals. Furthermore, only 27 reports have described cases of critical infections with this microorganism, which is notoriously difficult to identify.

Case presentation: We report the case of a 61-year-old male hemodialysis patient with diabetes mellitus, who developed severe septic arthritis that was associated with infectious endocarditis, which was identified using ^{18}F-fluorodeoxyglucose positron-emission tomography/computed tomography (FDG-PET-CT). *K. kristinae* was identified in two separate blood cultures. The patient recovered immediately after being treated using piperacillin followed by ampicillin/sulbactam and gentamicin.

Conclusions: To the best of our knowledge, this is the first case of *K. kristinae* septic arthritis associated with infectious endocarditis in a hemodialysis patient with diabetes mellitus. We suggest that physicians consider the pathogenic potential of *K. kristinae*, which can cause fatal infections, such as septic arthritis and infectious endocarditis, in immunocompromised patients. FDG-PET-CT is a useful and safe diagnostic tool for determining the cause of inflammatory disease in dialysis patients.

Keywords: *Kocuria kristinae*, Septic arthritis, Infectious endocarditis, Hemodialysis, FDG-PET-CT

Background

In Japan, the number of patients with diabetes is increasing every year, as is the rate of renal replacement therapy (RRT) for treating diabetic nephropathy. Both end-stage renal disease (ESRD) and diabetes mellitus are severe immunocompromised states, and dialysis patients are prone to infectious complications. Furthermore, we believe that patients with diabetes mellitus are predisposed to invasive infections. Therefore, we describe the case of a hemodialysis patient who had a wound infection and bacteremia with *Kocuria kristinae*, which is a microorganism that is considered non-pathogenic in healthy individuals. In addition, we provide a review of case reports regarding *K. kristinae* infections in humans.

* Correspondence: horinott@yahoo.co.jp
Department of Endocrinology, Metabolism and Nephrology, Kochi Medical School, Kohasu, Okoh-cho, Nankoku 783-8505, Kochi, Japan

Case presentation

A 61-year-old male hemodialysis patient with a history of diabetes mellitus and polyarthralgia was referred to our hospital. Two months before the referral, the patient had arthralgia of the right knee, which exhibited swelling, tenderness, and restricted motion. The patient subsequently experienced severe polyarthralgia that involved both shoulders, wrists, hip joints, foot joints, and the left knee joint, as well as rapidly progressing severe lumbago. At the admission, his temperature was 36.6 °C. A physical examination revealed swelling and warmth in all joints that the patient identified as being painful. The laboratory test results are shown in Table 1. A chest radiograph revealed mild cardiomegaly without other remarkable findings. Joint radiographs revealed no deformities. Magnetic resonance imaging (MRI) of the left hip joint revealed high-intensity lesions surrounding

Table 1 Laboratory data at admission

CBC (normal range)		Blood chemistry		Tumor markers		Blood culture	
RBC (400–552)	$239 \times 10^4/mm^3$	FBS (70–110)	179 mg/dL	CEA (<3.4)	0.8 ng/mL	*Kocuria kristinae*	(+)
Hb (13.2–17.2)	6.9 g/dL	Alp (104–338)	501 U/L	CA19-9 (<37)	2.8 U/mL	Antimicrobial susceptibilities (MIC)	μg/mL
Ht (40.4–51.1)	21.9 %	γ-GTP (5–70)	41 U/L	Infection		Penicillin	0.12
Plt (14.8–33.9)	$46.8 \times 10^4/mm^3$	t-Bil (0.2–1.2)	0.3 mg/dL	HBs Ag	(−)	Oxacillin	≤2.0
WBC (3.6–9.6)	$5.6 \times 10^3/mm^3$	d-Bil (0–0.4)	0.0 mg/dL	HCV Ab	(−)	Ampicillin	≤0.25
neu	73.0 %	ChE (168–470)	123 U/L	HTLV-I Ab	(−)	Cefazolin	≤8.0
lym	8.0 %	ALT (8–42)	24 U/L	EBV		Cefotaxime	≤8.0
mon	13.0 %	AST (13–33)	37 U/L	VCA-IgG	×640	cefepime	≤8.0
eos	6.0 %	LDH (119–229)	125 U/L	VCA-IgM	×<10	Cefotiam	≤8.0
bas	0.0 %	CPK (62–287)	10 U/L	EBNA	×20	Cefpirome	≤8.0
aty-ly	0.0 %	Crn (0.6–1.1)	10.3 mg/dL	Mumps	(−)	Cefozopran	≤8.0
Electrolytes		BUN (8–20)	52 mg/dL	Herpes zoster	(−)	Cefmetazole	≤16.0
Na (136–145)	137 mmol/L	UA (3.4–7.8)	8.5 mg/dL	Parvovirus B19	(−)	Cefdinir	≤1.0
K (3.4–4.5)	4.4 mmol/L	Amy (37–125)	71 U/L	Syphilis	(−)	Cefditoren	≤1.0
Cl (100–108)	99 mmol/L	TG (30–150)	106 mg/dL	QFT	(−)	Flomoxef	≤8.0
Ca (8.7–11.0)	10.2 mg/dL	H-Chol (>40)	17 mg/dL	Candida Ab	(−)	Imipenem/cilastatin	≤4.0
P (2.5–4.5)	4.7 mg/dL	L-Chol (<140)	61 mg/dL	β-D-glucan	(−)	Meropenem	≤4.0
Mg (1.8–2.4)	2.5 mg/dL	Serological examinations		Chlamydia trachomatis		Amoxicillin	≤4.0
Proteinogram		CRP (<0.3)	35.5 mg/dL	IgG	(−)	Gentamicin	≤4.0
TP (6.7–8.1)	7.1 g/dL	SAA (<8.0)	1843.9 mg/mL	IgA	(−)	Amikacin	≤16.0
Alb (3.9–4.9)	2.6 g/dL	MMP-3 (36.9–121.0)	586.4 ng/mL	Chlamydia pneumoniae		Arbekacin	≤4.0
Glb	4.5 g/dL	CH50 (30–45)	47.0 U/mL	IgG	(−)	Erythromycin	≤0.5
α1	11.2 %	C3 (65–135)	131.5 mg/dL	IgA	(−)	Clarithromycin	≤2.0
α2	16.6 %	C4 (13–35)	31.7 mg/dL	Synovial fluid		Clindamycin	≤0.5
β	10.7 %	ANA	(−)	Glossly purulent material		Minocycline	≤4.0
γ	34.3 %	ds-DNA Ab	(−)	WBC	$13,200 \times 10^3/mm^3$	Linezolid	≤2.0
IgG (870–1700)	2519 mg/dL	SSA Ab	(−)	neu	95.0 %	Vancomycin	≤2.0
IgA (110–410)	497 mg/dL	SSB Ab	(−)	pla	5.0 %	Teicoplanin	≤8.0
IgM (35–220)	87 mg/dL	RF	(−)	Crystals	(−)	Fosfomycin	≤4.0

Table 1 Laboratory data at admission *(Continued)*

M-protein	(–)	ACPA	(–)	Culture	(–)	Levofloxacin	≤1.0
HbA1c (4.6–6.2)	7.9 %	MPO-ANCA	(–)			Sulfamethoxazole/trimethoprim	≤2.0
ESR (<20)	>140 mm/h	PR3-ANCA	(–)			Rifampicin	≤1.0

Abbreviations: *CBC* complete blood cell count, *RBC* red blood cell count, *Hb* hemoglobin, *Ht* hematocrit, *Plt* platelet, *ESR* erythrocyte sedimentation rate, *WBC* white blood cell count, *neu* neutrophils, *lym* lymphocytes, *mon* monocytes, *eos*eosinophils, *bas* basophils, *aty-ly* atypical lymphocytes, *Na* sodium, *K* potassium, *Cl* chlorine, *Ca* calcium, *P* phosphorus, *Mg* magnesium, *TP* total protein, *Alb* albumin, *Glb* globulin, *IgG* immunoglobulin G, *IgA* immunoglobulin A, *IgM* immunoglobulin M, *FBS* fasting blood sugar, *Alp* alkaline phosphatase, *γ-GTP* γ-glutamyltransferase, *t-Bil* total bilirubin, *d-Bil* direct bilirubin, *ChE* cholinesterase, *ALT* alanine transaminase, *AST* aspartate aminotransferase, *LDH* lactate dehydrogenase, *CPK* creatine phosphokinase, *Crn* creatinine, *BUN* blood urea nitrogen, *UA* uric acid, *Amy* amylase, *TG* triglyceride, *H-Chol* high-density lipoprotein cholesterol,
L-Chol low-density lipoprotein cholesterol, *CRP* C-reactive protein, *SAA* serum amyloid A, *MMP-3* matrix metalloproteinase-3, *CH50* complement activity, *C3* complement 3, *C4* complement 4, *ANA* antinuclear antibody, *SSA Ab* anti-SS-A/Ro antibody,*SSB Ab* anti-SS-B/La antibody, *RF* rheumatoid factor, *ACPA* anti-cyclic citrullinated peptide antibody, *MPO-ANCA* myeloperoxidase-anti-neutrophil cytoplasmic antibody, *PR3-ANCA* serine proteinase3-anti-neutrophil cytoplasmic antibody, *HBs Ab* hepatitis B surface antigen, *HCV Ab* hepatitis C virus antibody, *HTLV-I Ab* human T-lymphotropic virus type 1 antibody,*pla* plasma cell, *EBV* Epstein-Barr virus, *VCA* viral capsid antigen, *EBNA* Epstein-Barr nuclear antigen, *QFT* QuantiFERON-TB, *pla* plasma cell

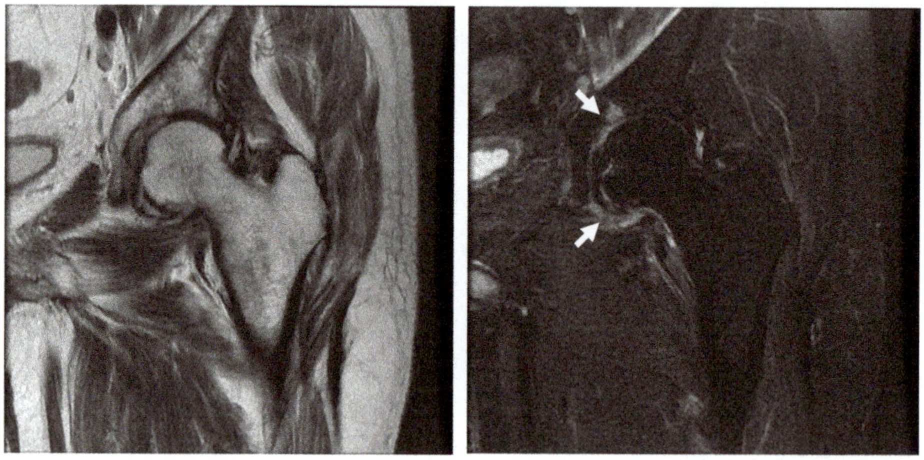

Fig. 1 The magnetic resonance imaging findings. The magnetic resonance findings from the left hip joint reveal high-intensity lesions (*white arrows*) surrounding the head of the femoral bone in the T2-weighted image (*right panel*)

the head of the femoral bone on the T2-weighted image (Fig. 1).^{18}F-fluorodeoxyglucose positron-emission tomography/computed tomography (FDG-PET-CT) revealed short segments of increased FDG uptake within the shoulders, wrists, hip joints, knees, and foot joints (Fig. 2). We had performed arthrocentesis at the admission, and an aspiration specimen from the right knee joint yielded grossly purulent material. Synovial fluid white cell counts were 13,200/mm^3, with 95 % polymorphonuclear leukocytes and 5 % monomorphonuclear leukocytes. Although the synovial fluid culture was negative, clusters of Gram-positive cocci were isolated from a blood specimen that was taken at the admission. Two blood cultures were both positive for *K. kristinae*, and these results were confirmed using the Vitek 2 system. The isolate was sensitive to all tested antibiotics (Table 1). We started treatment using intravenous piperacillin (2 g once per day), and the polyarthritis immediately improved. After 14 days of antibiotic treatment, the

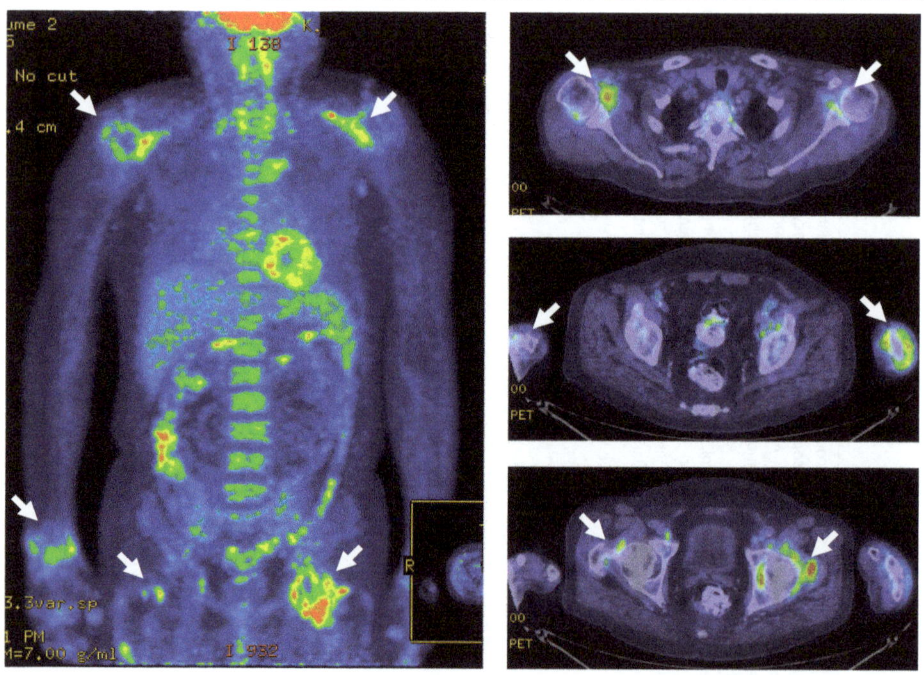

Fig. 2 The ^{18}F-fluorodeoxyglucose positron-emission tomography/computed tomography findings. ^{18}F-fluorodeoxyglucose positron-emission tomography/computed tomography reveals short segments of increased fluorodeoxyglucose uptake (*white arrows*) within the shoulders, wrists, hip joints, knees, and foot joints

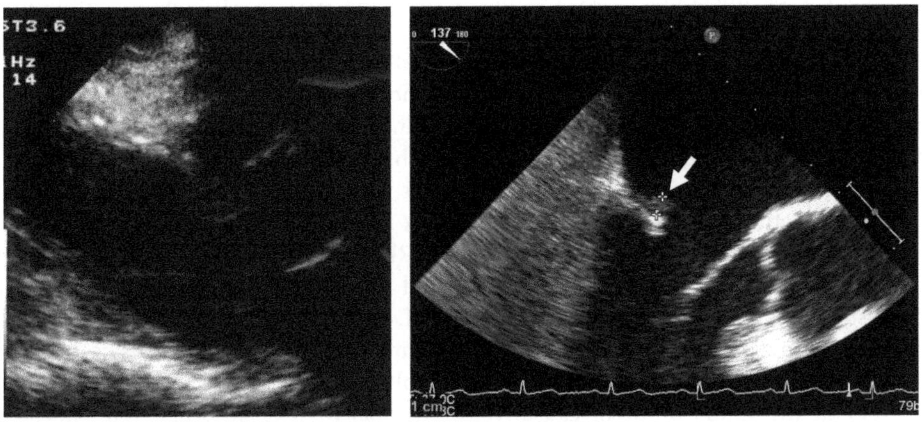

Fig. 3 The echocardiography findings. (*Left panel*) Echocardiography reveals no remarkable findings at 2 years before the presentation. (*Right panel*) Echocardiography at 1 month after the admission reveals mitral valve vegetation

patient's C-reactive protein levels were 0.8 mg/dL and the other laboratory data were normalized.

Electrocardiography detected no remarkable findings during his clinical course. However, 1 month after the admission, echocardiography detected vegetation on the mitral valve, which was compatible with infectious endocarditis (Fig. 3, right panel), although there had been no findings of vegetation at 2 years before the admission (Fig. 3, left panel). Physical examination after the echocardiography revealed Janeway's lesions, although we did not detect Osler's nodes or Roth's spots. Therefore, we stopped the intravenous piperacillin therapy and started treatment using intravenous ampicillin/sulbactam (1.5 g every other day) and intravenous gentamicin (100 mg every other day). The patient's clinical course was uneventful, and he was later discharged to our outpatient clinic (Fig. 4).

Discussion

K. kristinae was first described as *Micrococcus kristinae* in 1974 and was subsequently classified as *Micrococcus* spp., which is now separated into *Micrococcus*, *Nesterenkonia*, *Kytococcus*, *Dermacoccus*, and *Kocuria* [1, 2]. *K. kristinae* is a strictly aerobic species that is commonly identified among skin and oral flora [3]. Most physicians consider *Micrococcus* spp. (including *Kocuria*) nonpathogenic, and we initially assumed that the blood cultures from the present case were negative for pathogenic

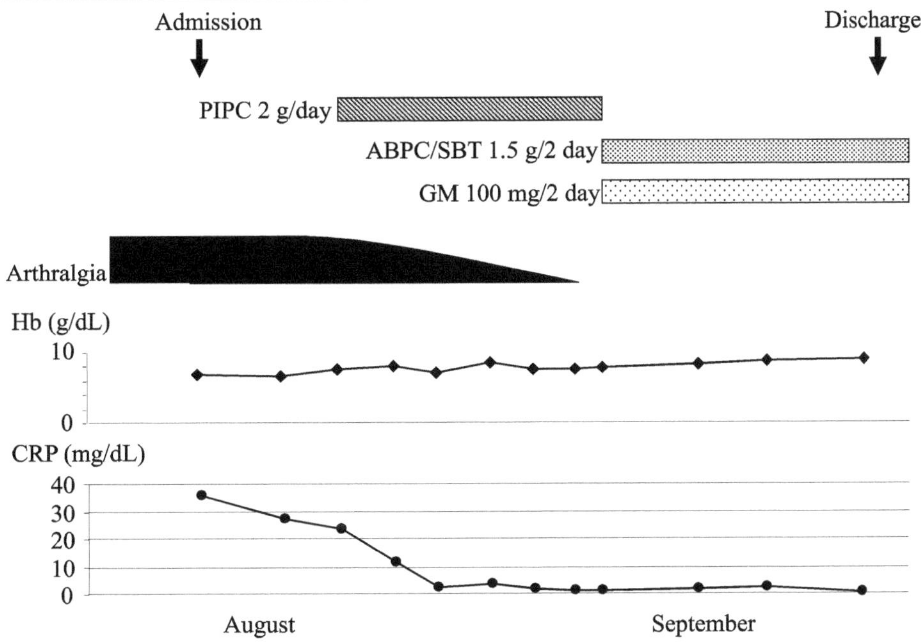

Fig. 4 The patient's clinical course. *PIPC* piperacillin, *APBC* ampicillin, *SBT* sulbactam, *GM* gentamicin, *Hb* hemoglobin, *CRP* C-reactive protein

bacteria. However, reports of infectious diseases that were caused by this species are gradually being published. The clinical characteristics of the 28 reported cases of *K. kristinae* infections are summarized in Tables 2 and 3 [4–16]. Most *K. kristinae* infections are reported as infections in immunocompromised hosts or patients with underlying malignancy, ESRD requiring dialysis, diabetes mellitus, and prematurity. Although published reports of *K. kristinae* infections are rare, the prevalence of this infection, especially among immunocompromised hosts, may be underestimated, as most physicians likely do not consider this organism as a pathogen.

Patients who are receiving RRT often have infectious diseases, although the identification of their causative microorganism(s) and focus of infection are difficult to accurately diagnose. Furthermore, patients who are receiving RRT are frequently immunocompromised and may have atypical infectious organisms that are considered normal bacterial flora in healthy individuals [17]. Among patients who are undergoing RRT, the host's immunity may be compromised by uremia that interferes with T cell and B cell function, macrophage phagocytosis, and antigen presentation, which can increase the risk of infection [17]. The population of patients with ESRD who receive RRT has been increasing worldwide, and this population included 314,180 Japanese patients in December 2013 [18]. Furthermore, the number of patients with diabetes mellitus is increasing, and diabetic nephropathy has recently become the leading cause (43.8 %) of RRT in Japan [18]. Because ESRD and diabetes mellitus can both lead to an immunocompromised status and increase susceptibility to unusual infections,

Table 2 Demographic data, treatments, and outcomes for 28 patients with *Kocuria kristinae* infections

Case	Antibiotic regimen	Course (days)	TPN	Outcome	Ref.	Year
1	Meropenem + glycopeptide → ciprofloxacin + clindamycin → catheter removal	NA	NA	Recovery	4	2002
2	Levofloxacin	14	No	Recovery	5	2005
3	Ceftriaxone + ofloxacin	16	NA	Death	6	2008
4	Azithromycin + ceftriaxone + vancomycin + oseltamivir → vancomycin + clindamycin → oxacillin	42	Yes	Recovery	7	2011
5	Vancomycin → teicoplanin → oxacillin	NA	Yes	Recovery	8	2011
6	Piperacillin/tazobactam → ciprofloxacin	NA	Yes	Recovery	8	2011
7	Oxacillin + vancomycin	NA	Yes	Recovery	8	2011
8	Oxacillin	NA	Yes	Recovery	8	2011
9	Tobramycin → cefotaxime + tazobactam → ciprofloxacin + teicoplanin + amoxicillin/clavulanic acid	24	No	Recovery	9	2011
10	Cefazolin + cefepime	14	No	Recovery	10	2011
11	Ceftriaxone + vancomycin	14	Yes	Recovery	11	2012
12	Ceftriaxone + metronidazole → sulbactam/ampicillin + gentamicin	25	No	Death	12	2013
13	No antibiotics	No	No	Unknown	13	2013
14	Dicloxacillin + vancomycin + levofloxacin	21	No	Recovery	14	2014
15	Ceftriaxone + amikacin + cefotaxime	16	No	Recovery	14	2014
16	Vancomycin	10	NA	Recovery	15	2014
17	Vancomycin	7	NA	Recovery	15	2014
18	Levofloxacin	7	NA	Recovery	15	2014
19	Linezolid	14	NA	Recovery	15	2014
20	Vancomycin	5	NA	Recovery	15	2014
21	Vancomycin + ceftazidime	10	Yes	Recovery	16	2015
22	Vancomycin	10	Yes	Recovery	16	2015
23	Vancomycin + ceftazidime	10	Yes	Recovery	16	2015
24	Oxacillin + vancomycin	9	Yes	Recovery	16	2015
25	Vancomycin + cefotaxime	12	Yes	Recovery	16	2015
26	Vancomycin + cefotaxime	10	Yes	Recovery	16	2015
27	Vancomycin + piperacillin/tazobactam	10	No	Recovery	16	2015
28	Piperacillin → ampicillin/sulbactam + gentamicin	30	No	Recovery	Current	2015

TPN total parenteral nutrition, *NA* not available

Table 3 Clinical, demographic, and bacterial data from 28 patients with *Kocuria kristinae* infections

Case	Age, year (month)	Sex	Country	Underlying disease	Isolation site	Catheters	Clinical presentation
1	51	F	Italy	Ovarian cancer, chemotherapy	Blood, catheter tip	CVC	Febrile neutropenia, sepsis
2	56	M	Hong Kong	Gallstones	Biliary fluid	No	Acute cholecystitis
3	68	M	France	MDS, acute myelogenous leukemia, tuberculosis, chemotherapy	Blood	CVC	Sepsis
4	29	F	USA	Pregnancy, hyperemesis gravidarum	Blood	CVC	Suppurative thrombosis
5	89	F	Taiwan	Post-resection ischemic bowel status, short bowel syndrome	Blood	CVC	Endocarditis
6	37	F	Taiwan	Gastric cancer	Blood	CVC	Bacteremia
7	2	M	Taiwan	Congenital short bowel syndrome, hypogammaglobulinemia	Blood	CVC	Bacteremia
8	68	F	Taiwan	Gastric cancer	Blood	CVC	Bacteremia
9	78	M	Italy	ESRD on CAPD	Peritoneal fluid	PDC	Peritonitis
10	69	M	China	ESRD on CAPD	Peritoneal fluid	PDC	Peritonitis
11	0 (4.0)	F	Turkey	Prolonged diarrhea, severe failure to thrive	Blood	CVC	Black hairy tongue, fever, bacteremia
12	74	M	Italy	Diabetes mellitus	Blood	No	Foot ulcer, endocarditis, sepsis
13	20	M	India	Urethral stricture	Urine	UC	Malaise
14	20	F	Mexico	ESRD on HD	Blood	CVC	Bacteremia
15	68	M	Mexico	ESRD on CAPD	Peritoneal fluid	PDC	Peritonitis
16	65	M	India	Lung small cell carcinoma	Sputum	NA	Leukocytosis (neutrophillia)
17	65	M	India	Carcinoma soft palate	Sputum	NA	Leukocytosis (neutrophillia)
18	41	F	India	Carcinoma lip and gingival sulcus	Sputum	NA	Leukocytosis (neutrophillia)
19	39	M	India	Squamous cell carcinoma of the buccal mucosa	pus	NA	Leukocytosis (neutrophillia)
20	42	F	India	Ductal carcinoma of the breast	pus	NA	Leukocytosis (neutrophillia)
21	0 (1.4)	M	Taiwan	Prematurity	Blood	CVC	Sepsis
22	0 (0.6)	M	Taiwan	Prematurity	Blood	CVC	Sepsis
23	0 (0.7)	F	Taiwan	Prematurity	Blood	CVC	Sepsis
24	0 (1.1)	F	Taiwan	Prematurity	Blood	CVC	Sepsis
25	0 (0.6)	F	Taiwan	Prematurity	Blood, catheter tip	CVC	Sepsis
26	0 (0.6)	F	Taiwan	Prematurity	Blood, catheter tip	CVC	Sepsis
27	0 (2.5)	F	Taiwan	Leukemia	Blood, catheter tip	CVC	Neutropenic fever
28	61	M	Japan	ESRD on HD, diabetes mellitus	Blood	No	Septic arthritis, endocarditis

Age is presented as year (month)
Abbreviations: *ESRD* end-stage renal disease, *CAPD* chronic ambulatory peritoneal dialysis, *HD* hemodialysis, *CVC* central venous catheter, *PDC* peritoneal dialysis catheter, *UC* urinary catheter

patients with ESRD and diabetes mellitus are likely very susceptible to uncommon and usually non-pathogenic microorganisms. However, *Kocuria* spp. infections are rarely reported among patients with diabetes and RRT. We speculate that there are two reasons for this phenomenon. First, most physicians believe that *Kocuria* spp., *Micrococcus* spp., and especially *K. kristinae* are non-pathogenic and might not consider these organisms as potentially causative organisms, despite observing positive culture results. Second, most *Kocuria* spp. and *Micrococcus* spp. are sensitive to almost all antibiotics (except ampicillin and erythromycin), and monotherapy often results in good outcomes [19]. In this context, Japanese investigators have reported that the causes of fever of unknown origin (FUO) are infection (27.7 %), non-infectious inflammatory disease (18.4 %), malignancy

(10.2 %), other conditions (14.8 %), and unknown causes (28.9 %) [20]. Thus, given the frequency of an unknown cause of FUO, we usually use empirical antibiotics to treat infections of unknown origin until culture results are available. Therefore, it is possible that repeating cultures will not identify the same microorganisms in each culture, as the empirical antibiotics might cure the infection without severe clinical events (e.g., sepsis) before the second sample is collected. Interestingly, infection is the primary cause of death among Japanese patients who are receiving RRT (26.5 %) [19], and it is likely that the number of patients with diabetes and RRT is going to continue increasing. Furthermore, the population of elderly Japanese patients is also increasing, which will likely result in a larger number of immunocompromised hosts. Based on these factors, it is possible that an increasing number of patients may have underlying *K. kristinae* infection that is not diagnosed until they develop severe complications, such as bacteremia and endocarditis. Therefore, it may be prudent to assess the pathogenic capacity of *K. kristinae* and any other unusual microorganisms, even if an infection of unknown origin improves after antibiotic monotherapy in patients who are elderly, have diabetes, or are receiving RRT. Moreover, clinicians should not underestimate the importance of a positive culture result for *K. kristinae*, as patients may experience repeated infections, develop severe infectious complications, and possibly die from this infection.

During recent years, many investigators have reviewed the diagnostic value of FDG-PET-CT. Although FDG was first developed to trace brain metabolism [21], FDG-PET-CT has subsequently been recognized as an early diagnostic tool that has high sensitivity for malignancies, such as melanoma and cervical, lung, breast, gastrointestinal, ovarian, and prostatic cancers [22]. Furthermore, recent studies have found that FDG-PET-CT could detect the existence of inflammatory diseases and determine their severity and extent [23]. Although contrast-enhanced CT and/or MRI are performed for diagnosing and examining malignancies, infections, and autoimmune diseases, the use of contrast agents for these techniques is often contraindicated in patients with severe renal insufficiency, as these agents increase the incidence of their adverse effects. In contrast, FDG-PET-CT is considered safer and simpler for dialysis patients, compared to contrast-enhanced CT or MRI. Therefore, we suggest that FDG-PET-CT should be used for diagnosing and evaluating dialysis patients if the origin of their disease is unclear and that physicians should not delay this diagnostic imaging, which can lead to a poor prognosis.

Conclusions

We report the first case of *K. kristinae* septic arthritis associated with infectious endocarditis in a chronic hemodialysis patient with diabetes mellitus. We suggest that physicians should consider the pathogenic potential of *K. kristinae*, as it can cause fatal infections (e.g., septic arthritis and infectious endocarditis) in immunocompromised patients or patients with diabetes and RRT. We also suggest that FDG-PET-CT is a very useful and safe diagnostic tool, which can help identify the focus of inflammatory disorders in dialysis patients.

Consent

Written informed consent was obtained from the patient for publication of this case report and the accompanying images. A copy of the written consent is available for review by the Editor-in-Chief of this journal.

Competing interests

The authors declare that they have no competing interests.

Authors' contributions

TH, YS, KO, and KI performed the laboratory testing. TH and YT drafted the manuscript. All authors read and approved the final manuscript.

References

1. Kloos WE, Tornabene TG, Schleifer KH. Isolation and characterization of micrococci from human skin, including two new species: *Micrococcus lylae* and *Micrococcus kristinae*. Int J Syst Evol Bacteriol. 1974;24:79–101.
2. Stackebrandt E, Koch C, Gvozdiak O, Schumann P. Taxonomic dissection of the genus *Micrococcus*: *Kocuria*gen. nov., *Nesterenkonia*gen. nov., *Kytococcus*gen. nov., *Dermacoccus* gen. nov., and *Micrococcus* Cohn 1872 gen. emend. Int J Syst Bacteriol. 1995;45:682–92.
3. Cordero MR, Zumalacárregui JM. Characterization of micrococcaceae isolated from salt used for Spanish dry-cured ham. Lett Appl Microbiol. 2000;31:303–6.
4. Basaglia G, Carretto E, Barbarini D, et al. Catheter-related bacteremia due to *Kocuria kristinae*in a patient with ovarian cancer. J Clin Microbiol. 2002;40:311–3.
5. Ma ES, Wong CL, Lai KT, et al. *Kocuria kristinae* infection associated with acute cholecystitis. BMC Infec Dis. 2005;5:60.
6. Martinaud C, Gaillard T, Brisou P, Gisserot O, de Jaureguiberry JP. Bacteremia caused by *Kocuria kristinae* in a patient with acute leukemia. Med Mal Infect. 2008;38:165–6 [in French].
7. Dunn R, Bares S, David MZ. Central venous catheter-related bacteremia caused by *Kocuria kristinae*: case report and review of the literature. Ann Clin Microbiol Antimicrob. 2011;10:31.
8. Lai CC, Wang JY, Lin SH, et al. Catheter-related bacteraemia and infective endocarditis caused by *Kocuria*species. Clin Microbiol Infect. 2011;17:190–2.
9. Calini A, Mattei R, Lucarotti I, Bartelloni A, Rosati A. *Kocuria kristinae*: an unusual cause of acute peritoneal dialysis-related infection. Perit Dial Int. 2011;31:105–7.
10. Cheung C, Cheng N, Chau C, Li CS. An unusual organism for CAPD related peritonitis: *Kocuria kristinae*. Perit Dial Int. 2011;31:107–8.
11. Karadag Oncel E, Boyraz MS, Kara A. Black tongue associated with *Kocuria* (*Micrococcus*) *kristinae* bacteremia in a 4-month-old infant. Eur J Pediatr. 2012;171:593.
12. Citro R, Prota C, Greco L, et al. *Kocuria kristinae* endocarditis related to diabetic foot infection. J Med Microbiol. 2013;62:932–4.
13. Tewari R, Dudeja M, Das AK, Nandy S. *Kocuria kristinae* in catheter associated urinary tract infection: a case report. J Clin Diagn Res. 2013;7:1692–3.
14. Chávez Valencia V, Orizaga de la Cruz C, Aguilar Bixano O, Huerta Ruíz MK, Sánchez Estrada EE. Infections due to *Kocuria kristinae*: case reports of two patients and review of the literature. Gac Med Mex. 2014;150 Suppl 2:183–5 [in Spanish].

15. Ahmed NH, Biswal I, Roy P, Grover RK. *Kocuria kristinae*, an unusual pathogen causing opportunistic infections in patients with malignancy. Indian J Med Microbiol. 2014;32:456–8.
16. Chen HM, Chi H, Chiu NC, Huang FY. *Kocuria kristinae*: a true pathogen in pediatric patients. J Microbiol Immunol Infect. 2015;48:80–4.
17. Leone S, Suter F. Severe bacterial infections in haemodialysis patients. Infez Med. 2010;18:79–85.
18. Masakane I, Nakai S, Ogata S, et al. An overview of regular dialysis treatment in Japan (as of 31 December 2013). Ther Apher Dial. 2015;19:540–74.
19. Szczerba I. Susceptibility to antibiotics of bacteria from genera *Micrococcus, Kocuria, Nesternkonia, Kytococcus* and *Dermacoccus*. Med Dosw Mikrobiol. 2003;55:75–80 [in Polish].
20. Yamanouchi M, Uehara Y, Yokokawa H, et al. Analysis of 256 cases of classic fever of unknown origin. Intern Med. 2014;53:2471–5.
21. Reivich M, Kuhl D, Wolf A, et al. The [18F] fluorodeoxyglucose method for the measurement of local cerebral glucose utilization in man. Circ Res. 1979;44:127–37.
22. Gallamini A, Zwarthoed C, Borra A. Positron emission tomography (PET) in oncology. Cancers (Basel). 2014;6:1821–89.
23. Balink H, Verberne HJ, Bennink RJ, van Eck-Smit BL. A rationale for the use of F18-FDG PET/CT in fever and inflammation of unknown origin. Int J Mol Imaging. 2012. doi: 10.1155/2012/165080.

Associations between fluid removal and number of B-lines, peak early mitral inflow wave velocity, and inferior vena cava dimensions in hemodialysis patients

Kazuo Kimura[1,2], Katsuya Kajimoto[3], Shigeru Otsubo[1,4*], Takashi Akiba[2] and Kosaku Nitta[1]

Abstract

Background: The inferior vena cava (IVC) dimensions represent the right ventricular preload, whereas the peak early mitral inflow wave velocity (peak E-velocity) represents the left ventricular preload. On the other hand, B-lines represent extravascular lung water. The aim of this study was to evaluate possible acute changes in the IVC dimensions, peak E-velocity, and number of B-lines during hemodialysis therapy.

Methods: A total of 55 consecutive patients receiving maintenance hemodialysis were enrolled in this study. We performed echo-graphic examinations at three time points (just after the start, during the middle, and just before the end of the hemodialysis therapy). We then investigated the changes in the IVC dimensions, peak E-velocity, and number of B-lines.

Results: The peak E-velocity decreased from 80 ± 26 cm/s at the start of the therapy to 58 ± 22 cm/s during the middle and 51 ± 21 cm/s at the end of the therapy. The IVC dimensions also decreased from 15 ± 4 mm at the start of the therapy to 12 ± 3 mm during the middle and 11 ± 3 mm at the end of the therapy. The number of B-lines also decreased from 12 ± 5 at the start of the therapy to 9 ± 4 during the middle and 5 ± 3 at the end of the therapy. The changes in the peak E-velocity and IVC dimensions were significantly greater during the first half of the dialysis period than during the second half of the dialysis period ($P < 0.0001$ and $P < 0.0001$, respectively). On the other hand, the changes in the number of B-lines during these periods were significantly smaller during the first half of the dialysis period than during the second half of the dialysis period ($P = 0.0016$).

Conclusions: We showed that the peak E-velocity and the IVC dimensions were reduced mainly during the first half of the dialysis period, while the number of B-lines showed a significant decrease mainly during the last half of the dialysis period. Even if the IVC dimensions are reduced sufficiently, caution is needed as lung congestion may still exist.

Keywords: B-lines, Early diastolic filling velocity, Early diastolic filling wave, Hemodialysis, Inferior vena cava, Lung ultrasound

* Correspondence: sotsubo@hb.tp1.jp
[1]Department of Medicine, Kidney Center, Tokyo Women's Medical University, Tokyo, Japan
[4]Department of Blood Purification, Tohto Sangenjaya Clinic, 2-13-2 Taishido, Setagaya-ku, Tokyo 154-0004, Japan
Full list of author information is available at the end of the article

Background

Chronic fluid overloading frequently occurs in hemodialysis patients, so volume assessment during hemodialysis is a primary, and often challenging, goal of nephrologists. Volume overload is directly associated with hypertension, increased arterial stiffness, left ventricular hypertrophy, heart failure, and ultimately higher rates of mortality and morbidity [1].

Lung ultrasound has recently been shown to be a useful, noninvasive technique for the assessment of extravascular lung water [2]. The most commonly observed finding was a comet tail artifact fanning out from the lung-wall interface and spreading upwards to the edge of the screen, previously named a "B-line" [3]. In patients with heart failure, the number of B-lines was correlated with the degree of extravascular lung water [4, 5]. Lung ultrasound is also reportedly useful for the accurate evaluation of dry weight and fluid status in hemodialysis patients [2, 6, 7].

The inferior vena cava (IVC) dimensions represent the right ventricular preload [8], whereas the peak early mitral inflow wave velocity (peak E-velocity) represents the left ventricular preload [9, 10]. On the other hand, B-lines represent extravascular lung water. The aim of this study was to evaluate possible acute changes in IVC dimensions, peak E-velocity, and B-lines during hemodialysis therapy.

Methods

A total of 55 patients receiving maintenance hemodialysis at Sekikawa Hospital and in whom more than 1 kg was removed during hemodialysis were enrolled in this study. Patients with lung disease or chest injury were excluded from this study.

Clinical data including age, sex, duration of hemodialysis therapy, presence of diabetes mellitus and/or hypertension and/or dyslipidemia complications, and the results of biological examinations were collected from the patients' clinical records. Hypertension was defined as a systolic blood pressure of 140 mmHg or higher, a diastolic blood pressure of 90 mmHg or higher, and/or the current use of antihypertensive drugs. Diabetes mellitus was defined as a fasting glucose level ≥ 126 mg/dL, a nonfasting glucose level ≥ 200 mg/dL, or the use of medication. Dyslipidemia was defined as a low-density lipoprotein cholesterol level ≥ 140 mg/dL, a high-density lipoprotein cholesterol level < 40 mg/dL, a triglyceride level ≥ 150 mg/dL, or the use of medication.

A peripheral blood sample was obtained before hemodialysis during the first session of the week. The serum N-terminal pro-brain natriuretic peptide (NT-proBNP) level in the pre-dialysis blood sample was measured using an electrochemiluminescence immunoassay on an Elecsys platform (Roche, Basel, Switzerland).

A lung ultrasound examination was performed during the first session of the week (at the same time as the peripheral blood sample preparation) using Vscan® (GE Healthcare, Japan), which is a hand-held ultrasound device with a wide-bandwidth phased-array probe (1.7–3.5 MHz) [11, 12]. Bilateral scanning of the anterior and lateral chest walls was performed with the patient in a supine position. An intercostal scan with a maximum extension of the visual pleural line was performed. The chest wall was divided into eight areas (two anterior and two lateral areas per side), and one scan was obtained for each area [13]. The anterior zone of the chest wall was designated from the sternum to the anterior axillary line and was then divided into upper and lower halves (from the clavicle to the third intercostal spaces and from the third space to the diaphragm). The lateral zone was positioned from the anterior axillary line to the posterior axillary line and was also divided into the upper and lower halves. The investigators attempted to detect comet tail artifacts fanning out from the lung-wall interface and spreading to the edge of the screen, which were previously named as B-lines (Fig. 1) [5, 6]. The total number of B-lines was estimated. Echocardiographic measurements were obtained at the same time, and the IVC dimensions and peak E-velocity were estimated. We performed echographic examinations three times (just after the start, just in the middle (for example, 2 h after the start of hemodialysis therapy if the treatment time is 4 h), and just before the end of the hemodialysis therapy). We then investigated the changes in the IVC dimensions, peak E-velocity, and B-lines. This study was conducted in accordance with the principles of the Declaration of Helsinki and was permitted by the research ethics committee of Sekikawa Hospital (Approved No. H2705). The data were expressed as the means ± SD or median (interquartile range, IQR). Paired t tests were used to examine changes in the variables.

All the statistical calculations were performed using JMP 5.1 software. P values less than 0.05 were considered statistically significant.

Results

The patient background characteristics are shown in Table 1. The mean age was 75 ± 11 years. Elderly patients were common in this study. Diabetic nephropathy was the major cause of end-stage kidney disease. Hypertension, diabetes mellitus, and dyslipidemia were present in 89.1, 47.3, and 16.4% of the study participants, respectively. The results of the biochemistry analyses,

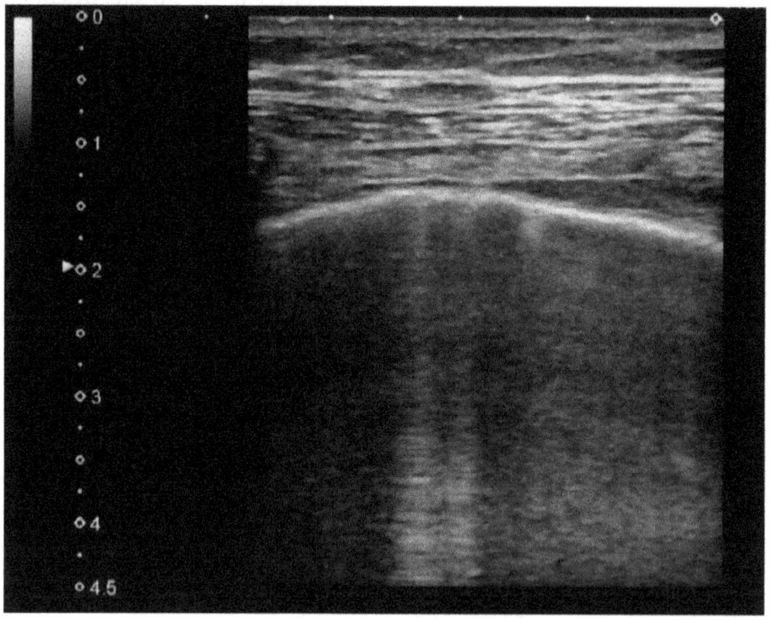

Fig. 1 B-lines—comet tail artifacts fanning out from the lung-wall interface and spreading upwards to the edge of the screen

Table 1 Background characteristics of the study participants

Characteristic	Quantity
Gender (M/F)	26/29
Age (year)	75 ± 11
Duration of HD (year)	6.5 ± 8.8
Primary cause of ESKD, *n* (%)	
Chronic glomerulonephritis	8 (14.5)
Diabetic nephropathy	26 (47.3)
Nephrosclerosis	13 (23.6)
Unknown and others	8 (14.5)
Hypertention, *n* (%)	49 (89.1)
Diabetes mellitus, *n* (%)	26 (47.3)
Dyslipidemia, *n* (%)	9 (16.4)
Atrial fibrillation, *n* (%)	8 (14.5)
History of PCI or CABG	8 (14.5)
History of valve replacement	2 (3.6)[a]
Body weight (kg)	52.0 ± 10.9
Systolic blood pressure (mmHg)	147 ± 25
Diastolic blood pressure (mmHg)	74 ± 15
Heart rate (beat/min)	75 ± 13

Mean ± SD, median (interquartile range)
HD hemodialysis, *ESKD* end-stage kidney disease, *PCI* percutaneous coronary intervention, *CABG* coronary artery bypass graft
[a]Both patients underwent aortic valve replacement therapy

including the NT-proBNP level, are shown in Table 2. The serum albumin level was relatively low (3.1 ± 0.5 g/dL), and the serum NT-proBNP level was relatively high (13,650 [4901–35,825] pg/mL) among the study participants. Table 3 shows the background characteristics of the echocardiographic indices. The mean ejection fraction was 60% ± 12%.

The treatment time was 3.7 ± 0.4 h, and 2.1 ± 0.9 kg water was removed. The blood pressure and pulse rate were 146 ± 25/74 ± 15 mmHg and 75 ± 13 beats/min at the first echo examination, 134 ± 24/72 ± 14 mmHg and 72 ± 16 beats/min at the second, 132 ± 27/73 ± 16 mmHg and 73 ± 15 beats/min at the final examination. Table 4 shows the changes in the echocardiographic indices. The peak E-velocity decreased from 80 ± 26 cm/s at the start of the therapy to 58 ± 22 cm/s during the middle and 51 ± 21 cm/s at the end of the therapy. The IVC dimensions also decreased from 15 ± 4 mm at the start of the

Table 2 Background characteristics of laboratory data

Characteristic	Quantity
Albumin (g/dL)	3.1 ± 0.5
Urea nitrogen (mg/dL)	50.2 ± 18.3
Creatinine (mg/dL)	7.36 ± 2.56
Sodium (mEq/L)	137 ± 4
C-reactive protein (mg/dL)	0.27 (0.10–0.86)
Hemoglobin (g/dL)	10.4 ± 1.2
NT-proBNP (pg/mL)	13,650 (4901–35,825)

Mean ± SD, median (interquartile range)
NT-proBNP N-terminal pro-brain natriuretic peptide

Table 3 Background characteristics of the echocardiographic indices

Parameter	Value
LVDd (mm)	46 ± 6
LVDs (mm)	31 ± 7
EF (%)	60 ± 14
Max WT (mm)	12 ± 2

Mean ± SD
LVDd left ventricular diastolic diameter, *LVDs* left ventricular systolic diameter, *EF* ejection fraction, *WT* wall thickness

therapy to 12 ± 3 mm during the middle and 11 ± 3 mm at the end of the therapy. The number of B-lines also decreased from 12 ± 5 at the start of the therapy to 9 ± 4 during the middle and 5 ± 3 at the end of the therapy (also shown in Fig. 2).

Table 5 shows a comparison of the changes in values between the middle to pre-dialysis periods and the post-dialysis to middle periods. The changes in the peak E-velocity and the IVC dimensions were significantly greater during the first half of the dialysis period than during the second half of the dialysis period ($P < 0.0001$ and $P < 0.0001$, respectively). On the other hand, the changes in the B-lines between these periods was significantly smaller during the first half of the dialysis period than during the second half of the dialysis period ($P = 0.0016$).

Figure 3 shows a representative case in this study. The peak E-velocity and IVC dimensions decreased mainly during the first half of the dialysis period, while the number of B-lines decreased steadily throughout the dialysis period.

Discussion

We found that the peak E-velocity and IVC dimensions decreased significantly mainly during the first half of the dialysis period, while the number of B-lines decreased significantly mainly during the last half of the dialysis period.

Lung ultrasound is a novel, well-validated technique that allows reliable estimates of lung water in clinical practice [14]. B-lines can be evaluated anywhere (including extreme environmental conditions using pocket-sized instruments to detect high-altitude pulmonary edema), anytime (during dialysis), by anyone (even a novice sonographer after 1 h of training), and on anybody (since the chest acoustic window usually remains patent even when an echocardiography is not feasible) [15].

The peak E-velocity represents the flow to the left ventricle, which occurs after the left ventricle diastole, reflecting the preload status [9, 10]. Ultrafiltration during hemodialysis results in a marked reduction in the circulating blood volume with a concomitant reduction in the left atrial pressure. Acharya et al. examined the parameters of left ventricular diastolic function among hemodialysis patients [16]. A comparison of the pre- and post-hemodialysis peak mitral E and A velocities showed a decrease in E-velocity, whereas the change in A velocity was not significant. Ultrafiltration during hemodialysis causes a rapid reduction in the preload, resulting in decreased early left ventricular diastolic filling without a change in the atrial phase of filling, thereby reducing the calculated E/A ratio [16]. We confirmed the change in the peak E-velocity and revealed a greater reduction during the first half of the dialysis period than during the second half of the dialysis period. We also confirmed that E/A ratio was declined during the hemodialysis therapy.

The IVC dimensions are strongly associated with the right atrial pressure and blood volume and therefore reflect the intravascular volume accurately.

Table 4 Changes in echocardiographic indices

Parameter	Just after the start (1st)	Middle (2nd)	Just before the end (3rd)	*P* (1st vs 2nd)	*P* (2nd vs 3rd)
E (cm/s)	80 ± 26	58 ± 22	51 ± 21	< 0.0001	< 0.0001
A (cm/s)[a]	87 ± 30	77 ± 22	72 ± 20	0.0006	0.0039
E/A	0.95 ± 0.39	0.72 ± 0.26	0.68 ± 0.26	< 0.0001	0.0083
Dct (msec)	255 ± 97	271 ± 92	281 ± 94	Ns	Ns
Ea (cm/s)	5.3 ± 1.7	5.4 ± 1.6	5.6 ± 1.6	0.0459	Ns
TRPG (mmHg)	4.5 ± 12.4	2.8 ± 9.5	2.4 ± 9.0	0.0237	Ns
IVC-ex (mm)	15 ± 4	12 ± 3	11 ± 3	< 0.0001	< 0.0001
IVC-in (mm)	11 ± 5	5 ± 3	3 ± 3	< 0.0001	< 0.0001
IVC collapsibility (%)	31 ± 19	61 ± 18	74 ± 20	< 0.0001	< 0.0001
B-lines	12 ± 5	9 ± 4	5 ± 3	< 0.0001	< 0.0001

Mean ± SD
E peak early diastolic filling velocity, *A* peak Atrial filling velocity, *Dct* deceleration time, *Ea* lateral early diastolic mitral annular velocities, *TRPG* tricuspid regurgitation pressure gradient, *IVC* inferior vena cava dimensions, *ex* exhalation, *in* inspiration
[a]Exclude eight atrial fibrillation

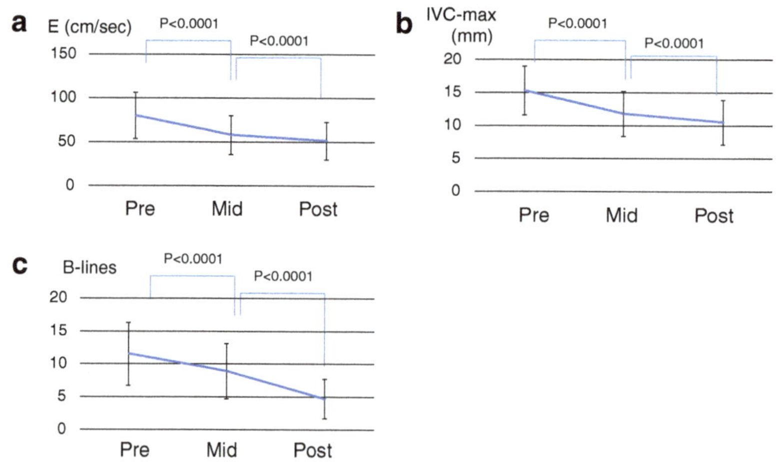

Fig. 2 Changes in echocardiographic indices. **a** Changes of peak E-velocity. **b** Changes of IVC dimensions. **c** Changes of B-lines. *Peak E-velocity* peak early mitral inflow wave velocity, *IVC* inferior vena cava

However, a major limitation of IVC dimension measurements is that ultrasound might not be sensitive enough to detect rapid volume decreases in HD patients because it reflects the intravascular filling grade [17, 18]. Indeed, similar to the change in the peak E-velocity, we showed that the IVC dimensions decreased mainly during the first half of the dialysis period, while the B-lines, which represent lung congestion, decreased significantly mainly during the last half of the dialysis period. This finding may be largely dependent on the time lag in plasma refilling. Alexiadis et al. reported that the number of B-lines has better discriminative power for predicting over- and underhydration, as determined by the IVC dimensions [2]. Mallamaci et al. suggested that the detection of extracellular water in the lung compartment constitutes a reliable tool for the prognosis of overhydration and is thus amenable to intervention [19]. So, we should be careful that even if the IVC dimensions are sufficiently reduced, lung congestion may still exist and should be treated.

Our study had some limitations. The sample size was relatively small, and the study was performed at a single institution. Activities of daily living of some patients were poor, so we could not examine height of patients. In addition, the limitations of lung ultrasound are essentially patient-dependent. Obese patients may be more difficult to examine because of the thickness of their ribcages and soft tissues. Furthermore, in this analysis, we performed ultrasound examinations only at the end of the hemodialysis therapy. However, it has been suggested that post-dialysis assessments should ideally occur 2 h after hemodialysis because of the re-equilibration of interstitial and intravascular compartments [20, 21]. Accordingly, further study is needed to evaluate the relationship between fluid removal and the timing of post-dialysis assessments in hemodialysis patients. Factors which could affect the change of the number of B-lines are important for the clinician. The change of B-lines was negatively related to the number of B-lines at the start of the hemodialysis therapy ($r^2 = 0.609$, $P < 0.0001$, data not shown). We should examine the association between the change of the number of B-lines and various factor under the same number of B-lines at the start of hemodialysis therapy, but we could not because of the small number of study participant. Even though ultrasound of extravascular lung water is reported as a new standard for pulmonary congestion [15], there is still no gold standard of examination to evaluate excess body water. In this study, we could not show other possible parameters such as chest X-ray or bioimpedance spectroscopy. Accordingly, further study will be needed to clarify this finding. Another limitation of this study is that we could not show the optimal number of B-lines after hemodialysis therapy. B-lines within physiological range may be present. We have previously reported that B-lines are associated with low serum level of albumin and low body weight [6]. So, optimal number of B-lines may be different among hemodialysis patients.

Table 5 Comparison of the changes in values between the middle to pre-dialysis periods and the post-dialysis to middle periods

	2nd–1st	3rd–2nd	*P* value
ΔE (cm/s)	− 23 ± 14	− 7 ± 6	< 0.0001
ΔIVC-ex (mm)	− 4 ± 3	− 1 ± 2	< 0.0001
ΔB-lines	− 3 ± 3	− 4 ± 2	0.0016

Mean ± SD
1st just after the start, *2nd* middle, *3rd* just before the end, *E* peak early diastolic filling velocity, *IVC* inferior vena cava dimensions, *ex* exhalation

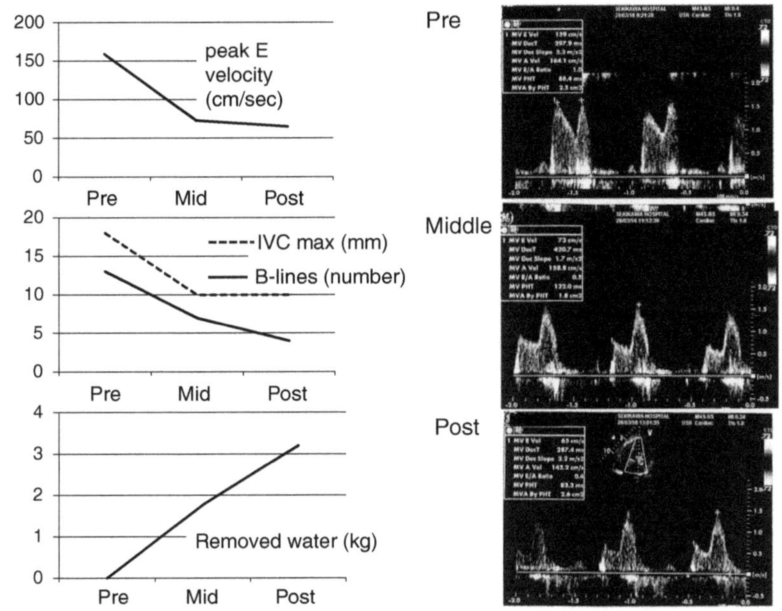

Fig. 3 Case of a 71 year-old female, chronic kidney disease 5D (due to diabetic nephritis). Change of peak E-velocity, IVC dimensions, and B-lines were shown. B-mode images of actual E and A velocity were also shown. Remarkable decrease of peak E-velocity was observed compared with peak atrial filling velocity. *Peak E-velocity* peak early mitral inflow wave velocity, *IVC* inferior vena cava

Conclusions

We showed that the peak E-velocity and IVC dimensions were reduced mainly during the first half of the dialysis period, while the number of B-lines decreased significantly mainly during the last half of the dialysis period. Even if the IVC dimensions are sufficiently reduced, caution is required as lung congestion may still exist.

Abbreviations

E-velocity: Peak early mitral inflow wave velocity; IVC: Inferior vena cava peak; NT-proBNP: N-terminal pro-brain natriuretic peptide

Acknowledgements

The authors are very grateful to the dialysis staff who understood the clinical importance of this study and who provided high-quality data in Sekikawa Hospital.

Funding

This study was not supported by any grants or funding.

Authors' contributions

KK planned the study, searched the literature, assessed the studies, extracted the data, analyzed the data, and prepared the article. KK and SO searched the literature, assessed the studies, and assisted in the article preparation. KK performed the lung echo. KN and TA assisted in the article preparation. All authors read and approved the final manuscript.

Competing interests

The authors declare that they have no competing interests.

Author details

[1]Department of Medicine, Kidney Center, Tokyo Women's Medical University, Tokyo, Japan. [2]Department of Nephrology, Sekikawa Hospital, Tokyo, Japan. [3]Department of Cardiology, Sekikawa Hospital, Tokyo, Japan. [4]Department of Blood Purification, Tohto Sangenjaya Clinic, 2-13-2 Taishido, Setagaya-ku, Tokyo 154-0004, Japan.

References

1. Tonelli M, Wiebe N, Culleton B, et al. Chronic kidney disease and mortality risk: a systematic review. J Am Soc Nephrol. 2006;17:2034–47.
2. Alexiadis G, Panagoutsos S, Roumeliotis S, Stibiris I, Markos A, Kantartzi K, et al. Comparison of multiple fluid status assessment methods in patients on chronic hemodialysis. Int Urol Nephrol. 2017;49:525–32.
3. Lichtenstein D. Pneumothorax and introduction to ultrasound signs in the lung. In: Heilmann U, Wilbertz H, Gosling A, editors. General ultrasound in the critically ill. 1st ed. Heidelberg: Springer-Verlag; 2005. p. 105–15.
4. Agricola E, Bove T, Oppizzi M, Marino G, Zangrillo A, Margonato A, et al. "Ultrasound comet-tail images": a marker of pulmonary edema: a comparative study with wedge pressure and extravascular lung water. Chest. 2005;127:1690–5.
5. Kajimoto K, Madeen K, Nakayama T, Tsudo H, Kuroda T, Abe T. Rapid evaluation by lung-cardiac-inferior vena cava (LCI) integrated ultrasound for differentiating heart failure from pulmonary disease as the cause of acute dyspnea in the emergency setting. Cardiovasc Ultrasound. 2012;10:49–51.
6. Kuzuhara S, Otsubo S, Kajimoto K, Akiba T, Nitta K. Association between B-lines detected during lung ultrasound and various factors in hemodialysis patients. Ren Replace Ther. 2017;3:17.
7. Noble VE, Murray AF, Capp R, Sylvia-Reardon MH, Steele DJ, Liteplo A. Ultrasound assessment for extravascular lung water in patients undergoing hemodialysis: time course for resolution. Chest. 2009;135:1433–9.

8. Simonson JS, Schiller NB. Sonospirometry: a new method for noninvasive estimation of mean right atrial pressure based on two-dimensional echographic measurements of the inferior vena cava during measured inspiration. J Am Coll Cardiol. 1988;11:557–64.
9. Triulzi MO, Castini D, Ornaghi M, Vitolo E. Effects of preload reduction on mitral flow velocity pattern in normal subjects. Am J Cardiol. 1990; 66:995–1001.
10. Sztajzel J, Ruedin P, Monin C, Stoermann C, Leski M, Rutishauser W, et al. Effect of altered loading conditions during haemodialysis on left ventricular filling pattern. Eur Heart J. 1993;14:655–61.
11. Cardim N, Fernandez Golfin C, Ferreira D, Aubele A, Toste J, Cobos MA, et al. Usefulness of a new miniaturized echocardiographic system in outpatient cardiology consultations as an extension of physical examination. J Am Soc Echocardiogr. 2011;24:117–24.
12. Liebo MJ, Israel RL, Lillie EO, Smith MR, Rubenson DS, Topol EJ. Is pocket mobile echocardiography the next-generation stethoscope? A cross-sectional comparison of rapidly acquired images with standard transthoracic echocardiography. Ann Intern Med. 2011;155:33–8.
13. Volpicelli G, Elbarbary M, Blaivas M, Lichtenstein DA, Mathis G, Kirkpatrick AW, et al. International liaison committee on lung ultrasound (ILC-LUS) for international consensus conference on lung ultrasound (ICC-LUS). International evidence-based recommendations for point-of-care lung ultrasound. Intensive Care Med. 2012;38:577–91.
14. Zoccali C. Lung ultrasound in the management of fluid volume in dialysis patients: potential usefulness. Semin Dial. 2017;30:6–9.
15. Picano E, Pellikka PA. Ultrasound of extravascular lung water: a new standard for pulmonary congestion. Eur Heart J. 2016;37:2097–104.
16. Acharya P, Ranabhat K, Trikhatri Y, Manandhar DN, Sharma SK, Karki P. Effect of preload reduction by haemodialysis on doppler indices of diastolic function in patients with end-stage renal disease. Kathmandu Univ Med J (KUMJ). 2008;6:98–101.
17. Feissel M, Michard F, Faller JP, Teboul JL. The respiratory variation in inferior vena cava diameter as a guide to fluid therapy. Intensive Care Med. 2004;30:1834–7.
18. Brennan JM, Ronan A, Goonewardena S, Blair JE, Hammes M, Shah D, et al. Handcarried ultrasound measurement of the inferior vena cava for assessment of intravascular volume status in the outpatient hemodialysis clinic. Clin J Am Soc Nephrol. 2006;1:749–53.
19. Mallamaci F, Benedetto FA, Tripepi R, Rastelli S, Castellino P, Tripepi G, et al. Detection of pulmonary congestion by chest ultrasound in dialysis patients. JACC Cardiovasc Imaging. 2010;3:586–94.
20. Katzarski KS, Nisell J, Randmaa I, Danielsson A, Freyschuss U, Bergstrom J. A critical evaluation of ultrasound measurement of inferior vena cava diameter in assessing dry weight in normotensive and hypertensive hemodialysis patients. Am J Kidney Dis. 1997;30:459–65.
21. Kouw PM, Kooman JP, Cheriex EC, Olthof CG, de Vries PM, Leunissen KM. Assessment of postdialysis dry weight: a comparison of techniques. J Am Soc Nephrol. 1993;4:98–104.

3

Effect of oral and intravenous iron therapy on hemoglobin levels in hemodialysis patients according to serum ferritin level

Shoichiro Daimon[1*] and Ichiro Mizushima[2]

Abstract

Background: For iron therapy in hemodialysis patients, intravenous rather than oral administration is recommended.

Methods: For hemodialysis patients with serum ferritin levels less than 200 ng/ml (less than 100 ng/ml: 67 patients, between 100 and 199 ng/ml: 20 patients) with no iron therapy for more than 3 months, iron was administered intravenously (40 mg of ferric oxide saccharate for ten times consecutively, $N = 40$) or orally (50 mg/day of sodium ferrous citrate $N = 31$, or 1500 mg/day of ferric citrate hydrate $N = 16$). We conducted the retrospective observational study to evaluate the changes in hemoglobin levels, the dose of erythropoietin-stimulating agents (ESAs), and the ratio of ESA dose/hemoglobin (Hb) levels for 28 weeks.

Results: During the first 8 weeks, hemoglobin levels increased and ESA/Hb ratio decreased uniformly with almost the same ESA dose. Subsequently, ESA/Hb ratio increased in patients with intravenous iron but decreased further in patients administered oral iron. ESA dose reduction at the end of the study in the patients receiving intravenous iron, sodium ferrous citrate, and ferric citrate hydrate were 12.2, 33.8, and 39.5 %, and ESA/Hb reduction ratios were 10.3, 34. 5, and 37.4 %, respectively. In patients with serum ferritin levels less than 100 ng/ml at baseline, ESA/Hb ratio decreased especially in those receiving oral rather than intravenous iron ($p < 0.05$), while it did not change with either oral or intravenous iron in patients with serum ferritin levels between 100 and 199 ng/ml.

Conclusions: In hemodialysis patients with serum ferritin levels less than 100 ng/ml, oral iron therapy is an effective method to treat anemia.

Keywords: Hemodialysis, Ferritin, Anemia, Iron, Erythropoietin-stimulating agents

Background

Anemia is common in hemodialysis patients, and a relative deficiency of erythropoietin (EPO) is the predominant cause [1]. Anemia management in hemodialysis patients was revolutionized by the introduction of erythropoietin-stimulating agents (ESAs) in the late 1980s and has become the mainstay of anemia treatment [2]. With the introduction of ESAs, iron deficiency has become an important component of anemia in hemodialysis patients [3]. Although intravenous (IV) iron administration can supply iron to hemodialysis patients irrespective of their condition, this method can enhance the risk of iron toxicity, and associations between high doses of IV iron and cardiovascular disease, infection, hospitalization, and death have been reported [4, 5]. Although oral iron supplementation is supposed to be more physiologic than that by the IV route, several studies have indicated that IV iron is superior to oral iron in hemodialysis patients [6, 7], and IV administration is widely recommended [8, 9]. Despite the copious evidences regarding the superiority of IV over oral iron for the treatment of anemia, some exceptions exist. In some centers in Canada, the efficacy of oral iron therapy in long-term hemodialysis patients was investigated, with equivalent efficacy between predominantly oral and IV iron administration reported [10].

* Correspondence: dai-clinic@m2.spacelan.ne.jp
[1]Department of Nephrology, Daimon Clinic for Internal Medicine, Nephrology and Dialysis, Oshino 1-400, Nonoichi 921-8802, Japan
Full list of author information is available at the end of the article

Here, we evaluated the effect of oral iron supplementation on anemia by comparing when iron is administered intravenously.

Methods

This study focused on stable hemodialysis patients in Daimon Clinic for Internal Medicine, Nephrology and Dialysis. Patients who had received blood transfusion or iron supplementation within 3 months were excluded. Serum ferritin levels were evaluated every 12 weeks, and 50 mg/day of sodium ferrous citrate was administered if serum ferritin levels were less than 200 ng/ml (less than 100 ng/ml in principle, but also between 100 and 199 ng/ml if serum ferritin levels were never below 100 ng/ml without iron administration for more than 3 months) and hemoglobin levels were less than 12 g/dl. When concomitant hyperphosphatemia was present, instead of sodium ferrous citrate, 1500 mg/day of ferric citrate hydrate was administered. Changes in hemoglobin levels, dose of continuous erythropoietin receptor activator (C.E.R.A.) (administered every 2 weeks) or darbepoetin alfa (every week), and ESA resistance (the ratio of dose of C.E.R.A. or darbepoetin alfa for 4 weeks/hemoglobin (Hb) levels) were compared retrospectively for 28 weeks. As a rule, darbepoetin alfa was administered for patients requiring a low dose (less than 50 μg/4 weeks) of ESA and C.E.R.A. for patients requiring higher doses. In 2012, we changed the iron supplementation policy for our hemodialysis patients from the IV to oral route. All the patients receiving sodium ferrous citrate or ferric citrate hydrate were treated after January 2012, during which period the oral iron supplementation policy was applied. As a reference, data of patients receiving IV iron were collected retrospectively: in 22 of 40 being obtained before we changed the iron supplementation policy for hemodialysis patients from the IV to oral route; in 18 of 40 being obtained from the patients after January 2012 who refused oral iron therapy; had a history of side effects from sodium ferrous citrate; or were suspected of poor drug compliance. As IV iron, 40 mg of ferric oxide saccharate was administered ten times consecutively. Patients with blood transfusion or iron supplementation within 3 months before IV iron therapy was initiated were excluded. Figure 1 shows the study design and Table 1 shows baseline characteristics of the patients. We evaluated the effect of oral iron supplementation on anemia by comparing when iron is administered intravenously. Furthermore, we compared the effect of iron therapy on anemia according to the serum ferritin level: less than 100 ng/ml and between 100 and 199 ng/ml.

Statistical analysis

Data were expressed as mean ± standard deviation. Differences in quantitative variables and categorical variables between three groups were compared by a t test and χ^2 test, respectively. Intergroup comparisons of repeatedly measured data in Fig. 3a–c were examined by repeated measures of analysis of variance (ANOVA). Statistical significance is defined as p less than 0.05. All statistical analyses were conducted using SPSS (version 19, Chicago, IL, USA).

Results

As shown in Fig. 2, mean hemoglobin levels increased uniformly in each of the IV, sodium ferrous citrate, and ferric citrate hydrate groups. The peak hemoglobin levels were noted at 10, 16, and 10 weeks, respectively, and after that, hemoglobin levels were controlled between 10 and 11 g/dl in each group. The control of hemoglobin levels after the steep increase in hemoglobin levels by iron administration was managed by a reduction of the ESA dose. ESA dose reduction at the end of the study in patients receiving IV iron, sodium ferrous citrate, and ferric citrate hydrate were 12.2, 33.8, and 39.5 %,

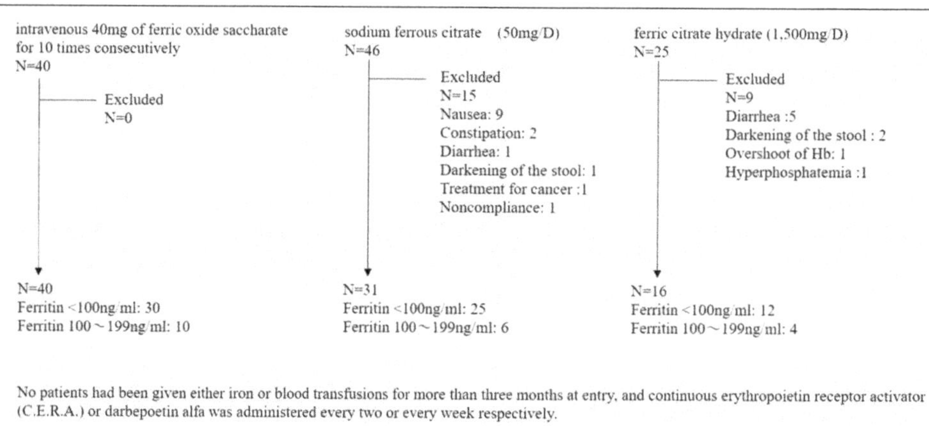

Fig. 1 Study design. No patients had been given either iron or blood transfusions for more than 3 months before entry, and continuous erythropoietin receptor activator (C.E.R.A.) or darbepoetin alfa was administered every 2 weeks and every week, respectively

Table 1 Baseline characteristics of the patients

	IV iron	Sodium ferrous citrate	Ferric citrate hydrate	IV iron	Sodium ferrous citrate	Ferric citrate hydrate	IV iron	Sodium ferrous citrate	Ferric citrate hydrate
	All	All	All	Serum ferritin <100 ng/ml	Serum ferritin <100 ng/ml	Serum ferritin <100 ng/ml	Serum ferritin 100~199 ng/ml	Serum ferritin 100~199 ng/ml	Serum ferritin 100~199 ng/ml
N	40	31	16	30	25	12	10	6	4
Female (%)	15 (37.5)	3 (9.7)[a]	6 (37.5)[b]	12 (40.0)	3 (25.0)[a]	5 (41.7)	3 (30.0)	0 (0.0)	1 (25.0)
Age (years)	70.9 ± 9.2	73.3 ± 9.6[a]	65.5 ± 10.9[b]	69.3 ± 8.5	65.8 ± 12.1[a]	76.0 ± 5.0[c]	75.6 ± 10.2	64.3 ± 3.7[a]	65.3 ± 15.8
Duration on dialysis (months)	87.5 ± 104.7	43.5 ± 58.3[a]	80.1 ± 107.2	92.2 ± 101.4	39.2 ± 51.6[a]	80.5 ± 120.3	73.4 ± 118.6	61.3 ± 84.7	79.0 ± 66.0
Diabetes (%)	15 (37.5)	17 (54.8)	8 (50.0)	10 (33.3)	14 (56.0)	6 (50.0)	5 (50.0)	3 (50.0)	2 (50.0)
Hemoglobin (g/dl)	9.8 ± 0.9	9.6 ± 1.2	10.0 ± 1.2	9.7 ± 0.9	9.8 ± 1.2	9.8 ± 1.1	10.0 ± 0.5	8.9 ± 1.1[a]	10.8 ± 1.5[b]
ESAs (μg/4 weeks)	104.6 ± 44.0	116.0 ± 44.6	101.9 ± 43.1	109.3 ± 45.5	120.6 ± 46.3	112.5 ± 43.3	90.5 ± 37.5	96.7 ± 32.7	70.0 ± 24.5
C.E.R.A. (*N*)	34	24	15	27	21	11	7	3	4
Darbepoetin alfa (*N*)	6	7	1	3	4	1	3	3	0
CRP (mg/dl)	0.18 ± 0.24	0.27 ± 0.45	0.31 ± 0.63	0.18 ± 0.26	0.20 ± 0.35	0.19 ± 0.31	0.17 ± 0.16	0.57 ± 0.69	0.68 ± 1.17
Serum alb (g/dl)	3.5 ± 0.3	3.6 ± 0.3	3.7 ± 0.2	3.6 ± 0.3	3.6 ± 0.3	3.6 ± 0.2	3.5 ± 0.2	3.6 ± 0.5	3.8 ± 0.3
p (mg/dl)	4.8 ± 1.0	5.0 ± 1.1	5.6 ± 1.3[a]	4.9 ± 1.1	5.1 ± 1.1	5.4 ± 1.2	4.6 ± 0.8	4.7 ± 0.7	6.3 ± 1.3[a, b]
Intact PTH (pg/ml)	173.6 ± 95.1	179.4 ± 115.3	160.8 ± 148.8	171.2 ± 103.5	156.1 ± 77.3	172.8 ± 168.1	180.8 ± 67.6	276.3 ± 192.4	124.5 ± 68.8
Ferritin (ng/ml)	79.4 ± 45.3	65.1 ± 35.7	74.4 ± 43.8	57.8 ± 25.2	51.3 ± 22.2	52.8 ± 20.4	144.4 ± 24.0	122.4 ± 19.9	139.1 ± 25.3
Fe (μg/dl)	N.A.	76.5 ± 23.4	73.3 ± 31.6	N.A.	80.4 ± 22.3	75.6 ± 33.0	N.A.	60.2 ± 22.5	66.8 ± 31.1

N.A. not available
[a]The difference is statistically significant versus IV iron group ($p < 0.05$)
[b]The difference is statistically significant versus sodium ferrous citrate group ($p < 0.05$)
[c]The difference is statistically significant versus sodium ferrous citrate group ($p < 0.001$)

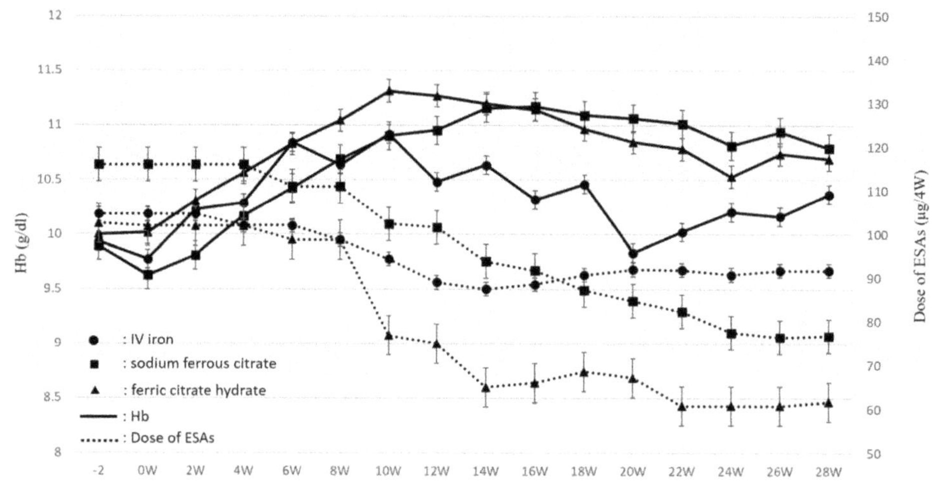

Fig. 2 Hemoglobin levels and dose of ESAs (C.E.R.A. or darbepoetin alfa) per 4 weeks during the study period. Data are expressed as mean ± SE

respectively. To compare the erythropoietic effect of iron administration under the simultaneous changes of hemoglobin levels and ESA dose, we evaluated the ratio of ESA dose for 4 weeks/Hb levels. In the first 10 weeks, ESA/Hb ratio decreased uniformly in the three groups but then started to increase in the IV group, whereas it decreased further in the sodium ferrous citrate and ferric citrate hydrate groups. At the end of study, ESA/Hb reduction ratios in patients receiving intravenous iron, sodium ferrous citrate, and ferric citrate hydrate were 10.3, 34.5, and 37.4 %, respectively (Fig. 3a). In patients with ferritin levels <100 ng/ml at the beginning of the study (Fig. 3b), ESA/Hb ratio decreased more by oral than IV iron ($p < 0.05$). By the multiple comparison of the groups, the ferric citrate hydrate group but not the sodium ferrous citrate group showed a significant tendency to decrease the ESA/Hb ratio as compared with the IV iron group ($p < 0.05$). In patients with ferritin levels 100~199 ng/ml at the beginning of the study, ESA/Hb ratio did not change with iron administration regardless of whether the IV or oral route was used (Fig. 3c). Table 2 shows the serum ferritin levels during the study. Serum ferritin levels at 24 weeks were almost the same as compared to those at 12 weeks in the IV iron group, while on the other hand, serum ferritin levels at 24 weeks were higher than those at 12 weeks in the oral iron groups.

Discussion

After the introduction of ESAs for the treatment of hemodialysis patients, iron deficiency became an important underlying component of anemia in hemodialysis patients [3]. Although oral iron supplementation is supposed to be more physiologic than the IV one, oral iron absorption is appreciable when serum ferritin concentration is less than 70 to 100 ng/ml and decreases when this exceeds 300 ng/ml [11]. Numerous studies have evaluated oral iron administration in hemodialysis patients, and overall, oral iron is not superior to IV iron [6, 7, 12], and thus, IV administration has been recommended [8, 9]. Although, compared with IV iron therapy, there is scarce evidence regarding the efficacy of oral iron for the treatment of anemia in hemodialysis patients, we obtained favorable effects with oral iron therapy. Possible explanations for this discrepancy include the following. In our study, the effectiveness of oral iron was recognized only in patients with serum ferritin levels less than 100 ng/ml at baseline and not in patients with higher ferritin levels. On the other hand, the mean serum ferritin levels in patients receiving oral iron reported by Fishbane et al. [6] and MacDougall et al. [7] were 178.9 and 309 ng/ml, respectively, and the former failed to demonstrate any efficacy of oral iron (ferrous sulfate or iron polysaccharide), while in the latter, although oral iron (ferrous sulfate) could increase hemoglobin levels with almost the same dose of ESA, serum ferritin levels decreased and efficacy was inferior to IV iron. These results indicate that oral iron therapy is effective predominantly in patients with low serum ferritin levels, with 100 ng/ml being a tentative border line to predict the efficacy of oral iron therapy.

Ferritin, together with transferrin saturation, is the recommended test to assess iron stores in dialysis patients [13]. IV iron administration is recommended when serum ferritin levels are less than 100 ng/ml in Japan [9], in contrast to 300 ng/ml in the European Best Practice (ERBP) group [14] and 500 ng/ml in the Kidney Disease: Improving Global Outcomes (KDIGO) [13]. Recently, there has been a tendency to increase the IV iron dose and mean serum ferritin levels of hemodialysis patients in many countries [15]. In the USA, the US Centers for Medicare and Medicaid Services instituted a partially capitated payment system for dialysis services that included both ESAs

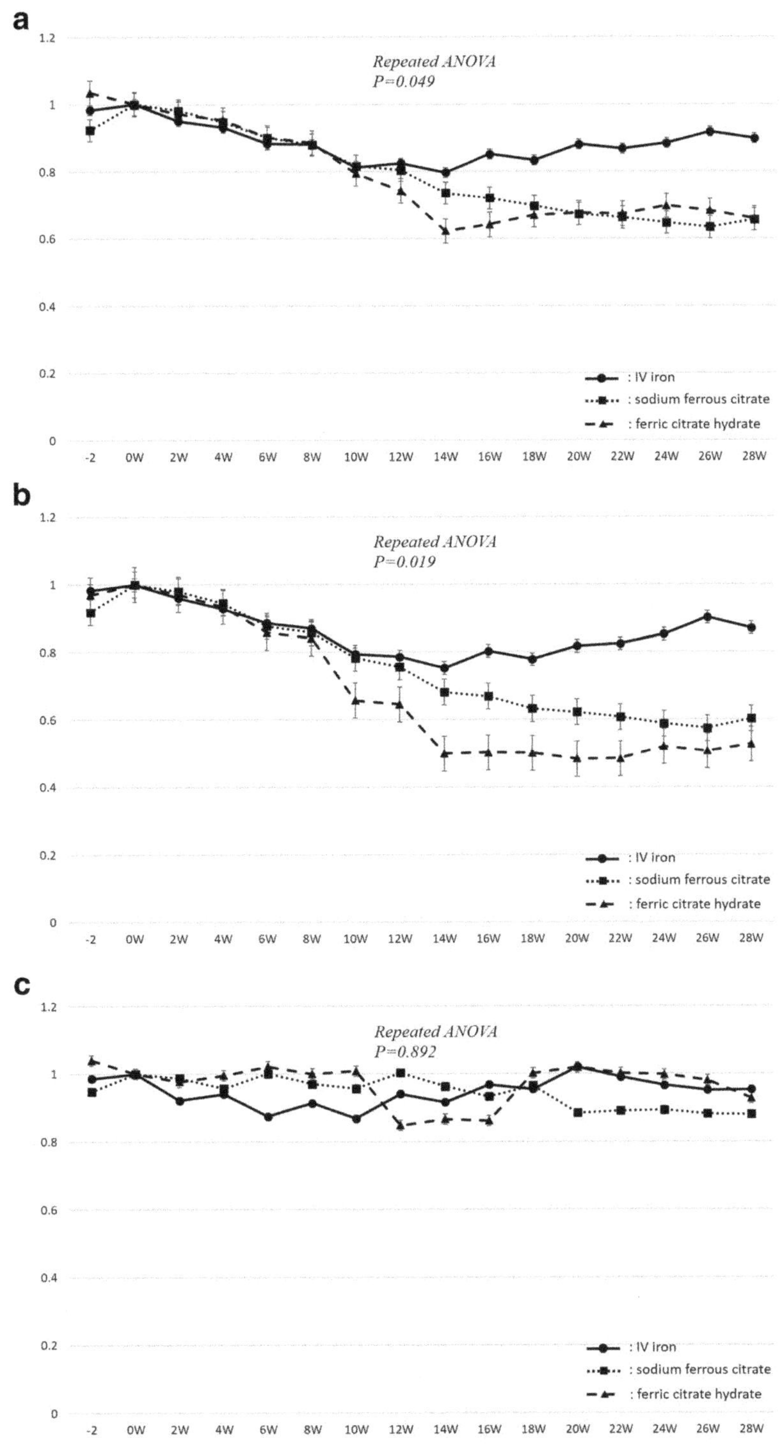

Fig. 3 **a** Ratio of dose of ESAs per 4 weeks/Hb during the study period (0W: reference). Data are expressed as mean ± SE. **b** Ratio of dose of ESAs per 4 weeks/Hb during the study period in patients with serum ferritin levels <100 ng/ml at baseline (0W: reference). Data are expressed as mean ± SE. **c** Ratio of dose of ESAs per 4 weeks/Hb during the study period in patients with serum ferritin levels 100~199 ng/ml at baseline (0W: reference). Data are expressed as mean ± SE

and IV iron in 2011, which further increased the use of low-cost IV iron and decreased the dose of high-cost ESAs, with the mean serum ferritin concentration exceeding 800 ng/ml in 2013 [16, 17]. A considerable variation in serum ferritin levels in hemodialysis patients is seen in individual countries [15], 144.49 ± 261.83 ng/ml

Table 2 Serum ferritin levels during the study period

	IV iron	Sodium ferrous citrate	Ferric citrate hydrate	IV iron	Sodium ferrous citrate	Ferric citrate hydrate	IV iron	Sodium ferrous citrate	Ferric citrate hydrate
	All	All	All	Serum ferritin <100 ng/ml	Serum ferritin <100 ng/ml	Serum ferritin <100 ng/ml	Serum ferritin 100~199 ng/ml	Serum ferritin 100~199 ng/ml	Serum ferritin 100~199 ng/ml
N	40	31	16	30	25	12	10	6	4
0 weeks	79.4 ± 45.3	65.1 ± 35.7	74.4 ± 43.8	57.7 ± 25.2	51.3 ± 22.2	52.8 ± 20.4	144.4 ± 24.0	122.4 ± 19.9	139.1 ± 25.3
12 weeks	92.9 ± 48.7	112.6 ± 56.4	128.9 ± 78.7	92.9 ± 48.7	98.5 ± 39.3	91.3 ± 48.0	N.A.	196.8 ± 76.3	232.4 ± 42.5
24 weeks	109.5 ± 71.3	140.9 ± 60.5	159.5 ± 57.3[a]	82.0 ± 41.8	130.7 ± 57.3[b]	153.6 ± 59.5[c]	164.5 ± 87.5	181.6 ± 60.2	189.0 ± 46.7

N.A. not available
[a]The difference is statistically significant versus IV iron group ($p < 0.05$)
[b]The difference is statistically significant versus IV iron group ($p < 0.005$)
[c]The difference is statistically significant versus IV iron group ($p < 0.001$)

in 2012 in Japan [18] which is the lowest in the countries participating in the Dialysis Outcomes and Practice Pattern Study (DOPPS). Lower ferritin levels in hemodialysis patients in Japan than in those in western countries which are proportional to IV iron dose [15] and low serum ferritin levels (median 72 ng/ml) in hemodialysis patients administered predominantly oral rather than IV iron reported from Canada [10] suggest that without IV iron administration, serum ferritin levels are low in many hemodialysis patients. The fact that with the oral iron supplementation policy which was initiated when serum ferritin levels are less than 200 ng/ml (in majority of them less than 100 ng/ml), 80 % of hemodialysis patients in our clinic receive oral iron also proves this.

Although iron is essential for hematopoiesis, the IV route bypasses regulation of iron absorption in the duodenum and intestine. It is speculated that nonphysiologic iron supplementation by IV iron easily increases the plasma nontransferrin-bound iron, which is readily accumulated in the liver and the reticuloendothelial system and increases iron stores. This induces hepcidin synthesis and limits further enteral iron absorption and release of iron from iron stores [19]. In this situation, oral iron therapy is less likely to be effective, which is supposed to be usual in patients receiving high-dose IV iron administration.

As an IV iron therapy, 40 mg of ferric oxide saccharate was administered ten times consecutively in our study, but this represents a relatively small dose and short duration of treatment and this may be the reason why the efficacy of IV iron ceased at around 16 weeks and also may be the reason for the lack of any apparent effect of IV iron in patients with serum ferritin levels 100~199 ng/ml at baseline. In one patient with IV iron therapy, serum ferritin levels were investigated frequently and showed that with a rapid increase in hemoglobin levels, in contrast, serum ferritin levels decreased and returned to the same level before IV iron at 16 weeks (data not shown). Changes in serum ferritin levels during the study (Table 2) also suggest the possibility of an insufficient dose of IV iron in this study. Nevertheless, in practice after changing the iron supplementation policy for hemodialysis patients from the IV to oral route, the ESA dose was halved with mean hemoglobin levels kept between 10.0 and 11.0 g/dl (data not shown). This proves the efficacy of oral iron in hemodialysis patients with low serum ferritin levels.

Regarding the study period, compared with our study, the observation periods of Fishbane et al. [6] and MacDougall et al. [7] were relatively short, 4 months and 16 weeks, respectively. Furthermore, Umanath et al. reported that serum ferritin levels increased through week 24, remaining relatively stable thereafter in hemodialysis patients treated with ferric citrate [20], which is in accordance with the information provided by pharmaceutical companies in Japan; it takes approximately 24 weeks by the time serum ferritin levels reach a plateau in patients receiving ferric citrate hydrate or sucroferric oxyhydroxide (data not shown). In our study, it took 24 weeks by the time ESA/Hb ratio reached plateaus in the oral iron groups (Fig. 3) and serum ferritin levels at 24 weeks were even higher than those at 12 weeks (Table 2) consistent with the above results. These results mean that it takes around half a year by the time oral iron exerts its maximum erythropoietic effect, while in patients receiving IV iron therapy, it takes a shorter time.

Our results suggest that for hemodialysis patients with serum ferritin levels less than 100 ng/ml, oral iron therapy can decrease the needed ESA dose which is equivalent or superior to that by IV iron. Moreover, although long-term safe range of serum ferritin levels is not known, oral iron therapy may also help to avoid iron toxicity and reduce the morbidity related to iron overload.

Although usually not severe, oral iron therapy has relatively frequent side effects including nausea, diarrhea, and constipation. From the standpoint of its efficacy as iron supplementation, oral instead of IV iron therapy is warranted for patients with serum ferritin levels less than 100 ng/ml and without side effects induced by oral iron therapy. On the other hand, in patients whose serum ferritin levels are never under 100 ng/ml, the absorption and utilization of oral iron are limited and in this situation, the use of a high dose of IV instead of oral iron may be warranted. However, because of the small number of patients; heterogeneity of distribution of age, sex, and Hb levels between groups; and retrospective nature of our study, our results cannot yet be considered conclusive. But in the meantime, our results suggest that for hemodialysis patients with ferritin levels less than 100 ng/ml, oral iron supplementation is an effective and likely safe method for the treatment of anemia and can decrease the ESA dose and may help to avoid iron toxicity.

Conclusions

Oral iron therapy without the use of IV iron is effective for the treatment of anemia in hemodialysis patients with low serum ferritin levels.

Abbreviations

C.E.R.A.: Continuous erythropoietin receptor activator; EPO: Erythropoietin; ESA: Erythropoietin-stimulating agent; Hb: Hemoglobin; IV: Intravenous

Acknowledgements

The authors thank all the staff members working at Daimon Clinic for Internal Medicine, Nephrology and Dialysis.

Funding

There is no funding to be disclosed.

Authors' contributions
IM was involved in the statistical analysis. Both authors read and approved the final manuscript.

Competing interests
The authors declare that they have no competing interests.

Author details
[1]Department of Nephrology, Daimon Clinic for Internal Medicine, Nephrology and Dialysis, Oshino 1-400, Nonoichi 921-8802, Japan. [2]Division of Rheumatology, Department of Internal Medicine, Kanazawa University Graduate School of Medicine, Kanazawa, Japan.

References

1. McGonigle RJ, Wallin JD, Shadduck RK, Fisher JW. Erythropoietin deficiency and inhibition of erythropoiesis in renal insufficiency. Kidney Int. 1984;25:437–44.
2. Kidney Disease Improving Global Outcomes (KDIGO). Clinical practice guideline for anemia in chronic kidney disease. Kidney Int. 2012;Suppl 2:292–8.
3. Eschbach JW, Egrie JC, Downing MR, Browne JK, Adamson JW. Correction of the anemia of end-stage renal disease with recombinant human erythropoietin. N Engl J Med. 1987;316:73–8.
4. Kuragano T, Matsumura O, Matsuda A, et al. Association between hemoglobin variability, serum ferritin levels, and adverse events/mortality in maintenance hemodialysis patients. Kidney Int. 2014;86:845–54.
5. Bailie GR, Larkina M, Goodkin DA, et al. Data from the Dialysis Outcomes and Practice Pattern Study validate an association between high intravenous iron doses and mortality. Kidney Int. 2015;87:162–8.
6. Fishbane S, Frei GL, Maesaka J. Reduction in recombinant human erythropoietin doses by the use of chronic intravenous iron supplementation. Am J Kidney Dis. 1995;26:41–6.
7. MacDougall IC, Tucker B, Thompson J, Tomson CRV, Baker LRI, Raine EG. A randomized controlled study of iron supplementation in patients treated with erythropoietin. Kidney Int. 1996;50:1694–9.
8. K/DOQI. K.DOQI clinical practice guidelines and clinical recommendation for anemia in chronic kidney disease. Am J Kidney Dis. 2006;47 Suppl 3:S58–70.
9. Tsubakihara Y, Nishi S, Akiba T, et al. 2008 Japanese Society for dialysis therapy: guidelines for renal anemia in chronic kidney disease. Ther Apher Dial. 2010;14:240–75.
10. Lenga I, Lok C, Marticorena R, Hunter J, Dacouris N, Goldstein M. Role of oral iron in the management of long-term hemodialysis patients. Clin J Am Soc Nephrol. 2007;2:688–93.
11. Eschbach JW, Cook JD, Scribner BH, Finch CA. Iron balance in hemodialysis patients. Ann Intern Med. 1977;87:710–3.
12. Wingard RL, Parker RA, Ismail N, Hakim RM. Efficacy of oral iron therapy in patients receiving recombinant human erythropoietin. Am J Kidney Dis. 1995;25:433–9.
13. Kidney Disease Improving Global Outcomes. KDIGO clinical practice guideline for anemia in chronic kidney disease: summary of recommendation statements. Kidney Int Suppl. 2012;2:283–7.
14. Locatelli F, Bárány P, Covic A, et al. Kidney disease: improving global outcomes guidelines on anaemia management in chronic kidney disease: a European renal best practice position statement. Nephrol Dial Transplant. 2013;28:1346–59.
15. Bailie GR, Larkina M, Goodkin DA, et al. Variation in intravenous iron use internationally and over time: the Dialysis Outcomes and Practice Pattern Study (DOPPS). Nephrol Dial Transplant. 2013;28:2570–9.
16. Weiner DE, Winkelmayer WC. Commentary on 'The DOPPS practice monitor for U.S. dialysis care: update on trends in anemia management 2 years into the bundle': iron(y) abounds 2 years later. Am J Kidney Dis. 2013;62:1217–20.
17. Charytan DM, Pai AB, Chan CT, on behalf of the Dialysis Advisory Group of the American Society of Nephrology, et al. Considerations and challenges in defining optimal iron utilization in hemodialysis. J Am Soc Nephrol. 2015;26:1238–47.
18. Nakai S, Hanafusa N, Masakane I, et al. An overview of regular dialysis treatment in Japan (as of 31 December 2012). Ther Apher Dial. 2014;18:535–602.
19. Young B, Zaritsky J. Hepcidin for clinicians. Clin J Am Soc Nephrol. 2009;4:1384–7.
20. Umanath K, Jalal DI, Greco BA, et al. Ferric citrate reduces intravenous iron and erythropoiesis-stimulating agent use in ESRD. J Am Soc Nephrol. 2015;26:2578–87.

4

Poor glycemic control attributable to insulin antibody in a fulminant type 1 diabetes patient under hemodialysis: successful treatment with double filtration plasmapheresis and prednisolone

Kentaro Wada[1*], Haruhito A. Uchida[2] and Yuko Wada[3]

Abstract

Background: Insulin antibody appears in approximately 40% of insulin users using human insulin and insulin analog formulations. Insulin antibody, characterized by high affinity and low insulin antibody binding capacity (% bound), rarely causes clinical problems including poor glycemic control. Recently, the insulin antibody against human insulin causing deterioration of glycemic control, characterized by low affinity and high insulin antibody binding capacity similar to those observed in insulin autoimmune syndrome, has been reported.

Case presentation: A 62-year-old male developing fulminant type 1 diabetes showing rapid hyperglycemia (602 mg/dL) and normal range of glycoalbumin (GA) (18.4%) in the introductory stage of hemodialysis (HD) was transferred to our hospital 3 weeks after the onset of diabetes. He had been administered insulin intensification therapy in other medical clinic; however, his glycemic control remained poor, showing ketoacidosis. After hospitalization, he was initially administered intravenous insulin for 2 days and then switched to subcutaneous intensification therapy (24 U/day); the dose was gradually increased maximum of 72 U/day within 2 months. His glycemic control deteriorated despite high-dose insulin administration and change in the insulin type. Insulin antibody was detected, insulin antibody binding capacity (% bound) was of a high value (89.5%), GA was 32.9%, and casual blood glucose widely changed in continuous glucose monitor, suggesting that unstable blood glucose fluctuations caused by insulin antibody; therefore, treatment with double filtration plasmapheresis (DFPP) and prednisolone (PSL) was performed. The insulin dose reduced, and glycemic control improved from 1 month after the commencement of treatment. Subsequently, insulin antibody level remained high; however, after 6 months, % bound declined (20.9%), and glycemic control improved (GA 23.7%) by PSL (gradually reduced to 5 mg/day). The Scatchard plots also indicated the effectiveness with DFPP and PSL therapy.

Conclusions: The authors present a unique case of fulminant type 1 diabetes developing during the HD introduction period. Although this is a rare complication, physicians specializing in dialysis therapy should also keep in mind that this is a life-threatening complication if the treatment is delayed and that concomitant therapy with apheresis such as DFPP and long-term steroids is effective in some cases when glycemic control deteriorates attributable to insulin antibody.

Keywords: Insulin antibody, Insulin antibody binding capacity, Fulminant type 1 diabetes, Hemodialysis, Double filtration plasmapheresis, Prednisolone

* Correspondence: kyw620@hotmail.co.jp
[1]Division of Nephrology and Dialysis, Department of Internal Medicine, Nippon Kokan Fukuyama Hospital, 1844, Tsunoshita, Daimon-cho, Fukuyama, Hiroshima 721-0927, Japan
Full list of author information is available at the end of the article

Background

Insulin antibody appear in approximately 40% of insulin users administered human insulin and insulin analog formulations. Insulin antibody, characterized by high affinity and low insulin antibody binding capacity (% bound), rarely causes clinical problems including glycemic control [1]. In contrast, insulin antibody against human insulin, characterized by low affinity and high insulin antibody binding capacity similar to those observed in insulin autoimmune syndrome, has been reported recently [2], with reports mentioning that glycemic control was difficult [3]. The authors herein report a case of fulminant type 1 diabetes developing during the hemodialysis (HD) introduction period complicated by renal cell carcinoma (RCC). Firstly, insulin therapy was introduced. Secondly, nephrectomy was performed. Glycemic control deteriorated thereafter. The cause of poor glycemic control could be associated with insulin antibody. Treatment with double filtration plasmapheresis (DFPP) and prednisolone (PSL) was performed for the case. The insulin antibody binding capacity decreased, as was also confirmed in Scatchard analysis. In the present case, DFPP and PSL successfully improved a long-term glycemic control.

Case presentation

A 62-year-old Japanese male under HD due to IgA nephropathy for approximately 1 week (at second HD session) with no previous history of diabetes mellitus was diagnosed and treated with insulin at other medical clinic. He had not been treated with corticosteroid for IgA nephropathy. His glycemic profile during the 2 years just before the introduction of HD was within normal range (fasting blood glucose level 78–98 mg/dL and hemoglobin A1c (HbA1c; NGSP) level 5.5–5.8%). The final monitoring for blood glucose and HbA1c levels were performed 3 months before onset of diabetes (fasting blood glucose 89 mg/dL, HbA1c 5.5%). Any precipitating event such as pancreatitis, sepsis, medication, or any traumatic event that might have caused impaired glucose tolerance did not appear. He complained of thirst, nausea, and vomiting; however, he did not show bronchitis. His body weight decreased 2.8 kg (height 163 cm, body weight 49.1 kg, body temperature 37.3 °C) compared with after the first HD session, and his blood glucose level was 602 mg/dL (HbA1c 5.9%, glycoalbumin (GA) 18.4%). Because his glycemic control was poor using insulin lispro and deemir, he was transferred to our hospital approximately 3 weeks after the onset of diabetes. On admission to our hospital, his blood glucose level was 642 mg/dL with ketoacidosis (HbA1c 8.3%, GA 32.9%, pH 7.04, HCO_3^- 12 mEq/L, plasma ketone 284 μmol/L, anion gap 19 mEq/L, plasma osmolality 331 mOsm/L). His diabetic ketoacidosis was managed using standard treatment protocols. The authors managed to keep his blood glucose concentrations within 150–200 mg/dL with continuous intravenous infusion (intravenous insulin therapy approximately 40 U/day for 2 days). Following recovery, he was introduced to an intensive insulin therapy (insulin glulisine and glargine) and maintained his blood glucose between 100 and 200 mg/dL (insulin glulisine as bolus 6-6-6 U, glargine as basal 0-0-6 U, a total of 24 U/day).

His blood count was as follows: white blood cells, 6900/μL; red blood cells, 328×10^4/μL; hemoglobin, 11.8 g/dL; hematocrit, 32.9%; platelet, 21.6×10^4/μL; using epoetin beta pegol 25 μg/2 weeks.

His serum albumin was 4.0 g/dL, alkaline phosphatase (ALP) 174 U/L, asparate aminotransferase (AST) 15 U/L, alanine aminotransferase (ALT) 14 U/L, gamma-glutamyl transpeptidase (γ-GTP) 17 U/L, blood urea nitrogen (BUN) 89, creatinine 7.54, and uric acid 5.9 mg/dL.

The glucagon, IgG, IgA, IgM, IgG4, carcinoembryonic antigen (CEA), and carbohydrate antigen (CA) 19-9 values were within normal limits. Serum interleukin-2 receptor level was slightly elevated at 1040 U/mL. Serum anti-glutamic acid decarboxylase (GAD) antibody, islet antigen 2 (IA-2) antibody, islet cell antibody (ICA), parathyroid hormone-related protein, anti-thyroid peroxidase (TPO) antibody, anti-thyroglobulin antibody, calcitonin, myeloperoxidase anti-neutrophil cytoplasmic antibody (MPO-ANCA), and protease 3 (PR3)-ANCA were not elevated. The serum C-peptide immunoreactivity (CPR) level was 0.04 ng/mL, and glucagon tolerance test revealed no elevation of CPR (Δ CPR 0 ng/mL).

Human leukocyte antigen (HLA) typing showed A2/24, B35/52, DR4(DRB1*04:01), DR15(DRB1*15:01), and DQB1*04:02:01/DQB1*06:02:01.

The pancreatic exocrine enzymes were slightly elevated as follows: pancreatic amylase, 155 U/l; elastase 1176 ng/dL; and lipase 65 U/L (slightly elevated compared with normal limits).

Abdominal ultrasonography revealed no remarkable findings, such as pancreatic enlargement, poorly defined edges, or ascites retention; however, it revealed a mass in the left kidney. Contrast computed tomography (CT) of the abdomen was subsequently performed and revealed a 43-mm mass in the left kidney (Fig. 1). Two months after admission, the mass was removed using a laparoscopic approach, and no gross metastasis was evident at surgery. Pathology of the mass was consistent with clear cell adenocarcinoma with no invasion of the capsule and renal pelvis. The margins of the resection were clear with no evidence of tumor in the renal veins.

Ultrasonography of the thyroid gland revealed no morphological defects, and the fundus findings of the patient were normal.

In the evaluation of glycemic daily profile using a continuous glucose monitor (CGM), his blood glucose level widely fluctuated, with a tendency for hyperglycemia

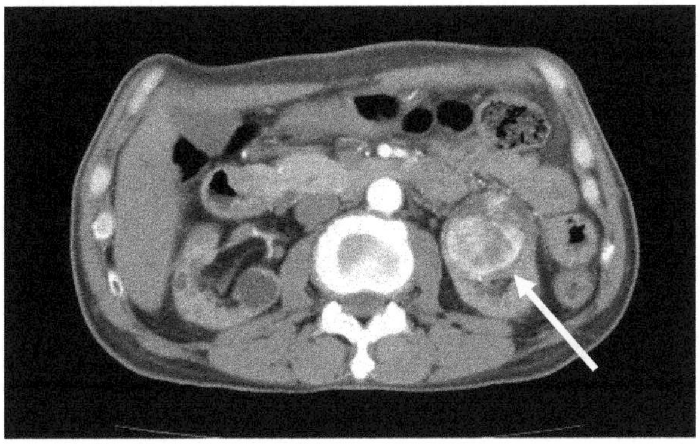

Fig. 1 A contrast computed tomography study of the abdomen revealed a 43 mm mass in the left kidney (*arrow, horizontal view*)

during the day and nocturnal hypoglycemia. Two weeks after admission, insulin antibody was detected, and the insulin antibody binding capacity was 89.1%.

First, insulin intensification therapy was introduced (at first, insulin lispro as bolus 6-6-6 U, detemir as basal 0-0-6 U, total of 24 U/day; and then changed insulin glulisine as bolus 6-6-6 U, glargine as basal 0-0-6 U, total of 24 U/day); however, maintaining his glycemic control in good condition was difficult. The dosage was therefore increased to a maximum of 72 U/day within 2 months (Fig. 2). His glycemic control deteriorated after nephrectomy despite treatment with high dose of insulin; therefore, he was introduced to insulin pump therapy (glulisine as bolus 22-18-20 U, glargine as basal; 12–7 am 0.1, 7–12 pm 0.8, 12–7 pm 0.4, 7–12 am 0.1 U/h, total of 8 U/day, grand total of 68 U/day). Because his casual blood glucose fluctuated widely at 246 ± 99 mg/dL in CGM (nocturnal hypoglycemia was frequently observed), insulin pump therapy was switched back to intensive insulin therapy (glulisine as bolus 18-17-18 U, glargine as basal; 8 U, a total of 61 U/day), resulting in an improvement in his casual blood glucose to 154 ± 55 mg/dL in CGM. Second, the insulin antibody and antibody binding capacity was high value; therefore, DFPP was performed twice a week for 3 h before HD for 5 weeks, totaling 10 times (concentration of replacement albumin fluid was 8%, plasma fractionator Evaflux 2A-20, Kawasumi Laboratories, Tokyo, Japan, and plasma separator Plasmacure PE-05, Kawasumi Laboratories, Tokyo, Japan), to eliminate the antibody. Third, PSL (Predonisolone, Takeda, Osaka, Japan) was commenced starting at 30 mg/day, after which the dosage was gradually decreased to 5 mg/day over 6 months. On comparing the insulin antibody binding capacity before treatment with that after treatment with DFPP and PSL, the value gradually decreased from 89.1 to 20.9% (6 months), while the casual blood glucose improved to 154 ± 55 mg/dL CGM, and the GA level declined from 36.5 to 23.7% (6 months). Furthermore, the frequency of hypoglycemia decreased, and the amount of insulin administered decreased from 61 to 38 U/day (6 months). These results suggested the long-term effectiveness of DFPP and PSL therapy (Fig. 2).

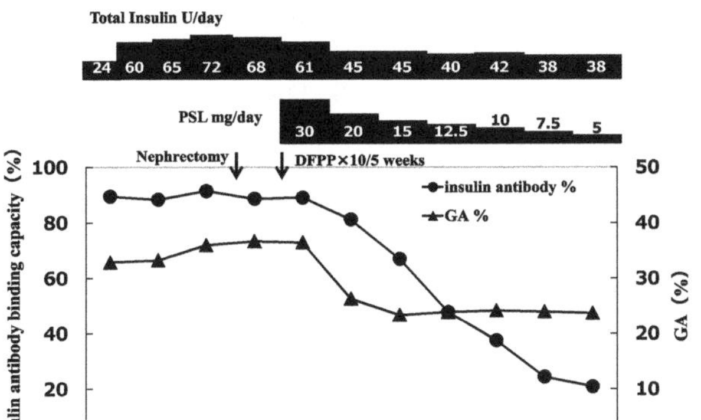

Fig. 2 The clinical course of the patient. DFPP was performed twice a week for 3 h before HD for 5 weeks, totaling 10 times. Abbreviations; *GA* glycoalbumin, *DFPP* double filtration plasmapheresis, *PSL* prednisolone

The insulin antibody binding capacity declined from 89.5% before treatment with DFPP and PSL to 23.7% at 6 months after introduction of the treatment. Further, using a Scatchard analysis to compare human insulin before with after treatment for qualitative evaluation of the antibody, low affinity and high binding capacity was indicated before treatment, at $k1 = 0.0034 \times 10^8\ M^{-1}$, $R1 = 112 \times 10^{-8}M$; however, the affinity elevated, and the number of binding capacity significantly declined after treatment, at $k1 = 0.04 \times 10^8\ M^{-1}$, $R1 = 9.1 \times 10^{-8}M$ (Fig. 3).

The patient has continued self-monitoring of blood glucose and self-administration of insulin and undergoing chronic maintenance HD 3 times a week in our hospital as an outpatient. He is clinically well, showing no signs of exacerbation of poor glycemic control, with a GA level of approximately 21%, even 12 months after the initiation of the treatment (total insulin of 32 U/day and PSL of 2.5 mg/day).

Discussion

The authors found out three important clinical issues in the present case: First, poor glycemic control following administration of insulin was attributable to insulin antibody during insulin treatment for rare fulminant type 1 diabetes developing shortly after the introduction of HD. Second, after the treatment with DFPP and PSL to reduce insulin antibody, the insulin antibody value was still high despite the results as follows: (1) a significant decrease in the insulin antibody binding capacity, (2) glycemic control improved, and (3) the amount of insulin administered was reduced. Third, a Scatchard analysis was useful for evaluating the qualitative changes in

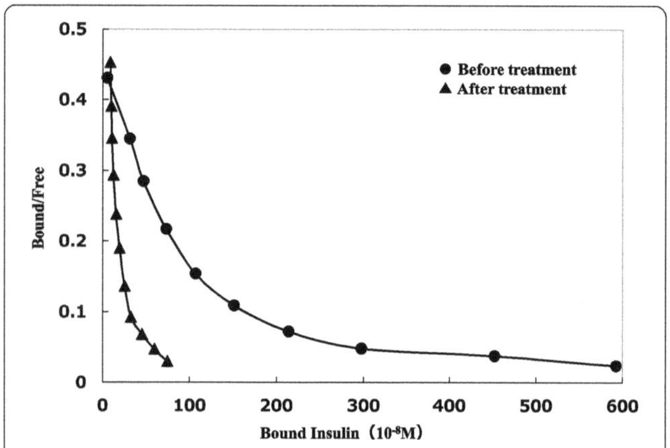

Fig. 3 Scatchard plots of insulin antibody in this patient. Before treatment of double filtration plasmapheresis and prednisolone (*circle*, $k1 = 0.0032 \times 10^8\ M^{-1}$, $R1 = 112 \times 10^{-8}$ M) and after treatment (*triangle*, $k1 = 0.0400 \times 10^8\ M^{-1}$, $R1 = 9.1 \times 10^{-8}$ M). Bound/free insulin at low concentration of bound insulin is thought to reflect the degree of affinity of the antibody. To assess the quantity of high-affinity antibody in relation to the level of affinity, the authors calculated the value of *X* intercept (R1) multiplied by the *Y* intercept (k1R1) of the Scatchard line for high-affinity binding sites, where k1 and R1 were affinity constant and binding capacity in high-affinity binding sites, respectively. These plots of after treatment indicate the degree of affinity of the antibody increased, whereas the degree of binding capacity dramatically decreased compared with before treatment

the insulin antibody level; high affinity and a decline in the number of binding sites were observed after treatment. These results indicated the effectiveness of the treatment with DFPP and PSL.

In general, while the pathogenesis of fulminant type 1 diabetes remains unknown, this is a subtype of non-autoimmune, fulminant disorder characterized by a remarkably abrupt onset (exhibiting hyperglycemia and ketoacidosis), elevated serum pancreatic enzyme concentrations, depletion of endogenous insulin secretion, and the absence of insulitis and diabetes-related antibody within several days after onset [4]. HbA1c level is often normal or slightly increased. The association between the disease and viral infections has been discussed as the cause [5], the pathogenesis is still unknown. Approximately 10% of new-onset type 1 diabetes cases in Japan has been reported to be fulminant type. Moreover, antecedent infection is observed in approximately 70%, along with complications of the upper respiratory symptoms and digestive symptoms [6]. Among HLA genes, several haplotypes constructing the DRB1 and DQB1 genes have been reported to relating to the susceptibility and resistance of the onset of type 1 diabetes [7]. However, it still remains unknown in detail. Fulminant type 1 diabetes is a fatal disease that requires rapid diagnosis and treatment. Regardless of the blood glucose level, patients under HD generally complain of dry mouth attributable to water restrictions. Moreover, they tend to cause as follows: (1) pseudo-hypo HbA1c values attributable to renal anemia and (2) shortened hemoglobin cycle. Moreover, to distinguish the present disease from dialysis disequilibrium syndrome might be difficult if the present disease developed shortly after introduction of HD. In patients under HD with no medical history of diabetes complicated with acute hyperglycemia and metabolic acidosis, HbA1c and diabetes-related auto-antibodies should be examined.

Next, regarding insulin antibody, it could be produced by two pathways as follows: (1) exogenous insulin formulations and (2) produced against the patient's own insulin, such as insulin autoimmune syndrome. In the present case, the clinical course suggested that insulin antibody were induced by exogenous insulin from the results as follows: (1) no characteristic HLA DR4 (DRB1*04:06) in the insulin autoimmune syndrome was observed, (2) the patient had no history of taking drugs that might induce the syndrome, and (3) the patient was undergoing exogenous insulin treatment.

Although there are no established treatments for insulin antibody, reports are available concerning the effectiveness of apheresis such as DFPP, steroids, and other immunosuppressive drugs [8]. As the molecular weight of insulin antibody has not been well known, DFPP was selected as an apheresis therapy to remove wide range of molecular weight in the present case. DFPP might be effective in HD patients complicated by fulminant type 1 diabetes with a high insulin antibody value and poor glycemic control, as well as HD patients complicated by other forms of insulin-dependent diabetes. Apheresis could be one of the most efficient therapies to eliminate antibodies; however, the therapeutic effect is temporary and disappears within a short-term of approximately 6 months; therefore, several reports are available mentioning the effectiveness of the long-term treatment with apheresis repeatedly, as well as the concomitant use of insulin-like growth factor (IGF) I for maintaining favorable glycemic control [8]. Discontinuation of insulin for the purpose of reducing insulin antibody is also one of the options [9].

Several reports in the literature describe the effectiveness of steroid therapy; however, the dosage of steroids at the time of introduction, methods for gradually reducing the dosage, and the presence of steroid pulse therapy (not performed in the present case) differ from reports. A certain consensus concerning the long-term prognosis of steroid treatment has not been obtained [10].

In the present case, since achieving good glycemic control was difficult due to the presence of insulin antibodies, the possibility remained that monotherapy (DFPP or steroid) might be insufficient; therefore, the authors performed two kinds of treatments (both DFPP and steroid) at the same time.

According to the laboratory results of the present case on admission, an abdominal CT scan revealed no findings such as pancreatic enlargement, poorly defined edges, or ascites retention. In contrast, a mild increase in pancreatic exocrine enzymes was observed. A thyroid gland ultrasound revealed no morphological defects. Despite severe hyperglycemia (602 mg/dL) at the onset of diabetes, HbA1c (5.9%) and GA (18.4%) poorly elevated. Three weeks later (when transferred to our hospital), his glycemic profile changed as follows: blood glucose 642 mg/dL, HbA1c 8.3, and GA 32.9%. Three weeks interval of acute onset of hyperglycemia and poor glycemic control might affect the deterioration of HbA1c and GA levels. Moreover, serum CPR level (0.04 ng/mL) and CPR value (0 ng/mL) by glucagon tolerance testing, indicating depletion of insulin secretion. Pancreatic islet-related auto-antibodies were negative.

In the present case, serological typing was DR15, and DNA typing was DR15 (DRB1*15:01), DQB1*04:02:01/DQB1*06:02:01 by HLA testing. These results showed the resistance to HLA associated with type 1 diabetes [7]. Moreover, HLA DRB1*04:05-DQB1*04:01 [11, 12] was not observed, which provided the potential association with fulminant type 1 diabetes. According to "the diagnostic criteria of fulminant type 1 diabetes [13]," association with HLA DRB1*04:05-DQB1*04:01 was not observed in the reference findings; however, the present case was diagnosed as fulminant type 1 diabetes that appeared almost simultaneously with the introduction of dialysis. No reports were available concerning fulminant type 1 diabetes complicated with dialysis therapy or renal disease. The relationship between fulminant type 1 diabetes and dialysis therapy was not clarified in this case. It seems accordingly that fulminant type 1 diabetes is merely an incidental complication in a HD patient.

In the present case, the clinical course suggested that poor glycemic control was attributable to insulin antibody after insulin administration; however, few reports were available showing the relationship between insulin antibody and poor glycemic control such as in the present case.

The patient did not require much insulin initially, but the insulin dose gradually increased from 24 U to a maximum of 72 U/day within 2 months. Insulin intensification therapy was introduced (at first, insulin lispro as bolus and detemir as basal and then changed insulin glulisine as bolus, glargine as basal); however, his glycemic control did not improve. This showed that changeness of the type of insulin did not effect in this case.

The number of daily exogenous insulin injections has been reported to be a factor influencing insulin antibody production [1]. Insulin intensification therapy could be related to the production of high amounts of insulin antibodies within a short period of time in this patient accordingly.

Hattori et al. reported as follows: (1) insulin antibody developed even in patients who have never used insulin (2.7%), (2) insulin glargine and aspart were more antigenic than other insulin analogs, (3) the time to produce insulin antibody after the start of insulin administration varied from several days to several months [14].

In the present case, the possibility remains as follows: (1) insulin antibody might be produced early after the start of the insulin treatment (he had been administered glargine at the beginning of the treatment), (2) the patient might have insulin antibody before insulin treatment; thereby, a large amount of insulin was required from the early stage of the treatment.

The insulin antibody value was remarkably elevated in the present case. Previous studies reported that insulin antibody observed among insulin users rarely effects on glycemic control [1]. In contrast, as in the present case, several reports in the literature describing poor glycemic control caused by insulin antibody have recently increased [3]. In the present case, glycemic control deteriorated despite strict self-administration of insulin. The main cause could be due to the involvement of insulin antibody as follows: (1) changes in the glycemic control and (2) the qualitative changes of the insulin antibody, as shown in the Scatchard analysis comparing the values before and after treatment with DFPP and PSL. A Scatchard analysis revealed that the patient had low affinity and high binding capacity before treatment, at k1 (affinity); 0.0034×10^8 M^{-1} and R1 (binding capacity), 112×10^{-8} M, characteristics that seemed similar to the insulin antibody findings in patients with insulin autoimmune syndrome [2]. In cases with poor glycemic control attributable to the appearance of insulin antibody after the administration of insulin, as in the present case, the Scatchard plot results showed insulin antibody characteristics similar to those in patients with insulin autoimmune syndrome [2]. Furthermore, previous reports also found that the insulin activity could be suppressed by increasing the insulin antibody binding capacity, thereby causing hyperglycemia in the daytime the large amount of insulin binding to the antibody in the daytime due to low affinity gradually dissociated in the nighttime, thereby causing nocturnal hypoglycemia [2]. The similar fluctuations of blood glucose concentration were also observed in the CGM in the present case.

A Scatchard analysis revealed "qualitative changes" in the insulin antibodies after DFPP and long-term PSL treatment in the present case, and significant improvement in the reduction of insulin dosage, blood glucose fluctuations (CGM), glycemic control (GA value), and the reduction of insulin antibody binding capacity was observed. The combination therapy of DFPP and long-term PSL treatment was effective. In contrast, the insulin antibody remained high value. These results show the effectiveness of treatment with DFPP, and PSL should be evaluated not only using the insulin antibody value but also using the CGM, GA value, and insulin antibody binding capacity in similar cases.

Although the present case has still been administered PSL with gradual reduction (5 mg/day), the possibility remains that glycemic control might deteriorate attributable to a reduction or discontinuation of PSL in the future. Insulin treatment is essential to the present case; therefore, monitoring long-term glycemic daily profile should be continued. Moreover, fulminant type 1 diabetes has been reported to be a high-risk group prone to the advancement of microvascular diseases attributable to poor glycemic control [15]. Long-term evaluation of daily glycemic profile is necessary for reducing the risk of cardiovascular disease.

Conclusions

In conclusion, the authors present a unique case of fulminant type 1 diabetes developing during the HD introduction period. The present case is rare; however, physicians specializing in endocrinology, nephrology, and dialysis therapy also should keep in mind that this is a life-threatening complication if the treatment is delayed and that concomitant therapy with apheresis such as DFPP and long-term PSL is effective in some cases when glycemic control deteriorates attributable to the appearance of insulin antibody. No established protocol concerning the dosage of steroids, gradual reduction method, or criteria for discontinuation has been available. Further accumulation and investigation of similar cases should be required.

Abbreviations

ALP: Alkaline phosphatase; ALT: Alanine aminotransferase; ANCA: Anti-neutrophil cytoplasmic antibody; AST: Asparate aminotransferase; BUN: Blood urea nitrogen; CA19-9: Carbohydrate antigen 19-9; CEA: Carcinoembryonic antigen; CGM: Continuous glucose monitor; CPR: C-peptide immunoreactivity; CT: Computed tomography; DFPP: Double filtration plasmapheresis; GA: Glycoalbumin; GAD: Glutamic acid decarboxylase; HbA1c: Hemoglobin A1c; HD: Hemodialysis; HLA: Human leukocyte antigen; IA-2: Islet antigen-2; ICA: Islet cell antibody; IGF: Insulin-like growth factor; MPO: Myeloperoxidase; PR3: Protease 3; PSL: Prednisolone; RCC: Renal cell carcinoma; TPO: Thyroid peroxidase; γ-GTP: Gamma-glutamyl transpeptidase.

Acknowledgements

The authors would like to express our sincere thanks to Dr Tomomi Hakoda for giving us valuable advice and the medical staffs of Nippon Kokan Fukuyama Hospital, Hiroshima, Japan for collecting samples of the patient and analyzing the samples. The authors also thank to Mr. Brain Quinn for his skillful English editing.

Funding

Not applicable. Our manuscript does not contain funding.

Authors' contributions

KW is responsible for the manuscript. KW and YW performed acquisition of data and interpretation of data, drafted, and revised manuscript. HAU helped to draft the manuscript. All authors read and approved the final manuscript.

Competing interests

The authors declare that they have no competing interests.

Author details

[1]Division of Nephrology and Dialysis, Department of Internal Medicine, Nippon Kokan Fukuyama Hospital, 1844, Tsunoshita, Daimon-cho, Fukuyama, Hiroshima 721-0927, Japan. [2]Department of Chronic Kidney Disease and Cardiovascular Disease, Okayama University Graduate School of Medicine, Dentistry and Pharmaceutical Sciences, Okayama, Japan. [3]Division of Nephrology and Dialysis, Department of Internal Medicine, Central Hospital, Hiroshima, Japan.

References

1. Van Haeften TW. Clinical significance of insulin antibodies in insulin-treated diabetic patients. Diabetes Care. 1989;12:641–8.
2. Uchigata Y, Eguchi Y, Takayama-Hasumi S, Omori Y. Insulin autoimmune syndrome (Hirata disease): clinical features and epidemiology in Japan. Diabetes Res Clin Pract. 1994;22:89–94.
3. Hoshina S, Kondo T, Fujioka M, Gocho N, Togawa A, Tanaka H, et al. A case of type 2 diabetes mellitus with polymyalgia rheumatica successfully treated with long-term corticosteroid administration for nocturnal hypoglycemia possibly caused by insulin antibody. J Japan Diab Soc. 2012;55:470–6 [in Japanese].
4. Imagawa A, Hanafusa T, Miyagawa J, Matsuzawa Y. A novel subtype of type 1 diabetes mellitus characterized by a rapid onset and an absence of diabetes-related antibodies. N Eng J Med. 2000;342:301–7.
5. Imagawa A, Hanafusa T. Fulminant type 1 diabetes—an important subtype in East Asia. Diabetes Metab Res Rev. 2011;27:959–64.
6. Imagawa A, Hanafusa T, Uchigata Y, Kanatsuka A, Kawasaki E, Kobayashi T, et al. Fulminant type 1 diabetes: a nationwide survey in Japan. Diabetes Care. 2003;26:2345–52.
7. Kawabata Y, Ikegami H, Kawaguchi Y, Fujisawa T, Shintani M, Ono M, et al. Asian-specific HLA haplotypes reveal heterogeneity of the contribution of HLA-DR and -DQ haplotypes to susceptibility to type 1 diabetes. Diabetes. 2002;51:545–51.
8. Koyama R, Nakanishi K, Kato M, Yamashita S, Kuwahara H, Katori H. Hypoglycemia and hyperglycemia due to insulin antibodies against therapeutic human insulin: treatment with double filtration plasmapheresis and prednisolone. Am J Med Sci. 2005;329:259–64.
9. Hara K, Tobe K, Uchigata Y, Nakazono M, Yasuda K, Terauchi Y, et al. Antibody-mediated insulin resistance treated by cessation of insulin administration. Intern Med. 2000;39:143–5.
10. Matsuyoshi A, Shimoda S, Tsuruzoe K, Taketa K, Chirioka T, Sakamoto F, et al. A case of slowly progressive type 1 diabetes with unstable glycemic control caused by unusual insulin antibody and successfully treated with steroid therapy. Diabetes Res Clin Pract. 2006;72:238–43.
11. Kawabata Y, Ikegami H, Awata H, Imagawa A, Maruyama T, Kawasaki E, et al. Differential association of HLA with three subtypes of type 1 diabetes: fulminant, slowly progressive and acute-onset. Diabetologia. 2009;52:2513–21.
12. Tsutsumi C, Imagawa A, Ikegami H, Makino H, Kobayashi T, Hanafusa T, on behalf of the Japan Diabetes Society Committee on Type 1 Diabetes Mellitus Research. Class II HLA genotype in fulminant type 1 diabetes: a nationwide survey with reference to glutamic acid decarboxylase antibodies. J Diabetes Investig. 2012;3:62–9.
13. Imagawa A, Hanafusa T, Awata T, Ikegami H, Uchigata Y, Osawa H, et al. Report of the Committee of the Japan Diabetes Society on the Research of Fulminant and Acute-onset Type 1 Diabetes Mellitus: new diagnositic criteria of fulminant type 1 diabetes mellitus. J Diabetes Investig. 2012;3:536–9.

5

Evaluating the association between walking speed and reduced cardio-cerebrovascular events in hemodialysis patients

Yoshifumi Abe[1], Atsuhiko Matsunaga[1*], Ryota Matsuzawa[2], Kei Yoneki[1,3], Manae Harada[1], Takaaki Watanabe[1], Toshiki Kutsuna[4], Masahiko Kimura[5], Kyo Shigeta[1], Yasuo Takeuchi[6] and Atsushi Yoshida[3]

Abstract

Background: Deterioration in walking ability characterized by slow walking speed is associated with an increased risk of mortality in patients on hemodialysis (HD), but few studies have examined the potential for walking speed to reduce the incidence of clinical events. In this study, we assessed a range of maximum walking speeds (MWS) with regard to their capacity to reduce cardio-cerebrovascular events in HD patients.

Methods: In total, 188 Japanese outpatients (90 men, 98 women; mean age, 65 years) undergoing maintenance HD three times a week were monitored for 7 years. We measured clinical characteristics and MWS at baseline and followed these patients to track any cardio-cerebrovascular events. Patients were divided into quartiles (Q1 = lowest, Q4 = highest) based on MWS for each sex. Cox proportional hazards regression and Kaplan-Meier estimates were used to assess the contribution of MWS to cardio-cerebrovascular events.

Results: During the follow-up period, cardio-cerebrovascular events occurred in 42 patients. After adjusting for potential confounders, the hazard ratio for events per 10 m/min increase in MWS was 0.77 (95 % confidence interval: 0.65–0.92; $P = 0.004$). Seven-year cumulative incidence rates were 36, 32, 13, and 9 % for Q1 through Q4, respectively, and a significant difference across MWS quartiles was observed ($P < 0.001$). While the incidence rates did not significantly differ between Q1 and Q2 or between Q3 and Q4, Kaplan-Meier curves clearly differed between Q2 and Q3.

Conclusions: Our findings suggest that more than the MWS level of Q3 (≥89 m/min in men and ≥85 m/min in women) may serve as important MWS values for disease management in ambulatory HD patients.

Keywords: Hemodialysis patient, Walking speed, Walking ability, Cardio-cerebrovascular event, Disease management

Background

Many recent clinical reports have demonstrated that motor function including walking ability can deteriorate significantly in patients with end-stage renal dysfunction who require hemodialysis (HD), compared to age-matched community-based healthy individuals [1, 2]. In particular, deterioration in walking ability characterized by slow walking speed is significantly associated with reduced physical activity, decline in instrumental activities of daily living, and overall lower quality of life [3–5]. Moreover, epidemiological cohort studies have found that slow walking speed is independently associated with mortality, hospitalization, and adverse events in healthy older individuals and in patients with heart disease, kidney disease, stroke, and other chronic diseases [4–7]. From a clinical perspective, it is necessary to evaluate and manage walking ability as a way to implement

* Correspondence: atsuhikonet@gmail.com
[1]Department of Rehabilitation Sciences, Kitasato University Graduate School of Medical Sciences, 1-15-1 Kitasato, Sagamihara, Kanagawa 252-0373, Japan
Full list of author information is available at the end of the article

effective disease management for patients (particularly the elderly) with chronic diseases that may require HD.

Overall, survival of patients with end-stage renal dysfunction has been improving annually over the past decade, regardless of whether HD or peritoneal dialysis is provided as treatment. This is because dialysis treatment technology and disease management for patients undergoing dialysis have made great progress in recent years [8]. Despite this, the percentage of elderly HD patients who are 60 years or older has reached 75 % in Japan [9]. Accordingly, HD patients are more likely to have decreased walking speed due to age-related loss of muscle mass (sarcopenia), as well as decreased muscle strength and balance function due to reduced physical activity [10]. In addition, patients who have undergone HD for 10 years or more comprise one third of all HD patients [9]. After regular HD treatment is initiated, these patients are also more likely to develop multiple comorbidities including ischemic heart disease, peripheral vascular disease, stroke, and orthopedic disease, to name a few, in addition to the primary cause of their end-stage renal dysfunction. Thus, HD patients have a 10 to 20 times higher risk for cardio-cerebrovascular events compared to age-matched healthy people [11]. However, very few studies have conducted longitudinal evaluations of walking speed associated with subsequent clinical events in HD patients, and optimal management techniques for walking speed in these patients remain unclear. Given the above, we conducted a 7-year cohort study to evaluate a range of walking speeds with regard to their capacity to reduce cardio-cerebrovascular events in HD patients.

Methods

Study population

This study was approved by the Ethics Committee of Kitasato University School of Allied Health Sciences and was conducted in accordance with the standards set forth by the latest revision of the Declaration of Helsinki. All patients received a detailed explanation of the study protocol and provided informed consent. From October 2002 to September 2014, clinically stable outpatients at the Hemodialysis Center at Sagami Junkanki Clinic were assessed for eligibility for inclusion in this prospective study. Patients were undergoing maintenance HD therapy three times a week according to the Japanese Society for Dialysis Therapy guidelines. In order to focus specifically on how walking ability impacts subsequent cardio-cerebrovascular events, subjects were excluded if they fulfilled the following criteria: duration of maintenance HD ≤3 months; hospitalization ≤6 months prior to study enrollment; history of recent myocardial infarction or angina pectoris; presence of uncontrolled cardiac arrhythmias, hemodynamic instability, or uncontrolled hypertension; require walking assistance; and the presence of any other conditions that limited walking (e.g., dementia, low vision or blindness, paralysis due to stroke, leg amputation).

Demographic and clinical factors

Information on demographic factors (age, sex, HD duration), physical characteristics (body mass index [BMI]), primary kidney disease, and comorbid conditions was collected at study entry. Blood hemoglobin, serum albumin, and serum C-reactive protein were obtained from patient hospital charts. To quantify comorbid illnesses in this study, we used a comorbidity index developed for dialysis patients (composed of primary causes of end-stage renal disease; atherosclerotic heart disease, congestive heart failure, cerebrovascular accident/transient ischemic attack, peripheral vascular disease, dysrhythmia, and other cardiac disease; chronic obstructive pulmonary disease; gastrointestinal bleeding; liver disease; cancer; and diabetes). This score was calculated using a previously described method that has been used to analyze survival among HD patients [12].

Maximum walking speed

Self-selected maximum walking speed (MWS) along a 10-m walkway was measured to assess patient walking ability before dialysis on a dialysis day. The validity and reliability of the 10-m walk test, which measures the time (in seconds or minutes) required for a patient to walk 10 m, have been investigated in several populations including healthy elderly, patients with neurological disorders, and those with orthopedic dysfunction [13]. First, patients were asked to walk down a 10-m walking lane with an acceleration area at their usual speed to prepare for the MWS measurement. They were then instructed to walk as fast as was safely possible, without running. MWS was defined as the higher value of two attempts and expressed as the ratio of distance to time (m/min) [13].

Cardio-cerebrovascular events

We assessed cardio-cerebrovascular events as an indicator of subsequent adverse outcomes for HD patients. Patients were followed until the following clinical events occurred during the 7-year cohort study: hospital admission for angina, myocardial infarction, heart failure, cerebral infarction, or cerebral hemorrhage. Diagnoses for primary admission were recorded using the International Classification of Disease, version 10 (ICD-10). Angina, myocardial infarction, and heart failure were defined as ICD-10 codes I20-I22 and I50, respectively, and cerebral infarction and cerebral hemorrhage as ICD-10 codes I60-I63. Angina was defined using ICD-10 codes as follows: I20, angina pectoris; I20.0, unstable angina; I20.1, angina pectoris with documented spasm; I20.8, other forms of angina pectoris; and I20.9, angina pectoris, unspecified. Myocardial infarction was defined using ICD-10 codes as follows: I21, acute myocardial infarction; I22, subsequent myocardial infarction; I21.0, acute transmural myocardial infarction of anterior wall; I21.1, acute transmural myocardial infarction of inferior wall; I21.2, acute transmural myocardial infarction of other sites; I21.3, acute transmural myocardial infarction of unspecified site; I21.4, acute subendocardial myocardial infarction; I21.9, acute myocardial infarction unspecified; I22.0, subsequent myocardial infarction of anterior wall; I22.1, subsequent myocardial infarction of inferior wall; I22.8, subsequent myocardial infarction of other sites; and I22.9, subsequent myocardial infarction of unspecified site. Heart failure was defined using ICD-10 codes as follows: I50, heart failure; I50.0, congestive heart failure; I50.1, congestive heart failure; and I50.9, heart failure, unspecified.

Statistical analysis

As there are no established MWS categories for HD patients, MWS was categorized into sex-specific quartiles based on previous studies that found a strong association between MWS and sex. Patients were divided into following quartiles, ranging from Q1 (slow MWS) to Q4 (fast MWS): <79, 79 to 89, 89 to 105, and ≥105 m/min in men and <72, 72 to 85, 85 to 100, and ≥100 m/min in women. Differences in clinical characteristics and MWS between quartiles were tested by one-way analysis of variance, Kruskal-Wallis test, or chi-squared test. A multivariable analysis was performed using the Cox proportional hazards regression model to estimate the independent prognostic effect of MWS on risk of subsequent cardio-cerebrovascular events after adjusting for confounders. We included the confounders (MWS, age, sex, BMI, HD duration, diabetic nephropathy of primary kidney disease, comorbidity score, hemoglobin, serum albumin, and serum C-reactive protein) in the models. Within the present study sample, there were 42 cardio-cerebrovascular events, which allowed for a maximum of four variables to be included in the multivariate Cox model. If the multivariate Cox model includes more than four covariates, it has the potential to cause overfitting. To avoid overfitting, all potential confounding factors were reduced to four composite characteristics with a significant ($P < 0.05$) association with subsequent cardio-cerebrovascular events in the univariate Cox model. We calculated the cumulative incidence of cardio-cerebrovascular events according to MWS quartiles. Kaplan-Meier analysis was used to estimate long-term effects. The log-rank test was used to examine differences in the risk of subsequent cardio-cerebrovascular events between MWS quartiles. The 7-year cumulative incidence probability was estimated using the life table method with the interval length set at 1 month. All analyses were performed using the Statistical Package for Social Sciences (SPSS Statistics 22.0 for Mac; IBM Corp., Armonk, NY, USA). Statistical significance was set at $P < 0.05$.

Results

Patient characteristics

Of the 465 Japanese outpatients assessed for their eligibility for inclusion, we excluded 119 patients who did not satisfy the inclusion criteria, and 158 patients declined to participate in the study. Ultimately, 188 HD patients were recruited (Fig. 1). Demographic and clinical characteristics of the patients are summarized in Table 1. The patients comprised 90 men and 98 women, aged 35–88 years (mean age, 65 years). The HD duration was 3.3 (25th, 75th percentiles, 1.4, 9.5) years at baseline. The most common underlying kidney diseases were diabetic nephropathy (33.5 %), followed by glomerulonephritis (32.4 %). Mean comorbidity score was 4.8 ± 3.0, and MWS for all patients was 87.5 ± 19.6 m/min. Table 1 shows the baseline characteristics of the patients according to MWS quartiles 1–4. We found significant quartile-dependent differences in age, comorbidity score, serum albumin, and MWS ($P < 0.01$, $P < 0.01$, $P = 0.02$, $P < 0.001$ respectively). Other baseline characteristics did not differ significantly across the four quartiles.

Outcomes

Patients were followed for up to 7 years. The overall follow-up durations ranged from 1 to 84 months (median, 53 months). During the follow-up period, cardio-cerebrovascular events occurred in 42 patients (22 %): 8 of angina, 12 of myocardial infarction, 16 of heart failure, 1 of subarachnoid hemorrhage, 1 of intracerebral hemorrhage, and 4 of cerebral infarction. Twenty-five percent of the patients with Q1 and Q2 group occurred events after 21 and 40 months. On the other hand, the events rate of patients with Q3 and Q4 at the end of the follow-up was less than 25 %.

The relationship between outcomes and MWS as continuous variables

According to the Cox proportional hazards model, the increase in crude hazard ratio (HR) of MWS per 10 m/min was 0.74 (95 % confidence interval [CI], 0.63–0.86; $P < 0.001$), which indicated that maintaining a higher MWS was associated with a reduction in cardio-cerebrovascular events (Table 2). After adjusting for the effects of age, diabetic nephropathy, and comorbidity score, the HR was 0.77 (95 % CI, 0.65–0.92; $P = 0.004$) (Table 2).

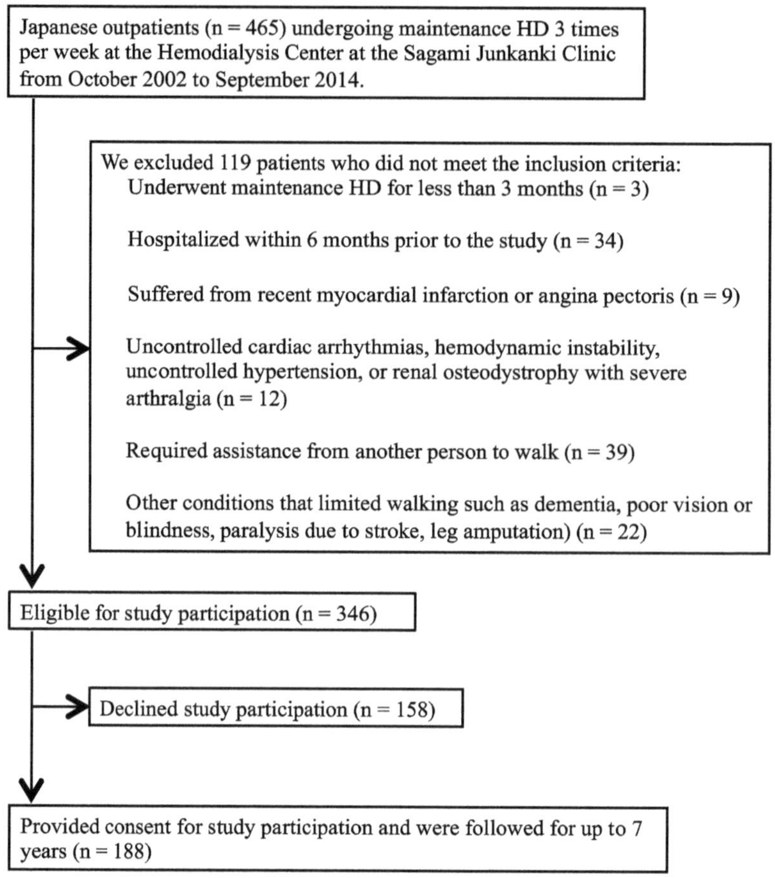

Fig. 1 Flow diagram for patient selection and exclusion

The relationship between outcomes and MWS as categorical variables

Seven-year cumulative incidence rates were 36, 32, 13, and 9 % for Q1 through Q4, respectively ($P < 0.001$). The cumulative incidence rates of cardio-cerebrovascular events in Q1 were significantly higher than those in Q3 and Q4 ($P = 0.003$, $P < 0.001$, respectively). Cumulative incidence rates of cardio-cerebrovascular events in Q2 were also significantly higher than rates in Q3 and Q4 ($P = 0.03$, $P = 0.004$, respectively). While incidence rates did not significantly differ between Q1 and Q2 or between Q3 and Q4, Kaplan-Meier curves showed clear differences between Q2 and Q3 (Fig. 2).

Discussion

The main finding of this study is that the initial MWS at the time of study entry significantly influenced the 7-year cumulative incidence of cardio-cerebrovascular events in ambulatory patients on hemodialysis (HD), independent of age, sex, BMI, HD duration, diabetic nephropathy of primary kidney disease, comorbid conditions, and markers of anemia, nutrition, and inflammation. To our knowledge, this is the first study to demonstrate an association between walking ability and subsequent cardio-cerebrovascular events in an Asian population of patients with chronic kidney disease undergoing HD. Based on our findings, the hazard ratio for clinical events per 10-m/min increases in MWS was 0.77. Our study also revealed that male HD patients with MWS ≥89 m/min and female HD patients with MWS ≥85 m/min at baseline had a significantly lower cumulative incidence of cardio-cerebrovascular events compared to other patients during the 7-year follow-up period. These different walking speeds had not yet been evaluated for their potential to reduce subsequent clinical events in ambulatory HD patients. As such, our present study findings have important implications with regard to effective disease management in Japanese HD populations.

Recent studies have shown that walking speed is gaining interest for the prognosis of adverse health-related events, particularly for elderly individuals. Montero-Odasso et al. showed that a slow walking speed alone in otherwise well-functioning elderly individuals was enough to predict the risk for future adverse events during a 2-year follow-up study [5]. A recent 7-year cohort

Table 1 Baseline characteristics based on levels of maximum walking speed

Characteristic	Overall (*n* = 188)	Maximum walking speed				*P* value
		Q1 (*n* = 47)	Q2 (*n* = 47)	Q3 (*n* = 47)	Q4 (*n* = 47)	
Age (years)	65 (10)	73 (10)	64 (8)	63 (9)	60 (9)	<0.001
Women	98 (52.1)	24 (51)	25 (53)	24 (51)	25 (53)	0.99
Body mass index (kg/m^2)	21.2 (3.2)	20.3 (3.2)	21.7 (3.3)	20.7 (3.3)	21.9 (2.8)	0.42
Hemodialysis duration (years)	3.3 (1.4, 9.5)	2.5 (1.2, 8.1)	3.8 (2.0, 12.6)	3.2 (1.8, 7.3)	3.3 (1.0, 8.5)	0.35
Primary kidney disease						0.19
Diabetic nephropathy	63 (33.5)	17 (36.2)	17 (36.2)	16 (34.0)	13 (27.7)	
Glomerulonephritis	61 (32.4)	9 (19.1)	15 (31.9)	18 (38.3)	19 (40.4)	
Hypertension	16 (8.5)	4 (8.5)	5 (10.6)	4 (8.5)	3 (6.4)	
Polycystic renal disease	7 (3.7)	1 (2.1)	0 (0)	4 (8.5)	2 (4.3)	
Other nephropathies	41 (21.8)	16 (34.0)	10 (21.3)	5 (10.6)	10 (21.3)	
Comorbid condition						
Presence of cardiac disease[a]	91 (48.4)	31 (66.0)	20 (42.6)	26 (55.3)	14 (29.8)	0.003
Peripheral vascular disease	20 (10.6)	7 (3.7)	5 (2.7)	4 (2.1)	4 (2.1)	0.72
Presence of diabetes mellitus	76 (40.4)	19 (40.4)	22 (46.8)	18 (38.3)	17 (36.2)	0.74
Comorbidity score	4.8 (3.0)	6.3 (2.8)	4.7 (3.0)	4.4 (2.9)	3.6 (2.7)	<0.001
Laboratory values						
Hemoglobin (g/dL)	10.3 (1.0)	10.2 (0.9)	10.0 (1.0)	10.3 (0.9)	10.4 (1.0)	0.34
Serum albumin (g/dL)	3.9 (0.3)	3.8 (0.3)	3.8 (0.3)	3.9 (0.3)	4.0 (0.3)	0.02
Serum C-reactive protein (mg/dL)	0.3 (0.7)	0.4 (0.8)	0.3 (0.7)	0.3 (0.7)	0.3 (0.4)	0.61
Walking ability						
Maximum walking speed (m/min)	87.5 (19.6)	62.7 (11.6)	81.4 (4.9)	94.1 (5.6)	111.9 (8.1)	<0.001

Values are expressed as mean (standard deviation), median (25th, 75th percentiles), or number (percentage of total). The cutoff values defining the maximum walking speed quartiles were <79, 79–89, 89–105, and ≥105 m/min in men and <72, 72–85, 85–100, and ≥100 m/min in women
[a]History of coronary disease, congestive heart failure, myocardial infarction, or other cardiac disease

Table 2 Univariate and multivariate Cox models for the effects of maximum walking speed on cardio-cerebrovascular events

Factors	Units of increase	Univariate Cox model[a]		Multivariate Cox model[b]	
		HR (95 % CI)	*P*	HR (95 % CI)	*P*
Maximum walking speed	10 m/min	0.74 (0.63–0.86)	<0.001	0.77 (0.65–0.92)	0.004
Age (years)	1 year	1.05 (1.01–1.08)	0.006	1.03 (0.99–1.07)	0.16
Men (vs. women)	–	0.60 (0.33–1.11)	0.10		
Body mass index	1 kg/m^2	1.03 (0.93–1.13)	0.61		
Hemodialysis duration	1 year	1.01 (0.97–1.05)	0.70		
Diabetic nephropathy (presence)	1 presence	1.96 (1.06–3.60)	0.03	1.93 (1.02–3.64)	0.04
Comorbidity score	1	1.11 (1.01–1.21)	0.04	1.02 (0.92–1.14)	0.70
Hemoglobin	0.1 g/dL	1.15 (0.85–1.56)	0.35		
Serum albumin	0.1 g/dL	0.42 (0.17–1.05)	0.06		
Serum C-reactive protein	0.1 mg/dL	1.21 (0.85–1.73)	0.30		

Analyses were performed using a Cox proportional hazards regression model
HR hazard ratio, *CI* confidence interval
[a]Unadjusted for clinicopathological factors of cardio-cerebrovascular events
[b]Adjusted for age, diabetic nephropathy, and comorbidity score

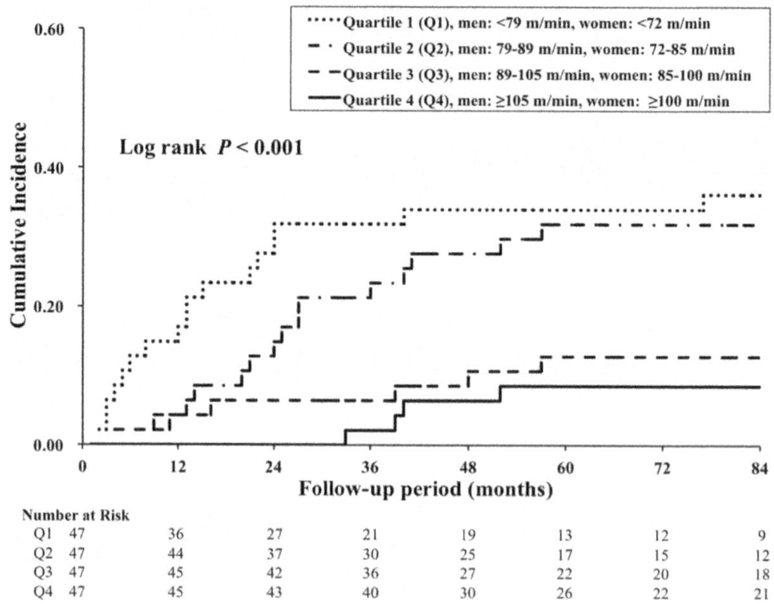

Fig. 2 Kaplan-Meier estimates for cumulative incidence rates of subsequent cardio-cerebrovascular events according to maximum walking speed quartiles

study of MWS in community-dwelling elderly reported that those who walked slowly had an almost threefold higher risk for cardiovascular mortality compared to those who walked faster [6]. Several clinical studies have found that a slow walking speed is significantly associated with an increased risk of subsequent cardiovascular events in elderly patients with ischemic heart disease, independent of cardiac function and comorbid conditions [14–17]. In addition, a slow walking speed was used as an indicator of frailty or geriatric conditions as well as decreased muscle strength (weak grip), cognitive impairment, and depression [16, 17]. Our findings are consistent with those reported by previous studies of elderly patients with chronic heart disease. Characteristics of HD patients enrolled in our present study were as follows: elderly with a mean age of 65 years (range 35–88 years), long disease duration with a median time on HD of 3.3 years (range 0.3–31.2 years), and decreased physical function with a mean MWS of 87.5 m/min (range 33.2–139.2 m/min) as much as patients with chronic heart disease [14]. Physical function including walking speed among HD patients reportedly decreases year after year and tends to have already deteriorated somewhat since before the initiation of HD treatment [18, 19]. Therefore, it is clinically necessary to evaluate and manage walking speed in order to implement effective disease management for HD patients.

The association of slow walking speed with increased risk of cardio-cerebrovascular events in the present study can be explained primarily in terms of the relationship between walking speed and physical activity. Those who walk fast likely tend to maintain high levels of habitual physical activity of daily living. Kumahara et al. reported that walking speed was significantly associated with daily physical activity in healthy people aged 18–64 years [3]. Several other studies indicated that high levels of physical activity were associated with a decreased risk of subsequent cardio-cerebrovascular events in healthy older adults [20, 21]. We found in previous studies that a lower level of habitual physical activity is an independent risk factor for all-cause mortality and is closely associated with slow MWS in maintenance HD patients [13, 22]. Several previous studies also revealed that HD patients who increased their level of physical activity were able to improve risk factors for cardio-cerebrovascular disease, such as hypertension, arterial stiffness, inflammatory reaction, vascular endothelial function, high levels of plasma triglycerides and low levels of high-density lipoprotein cholesterol, dysfunction of the cardiac autonomic nervous system, and reduced maximal oxygen consumption [22–24]. These reports suggest that maintaining high levels of habitual physical activity by walking at a fast speed can help prevent the development of atherosclerotic vascular disease and avoid complications from atherosclerotic vascular disease. The main findings of the present study regarding the association between slow walking speed and subsequent poor outcomes are consistent with findings noted in previous reports.

In our 7-year follow-up study, we also assessed the relationship between levels of MWS (divided into quartiles for each sex) and subsequent cardio-cerebrovascular events in order to clarify whether or not walking speed may comprise a part of effective disease management for the prevention of events. Kaplan-Meier curves clearly differed between Q2 and Q3 (regardless of an MWS ≥89 m/min in men and ≥85 m/min in women), while no significant difference was found between Q3 and Q4 (regardless of an MWS ≥105 m/min in men and ≥100 m/min in women). A recent cohort study of walking speed with a 5-year follow-up period reported that community-dwelling elderly people (aged ≥65 years) with a slow walking speed (≤90 m/min for men and ≤ 81 m/min for women) had a higher risk for cardiovascular mortality compared to those with a fast walking speed [6]. Yamamoto et al. also showed that ischemic heart disease patients with a fast walking speed (>90 m/min for men and >81 m/min for women) at baseline had a significantly lower cumulative incidence of cardiac events compared to other participants during a 3-year follow-up study [15]. Findings from these studies are fairly consistent with our results. We would therefore surmise that MWS above that for Q3 (MWS ≥89 m/min in men and ≥85 m/min in women) would be a suitable walking speed for disease management in HD patients. A colleague of ours and Yamamoto have reported that the walking speed of age- and sex-matched healthy elderly people from the same geographic region as the present study was almost more than the MWS level of Q3; specifically, no healthy males had a MWS less than 90 m/min, and no healthy females had a MWS less than 81 m/min [14]. Accordingly, anything above the Q3 MWS was thought to be a relatively attainable MWS for elderly HD patients because the lowest value within Q3 is likely to represent the lower limit for MWS among healthy elderly people. MWS above that for Q3 is also a reasonable MWS that should be achieved in order to walk to regular visits at an outpatient clinic for successful and continual HD treatment, maintain instrumental activities of daily living (e.g., outside social activities, outings, etc.), and maintain quality of life for an elderly HD outpatient. In addition, previous studies have found that leg strength and standing balance function are independently associated with walking speed in ambulatory HD patients [25]. Therefore, improvements in MWS could be achieved in HD patients showing a low MWS with exercising guidance aimed at promoting improved daily physical activity, and/or resistance training to improve leg strength and balance function.

This study had some limitations. First, because it was an observational study, residual confounders may remain. Second, given the study design, causality cannot be established. Thus, additional randomized and controlled studies are needed. To the best of our knowledge, this is the first study to show the correlation between cardio-cerebrovascular events and MWS in HD patients. Third, because we evaluated MWS of HD patients only at baseline, temporal fluctuations in walking abilities were not evaluated. However, because we recruited clinically stable and adequately dialyzed patients, their walking ability was assumed not to fluctuate dramatically. Fourth, we excluded patients who needed assistance with walking. As a result, comorbid conditions in the patients were relatively mild. These limitations should be considered when generalizing our study results to more severely limited patients. Finally, this was a small-scale observational study, so our results may lack general applicability.

Conclusions

Our 7-year follow-up study revealed that a slow walking speed was significantly and independently associated with an increased risk of subsequent cardio-cerebrovascular events. In addition, we found that MWS ≥89 m/min for males and MWS ≥85 m/min for females might serve as important MWS values for disease management in HD patients.

Abbreviations

HD: Hemodialysis; MWS: Maximum walking speed; BMI: Body mass index; ICD: International Classification of Disease; HR: Hazard ratio; CI: confidence interval

Acknowledgements

The authors wish to thank all patients who participated in this study. The authors also thank Dr. Yutaka Takagi, Dr. Junko Horiguchi, Ms. Junko Yoneyama, Ms. Kaoru Uemura, Ms. Fusayo Hemmi, Mr. Naoki Murouchi, and Mr. Toshiya Minowa for performing experiments and the HD treatment staff at the Sagami Junkanki Clinic for their contributions to this study.

Funding

This research was supported by JSPS KAKENHI Grant Numbers 23500614 and 26350631.

Authors' contributions

This article has 11 authors. Our study needed a planner of the study (YA), three persons for the measurement (KY, MH, TW), two persons of study explainer (YT, AY), two persons for data entry (RM, TK), two persons analyst (MK, KS), and the head of research (AM). All authors read and approved the final manuscript.

Competing interests

The authors declare that they have no competing interests.

Author details

[1]Department of Rehabilitation Sciences, Kitasato University Graduate School of Medical Sciences, 1-15-1 Kitasato, Sagamihara, Kanagawa 252-0373, Japan. [2]Department of Rehabilitation, Kitasato University Hospital, Sagamihara, Kanagawa, Japan. [3]Sagami Junkanki Clinic, Sagamihara, Kanagawa, Japan. [4]Department of Rehabilitation, Kitasato University East Hospital, Sagamihara, Kanagawa, Japan. [5]School of Allied Health Sciences, Kitasato University, Sagamihara, Kanagawa, Japan. [6]School of Medicine, Kitasato University, Sagamihara, Kanagawa, Japan.

References

1. Painter P, Carlson L, Carey S, Paul SM, Myll J. Physical functioning and health-related quality-of-life changes with exercise training in hemodialysis patients. Am J Kidney Dis. 2000;35(3):482–92.
2. Johansen KL, Painter P, Kent-Braun JA, Ng AV, Carey S, Da Silva M, et al. Validation of questionnaires to estimate physical activity and functioning in end-stage renal disease. Kidney Int. 2001;59(3):1121–7.
3. Kumahara H, Schutz Y, Ayabe M, Yoshioka M, Yoshitake Y, Shindo M, et al. The use of uniaxial accelerometry for the assessment of physical-activity-related energy expenditure: a validation study against whole-body indirect calorimetry. Br J Nutr. 2004;91(2):235–43.
4. Shinkai S, Watanabe S, Kumagai S, Fujiwara Y, Amano H, Yoshida H, et al. Walking speed as a good predictor for the onset of functional dependence in a Japanese rural community population. Age Ageing. 2000;29(5):441–6.
5. Montero-Odasso M, Schapira M, Soriano ER, Varela M, Kaplan R, Camera LA, et al. Gait velocity as a single predictor of adverse events in healthy seniors aged 75 years and older. J Gerontol A Biol Sci Med Sci. 2005;60(10):1304–9.
6. Dumurgier J, Elbaz A, Ducimetière P, Tavernier B, Alpèrovitch A, Tzourio C. Slow walking speed and cardiovascular death in well functioning older adults: prospective cohort study. BMJ. 2009;339:b4460. doi:10.1136/bmj.b4460.
7. Creaby MW, Bennell KL, Hunt MA. Gait differs between unilateral and bilateral knee osteoarthritis. Arch Phys Med Rehabil. 2012;93(5):822–7. doi:10.1016/j.apmr.2011.11.029.
8. Nakai S, Masakane I, Shigematsu T, Hamano T, Yamagata K, Watanabe Y, et al. An overview of regular dialysis treatment in Japan (as of 31 December 2007). Ther Apher Dial. 2009;13(6):457–504. doi:10.1111/j.1744-9987.2009.00789.x.
9. Hanafusa N, Nakai S, Iseki K, Tsubakihara Y. Japanese society for dialysis therapy renal data registry—a window through which we can view the details of Japanese dialysis population. Kidney Int Suppl (2011). 2015;5(1):15–22.
10. Cheema B, Abas H, Smith B, O'Sullivan AJ, Chan M, Patwardhan A, et al. Investigation of skeletal muscle quantity and quality in end-stage renal disease. Nephrology (Carlton). 2010;15(4):454–63. doi:10.1111/j.1440-1797.2009.01261.x.
11. Foley RN, Parfrey PS, Harnett JD, Kent GM, O'Dea R, Murray DC, et al. Mode of dialysis therapy and mortality in end-stage renal disease. J Am Soc Nephrol. 1998;9(2):267–76.
12. Liu J, Huang Z, Gilbertson DT, Foley RN, Collins AJ. An improved comorbidity index for outcome analyses among dialysis patients. Kidney Int. 2010;77(2):141–51. doi:10.1038/ki.2009.413.
13. Kutsuna T, Matsunaga A, Matsumoto T, Ishii A, Yamamoto K, Hotta K, et al. Physical activity is necessary to prevent deterioration of the walking ability of patients undergoing maintenance hemodialysis. Ther Apher Dial. 2010; 14(2):193–200. doi:10.1111/j.1744-9987.2009.00750.x.
14. Yamamoto S, Matsunaga A, Kamiya K, Miida K, Ebina Y, Hotta K, et al. Walking speed in patients with first acute myocardial infarction who participated in a supervised cardiac rehabilitation program after coronary intervention. Int Heart J. 2012;53(6):347–52.
15. Yamamoto S, Matsunaga A, Wang G, Hoshi K, Kamiya K, Noda C, Kimura M, et al. Effect of balance training on walking speed and cardiac events in elderly patients with ischemic heart disease. Int Heart J. 2014;55(5):397–403.
16. Matsuzawa Y, Konishi M, Akiyama E, Suzuki H, Nakayama N, Kiyokuni M, et al. Association between gait speed as a measure of frailty and risk of cardiovascular events after myocardial infarction. J Am Coll Cardiol. 2013; 61(19):1964–72. doi:10.1016/j.jacc.2013.02.020.
17. Chaudhry SI, McAvay G, Chen S, Whitson H, Newman AB, Krumholz HM, et al. Risk factors for hospital admission among older persons with newly diagnosed heart failure: findings from the Cardiovascular Health Study. J Am Coll Cardiol. 2013;61(6):635–42. doi:10.1016/j.jacc.2012.11.027.
18. Painter P, Marcus RL. Assessing physical function and physical activity in patients with CKD. Clin J Am Soc Nephrol. 2013;8(5):861–72.
19. Roshanravan B, Robinson-Choen C, Patel KV, Ayers E, Littman AJ, de Boer IH, et al. Association between physical performance and all-cause mortality in CKD. J Am Soc Nephrol. 2013;24(5):822–30. doi:10.1681/ASN.2012070702.
20. Nocon M, Hiemann T, Müller-Riemenschneider F, Thalau F, Roll S, Willich SN. Association of physical activity with all-cause and cardiovascular mortality: a systematic review and meta-analysis. Eur J Cardiovasc Prev Rehabil. 2008; 15(3):239–46. doi:10.1097/HJR.0b013e3282f55e09.
21. Kono Y, Yamada S, Kamisaka K, Araki A, Fujioka Y, Yasui K, et al. Recurrence risk after noncardioembolic mild ischemic stroke in a Japanese population. Cerebrovasc Dis. 2011;31(4):365–72. doi:10.1159/000323233.
22. Matsuzawa R, Matsunaga A, Wang G, Kutsuna T, Ishii A, Abe Y, et al. Habitual physical activity measured by accelerometer and survival in maintenance hemodialysis patients. Clin J Am Soc Nephrol. 2012;7(12): 2010–6. doi:10.2215/CJN.03660412.
23. Deligiannis A, Kouidi E, Tourkantonis A. Effects of physical training on heart rate variability in patients on hemodialysis. Am J Cardiol. 1999;84(2):197–202.
24. Mustata S, Chan C, Lai V, Miller JA. Impact of an exercise program on arterial stiffness and insulin resistance in hemodialysis patients. J Am Soc Nephrol. 2004;15(10):2713–8.
25. Abe Y, Matsunaga A, Matsuzawa R, Kutsuna T, Yamamoto S, Yoneki K, et al. Determinants of slow walking speed in ambulatory patients undergoing maintenance hemodialysis. PLoS ONE. 2016;11(3):e0151037. doi:10.1371/journal.pone.0151037.

6

Clinical advantage and tolerability of ibandronate in hemodialysis patients

Satoru Mitsuboshi[1*], Hitoshi Yamada[1], Kazuhiko Nagai[1] and Hideo Okajima[2]

Abstract

Background: Tartrate-resistant acid phosphatase-5b (TRACP-5b) and bone-specific alkaline phosphatase (BALP) levels have not been evaluated following ibandronate treatment in hemodialysis (HD) patients.

Methods: To evaluate the efficacy and tolerability of ibandronate, including TRACP-5b and BALP levels, in patients on HD, we conducted a 6-month retrospective study of 13 HD patients who were administered ibandronate at Kaetsu Hospital in Japan. All enrolled patients were placed on a regimen of intravenous ibandronate at a dose of 1 mg once every 4 weeks, from August 2015 to October 2016. Baseline and end-of-study levels of TRACP-5b and BALP were determined 1 month before and 6 months after the start of ibandronate treatment.

Results: TRACP-5b levels were significantly decreased from 785.3 ± 385.8 mU/dL at baseline to 638.2 ± 423.4 mU/dL at end of study ($P = 0.03$). Additionally, the changing levels of TRACP-5b were positively associated with baseline hip bone mineral density (BMD) ($P = 0.02$, $r = 0.65$). In contrast, BALP levels were not significantly changed. Moreover, hip BMD tended to decrease from 0.51 ± 0.10 g/cm^2 at baseline to 0.47 ± 0.11 g/cm^2 at end of study ($P = 0.07$). The tolerability index showed no statistical difference between baseline and end of study.

Conclusion: Our results indicate that ibandronate treatment in HD patients—especially those with low BMD—might sufficiently reduce TRACP-5b levels with no long-term changes in other clinical laboratory parameters. Therefore, ibandronate might be a feasible treatment option for HD patients who develop low BMD.

Keywords: Ibandronate, Tartrate-resistant acid phosphatase-5b, Bone-specific alkaline phosphatase, Bone mineral density, Hemodialysis

Background

Hemodialysis (HD) patients have a fourfold higher incidence of hip fracture compared with the general population [1]. Also, hip fractures are associated with low bone mineral density (BMD) [2] and increasing risk of mortality [3]. Thus, proper treatment is important in HD patients with low BMD.

Bisphosphonates are valuable agents for the treatment of low BMD [4] and provide vertebral and non-vertebral anti-fracture efficacy [5]. Ibandronate is a bisphosphonate that is available for intravenous use. A study in HD patients showed that about 36% of intravenously administered ibandronate 1 mg was removed from the plasma after one HD session, and plasma ibandronate concentrations were close to the lower quantification limit after three HD sessions [6]. Thus, in HD patients, a suggested monthly dose of 1 mg ibandronate should not result in plasma accumulation of ibandronate. Additionally, in HD patients, ibandronate 2 mg every 4 weeks was shown to significantly increase BMD and decrease bone turnover after 48 weeks [7]. However, little information is available regarding the efficacy and safety of ibandronate in HD patients.

In HD patients, bisphosphonate treatment is evaluated using the following markers of bone metabolism: tartrate-resistant acid phosphatase-5b (TRACP-5b) as a bone resorption marker and bone-specific alkaline phosphatase (BALP) as a bone formation marker because these markers showed no influence on renal dysfunction during an HD session [8].

* Correspondence: ccrtyo34057@gmail.com
[1]Department of Pharmacy, Kaetsu Hospital, 1459-1 Higashikanazawa, Akiha-ku, Niigata-shi, Niigata 956-0814, Japan
Full list of author information is available at the end of the article

Table 1 Patient profiles

Patient characteristics	$N = 13$
Mean age, years ± SD	78 ± 10
Sex, female/male	4/9
Mean dry weight, kg ± SD	47 ± 7
Mean years of hemodialysis ± SD	13 ± 9
Etiology of renal disease, *n*	
Glomerulonephritis	6
Nephrosclerosis	3
Diabetic kidney disease	2
Other	2
Mean hip BMD, g/cm ± SD	0.52 ± 0.12

SD standard deviation, *BMD* bone mineral density

However, although TRACP-5b markers are useful for monitoring bisphosphonate treatment [9, 10], no data have been examined for TRACP-5b and BALP levels following ibandronate treatment in HD patients. Therefore, this study aimed to evaluate the efficacy and tolerability of ibandronate in HD patients, including the TRACP-5b and BALP levels.

Methods

This 6-month retrospective study involved HD patients who had been receiving ibandronate at Kaetsu Hospital. All enrolled patients whose BMD was less than 80% of the mean BMD for young adults were started on intravenous ibandronate at a dose of 1 mg once every 4 weeks from August 2015 to October 2016. Baseline and the end of the study were defined as 1 month before and 6 months after the start of ibandronate treatment, respectively.

Hip BMD, TRACP-5b, and BALP representing the efficacy indexes were assessed at baseline and end of study. Additionally, to evaluate factors influencing changing levels of TRACP-5b, we examined the relationship between changes in the levels of TRACP-5b and the patients' backgrounds.

Table 2 Drug treatments administered to patients at baseline and at the end of the study period

	Baseline	End of study
Anti-hypertensive agents		
Angiotensin receptor blocker	5	5
Calcium channel blocker	6	6
Alpha adrenergic blocker	2	2
Beta blockers	2	2
HMG-CoA reductase inhibitors	0	0
Cinacalcet, *n*	2	2
Oral vitamin D	3	3
Intravenous vitamin D	8	8
Calcium polystyrene sulfonate	1	1

Values represent number of medicines, *n*
HMG-CoA hydroxymethylglutaryl-coenzyme A

Moreover, the levels of the following clinical parameters were considered as an overall tolerability index and were measured at baseline and end of study: hemoglobin, hematocrit, platelet count, blood urea nitrogen, serum creatinine, serum sodium, serum potassium, serum chloride, serum calcium, serum inorganic phosphorus, aspartate transaminase (AST), alanine aminotransferase (ALT), alkaline phosphatase, lactate dehydrogenase, total protein, and intact parathyroid hormone (iPTH). Serum calcium was adjusted when the serum albumin level was less than 4.0 g/dL (adjusted serum calcium = serum calcium − serum albumin + 4.0 g/dL) [11]. Hepatotoxicity was defined as a threefold increase in AST or ALT levels from the upper limit of baseline [12]. Also, blood samples were obtained via vascular access before HD sessions.

Continuous values were expressed as means ± standard deviation. Statistical analysis was performed using paired t test, Mann-Whitney U test, and Pearson's correlation coefficient test. Significance was set at $P < 0.05$. The software package JMP 9 (SAS Institute Inc., Cary, NC) was used for all statistical analysis.

Results

Fourteen HD patients were started on ibandronate treatment between August 2015 and October 2016. However, data from only 13 patients were included in this study because 1 patient was excluded following hospitalization for severe infectious disease during the observation period. Thirteen HD patients continued ibandronate treatment during the observation period. All 13 patients had oliguria or anuria and did not undergo bone biopsy. One patient had been receiving monthly intraarticular injections of 8 mg dexamethasone for 3 years before the study period.

Patient profiles are shown in Table 1, and drug treatments are listed in Table 2. During the study period, HD background, cinacalcet, oral and intravenous vitamin D, and administration of calcium polystyrene sulfonate remained unchanged. In phosphate binders, 2 patients added lanthanum carbonate and 1 patient added ferric citrate hydrate. Hematinics (iron and other erythropoiesis-stimulating agents) were adjusted according to patient status during the study period.

Changes in markers of bone metabolism and hip BMD during the observation period are shown in Table 3.

Table 3 Changes in markers of bone metabolism and hip BMD during the observation period

	Baseline	End of study	P*
TRACP-5b (mU/dL)	785.3 ± 385.8	638.2 ± 423.4	0.03
BALP (μg/L)	18.1 ± 11.4	17.4 ± 10.3	0.55
Hip BMD (g/cm^2), $n = 9$	0.51 ± 0.10	0.47 ± 0.11	0.07

Values represent mean ± standard deviation
TRACP-5b tartrate-resistant acid phosphatase-5b, *BALP* bone-specific alkaline phosphatase, *BMD* bone mineral density
*Paired t test ($P < 0.05$)

TRACP-5b levels significantly decreased from 785.3 ± 385.8 mU/dL at baseline to 638.2 ± 423.4 mU/dL at end of study ($P = 0.03$). Levels of TRACP-5b decreased in 11 patients and increased in 2 patients (Table 4). Additionally, we examined the relationship between changing levels of TRACP-5b and the patients' backgrounds. As a result, the changing levels of TRACP-5b were positively associated with the baseline hip BMD ($P = 0.02$, $r = 0.65$; Fig. 1). Levels of TRACP-5b were significantly decreased in female patients compared with male patients (− 359.8 ± 94.9 vs − 52.7 ± 172.2, $P < 0.01$, Mann-Whitney U test). In contrast, BALP levels were not significantly changed from 18.1 ± 11.4 μg/L at baseline to 17.4 ± 10.3 μg/L at end of study ($P = 0.55$). Moreover, hip BMD tended to decrease from 0.51 ± 0.10 g/cm^2 at baseline to 0.47 ± 0.11 g/cm^2 at end of study ($P = 0.07$). However, hip BMD could not be assessed in 4 patients. One patient died as a result of an accident outside of the hospital, and 3 patients had not yet undergone hip BMD measurement during the observation period.

Changes in clinical laboratory data (representing the tolerability index) during the observation period are shown in Table 5. AST and ALT were significantly decreased from 11.8 ± 4.1 U/L and 8.6 ± 2.8 U/L at baseline to 9.4 ± 3.0 U/L and 6.7 ± 2.6 U/L at end of study, respectively ($P = 0.03$ and $P < 0.01$). The other tolerability index showed no statistical difference at baseline compared with 6 months after the start of ibandronate treatment. Serum calcium levels < 8.4 mEq/L were seen in 2 patients at baseline and in 5 patients at end of study. In contrast, in 1 patient, AST and ALT levels were increased threefold from the upper limit of baseline at 3 months after start of ibandronate treatment. However, although the patient continued ibandronate treatment, AST and ALT levels were decreased to baseline. Additionally, none of the other patients had laboratory values indicating hepatotoxicity during the observation period. Also, none withdrew from the study due to adverse effects or allergic reactions.

Discussion

TRACP-5b levels were significantly decreased after administration of ibandronate, and the baseline hip BMD and changing levels of TRACP-5b showed a statistically significant correlation. Thus, we have shown that ibandronate treatment decreases TRACP-5b levels in HD patients, and that HD patients who had lower hip BMD might demonstrate improved TRACP-5b levels. Also, levels of TRACP-5b were significantly decreased in female patients compared with male patients because female patients had lower BMD compared with male patients (Fig. 1). Both sexes lose BMD at relatively slow rates starting at around age 40, with women showing a more rapid BMD decline than men with the onset of menopause in their late 40s or early 50s [13]. Thus, female patients might demonstrate improved TRACP-5b levels. The mechanism underlying the association between the baseline hip BMD and changing levels of TRACP-5b is unclear. However, elevated bone turnover was associated with low BMD [14] and was associated with efficacy of bisphosphonate treatment [15]. Therefore, these results suggest that patients with lower hip BMD might respond more effectively to ibandronate treatment. Additionally, although 2 patients did not take vitamin D3 and 1 patient received steroids during the study period, all 3 of these patients had decreased TRACP-5b levels. Therefore, these patients might be expected to have a demonstrable effect of ibandronate treatment.

Table 4 Changes in TRACP-5b levels during the study period

Patient	Sex	Age (years)	Baseline iPTH (pg/mL)	Baseline serum calcium (mEq/L)	Baseline BALP (μg/L)	Baseline TRACP-5b (mU/dL)	End of study TRACP-5b (mU/dL)	Changing levels of TRACP-5b (mU/dL)
1	Female	80	69	8.5	12.6	1110	656	− 454
2	Male	68	279	9.4	15.5	656	754	+ 98
3	Male	89	478	9.2	9.6	346	256	− 90
4	Male	57	246	8.8	12.1	641	584	− 57
5	Male	67	238	8.8	17.6	1070	946	− 124
6	Female	71	474	8.4	19.3	633	366	− 267
7	Male	92	280	8.2	11.5	933	684	− 249
8	Male	83	50	9.3	6.5	425	195	− 230
9	Male	78	42	8.6	9.7	301	179	− 122
10	Female	85	773	10.1	36.8	1400	1110	− 290
11	Female	88	167	8.4	31.9	986	558	− 428
12	Male	78	65	8.7	10.1	338	328	− 10
13	Male	79	542	8.1	41.6	1370	1680	+ 310

iPTH intact parathyroid hormone, *TRACP-5b* tartrate-resistant acid phosphatase-5b, *BALP* bone-specific alkaline phosphatase

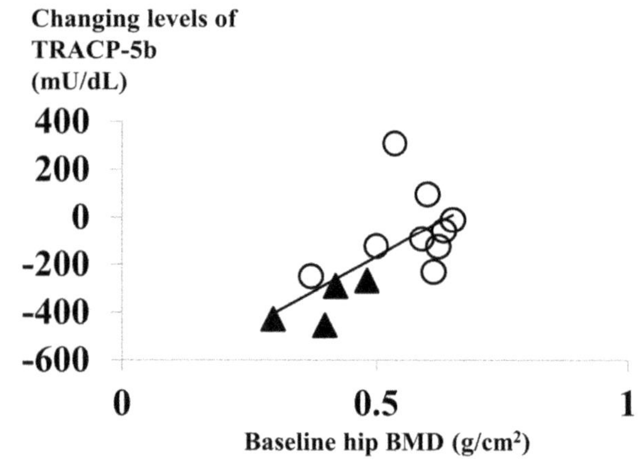

Fig. 1 Relationship between baseline hip BMD and changing levels of TRACP-5b. Pearson's correlation coefficient test. A statistically significant correlation was observed ($r = 0.65$; $P = 0.02$). TRACP-5b, tartrate-resistant acid phosphatase-5b; BMD, bone mineral density. White circle: male; black triangle: female

In this study, BALP levels were not significantly changed, and hip BMD tended to decrease. However, no data are available regarding the BALP levels in HD patients on ibandronate treatment. Conversely, Bergner et al. reported that 48 weeks of ibandronate treatment significantly increased lumbar spine BMD in HD patients [7]. Additionally, in non-HD patients, percent decreases in median BALP levels from baseline were significantly greater with ibandronate versus placebo for 1 year [16]. Moreover, a meta-analysis demonstrated that 2 years of ibandronate treatment improved hip BMD [17]. Further, short-term BMD monitoring (less than 5 years) cannot achieve a high degree of explained variation in BMD change at current levels of DXA performance [18]. Therefore, BALP levels might be decreased and hip BMD might be increased when the treatment period is extended for more than 1 year.

Table 5 Changes in clinical laboratory data during the observation period

	Baseline	End of study	P*
Hemoglobin (g/dL)	10.2 ± 1.3	10.1 ± 0.8	0.75
Hematocrit (%)	31.7 ± 3.9	31.2 ± 2.5	0.66
Platelet count (× 10^4 cells/mm^3)	16.2 ± 5.7	16.1 ± 5.3	0.86
Blood urea nitrogen (mg/dL)	57.0 ± 13.3	60.7 ± 11.8	0.31
Serum creatinine (mg/dL)	9.6 ± 2.2	10.0 ± 2.5	0.55
Serum sodium (mEq/L)	137.7 ± 2.2	137.0 ± 2.4	0.09
Serum potassium (mEq/L)	4.8 ± 0.6	5.2 ± 0.9	0.08
Serum chloride (mEq/L)	107.1 ± 2.4	107.0 ± 2.0	0.93
Serum calcium (mEq/L)	8.8 ± 0.6	8.8 ± 0.7	0.84
Serum inorganic phosphorus (mEq/L)	5.2 ± 1.1	5.2 ± 1.5	0.99
Aspartate transaminase (U/L)	11.8 ± 4.1	9.4 ± 3.0	0.03
Alanine aminotransferase (U/L)	8.6 ± 2.8	6.7 ± 2.6	< 0.01
Alkaline phosphatase (U/L)	278.8 ± 102.1	265.2 ± 111.6	0.34
Lactate dehydrogenase (U/L)	176.1 ± 24.1	170.6 ± 35.4	0.41
Total protein (g/dL)	6.2 ± 0.5	6.2 ± 0.6	0.95
Intact PTH (pg/mL)	284.8 ± 224.4	306.1 ± 355.1	0.71

Values represent mean ± standard deviation
PTH parathyroid hormone
*Paired *t* test ($P < 0.05$)

In 1 patient, AST and ALT levels were increased threefold from the upper limit of baseline at 3 months after the start of ibandronate treatment. However, the possibility of hepatotoxicity as an adverse event was considered low. Because of this, the patient continued ibandronate treatment, so AST and ALT levels eventually decreased to baseline. Also, none of the other patients had laboratory findings suggestive of hepatotoxicity during the observation period; AST and ALT were significantly decreased after the observation period. On the other hand, serum calcium levels were not significantly changed, and patients with serum calcium levels < 8.4 mEq/L tended to show increased levels after the observation period. However, other clinical laboratory data such as the tolerability index showed no significant changes from the baseline to end of study. These results suggest that 6 months of ibandronate treatment was well tolerated in the HD patients in our study because no patients experienced hepatotoxicity, allergic reactions, or other adverse effects. Nevertheless, it may be important to monitor serum calcium in HD patients receiving ibandronate therapy.

Liu et al. reported that bisphosphonates should be carefully considered with specific requirements in HD patients because the use of bisphosphonates may aggravate clinical symptoms in patients with low bone turnover (BALP < 20 ng/mL and iPTH < 100 pg/mL) [19, 20]. However, our study did not examine bone biopsy. Additionally, although this study included 4 patients with low bone turnover (BALP < 20 ng/mL and iPTH < 100 pg/mL), all 4 patients demonstrated decreased TRACP-5b levels (maximum value and minimum values changed by − 454 and − 10, respectively). Therefore, in these patients, bisphosphonate efficacy should be carefully monitored.

Our study has some limitations. These include the small sample size, lack of a control group, and no bone biopsy. Additionally, the study period was too short to evaluate changes in BMD and patients who had a tendency toward high iPTH were included. Therefore, more robust long-term studies are needed to confirm these findings.

Conclusions

Taken together, our results indicate that ibandronate treatment in HD patients—especially those with low BMD—might sufficiently reduce TRACP-5b levels, with no long-term changes in other clinical laboratory parameters. Therefore, ibandronate might be a feasible treatment option for HD patients who develop low BMD.

Abbreviations

ALT: Alanine aminotransferase; AST: Aspartate transaminase; BALP: Bone-specific alkaline phosphatase; BMD: Bone mineral density; HD: Hemodialysis; iPTH: Intact parathyroid hormone; TRACP-5b: Tartrate-resistant acid phosphatase-5b

Acknowledgements

The authors thank the hospital staff and patients who participated in this study.

Funding

The authors have received no research funds.

Authors' contributions

SM and HO designed the study. SM performed the statistical analysis and wrote the manuscript. HY and KN performed the data analysis and critical review of manuscript. All authors participated in the care of the patients. All authors read and approved the final manuscript.

Competing interests

The authors declare that they have no competing interests.

Author details

[1]Department of Pharmacy, Kaetsu Hospital, 1459-1 Higashikanazawa, Akiha-ku, Niigata-shi, Niigata 956-0814, Japan. [2]Department of Internal Medicine, Kaetsu Hospital, 1459-1 Higashikanazawa, Akiha-ku, Niigata-shi, Niigata 956-0814, Japan.

References

1. Alem AM, Sherrard DJ, Gillen DL, Weiss NS, Beresford SA, Heckbert SR, Wong C, Stehman-Breen C. Increased risk of hip fracture among patients with end-stage renal disease. Kidney Int. 2000;58(1):396–9.
2. Atsumi K, Kushida K, Yamazaki K, Shimizu S, Ohmura A, Inoue T. Risk factors for vertebral fractures in renal osteodystrophy. Am J Kidney Dis. 1999;33(2):287–93.
3. Fisher ES, Baron JA, Malenka DJ, Barrett JA, Kniffin WD, Whaley FS, Bubolz TA. Hip fracture incidence and mortality in New England. Epidemiology. 1991;2(2):116–22.
4. Perazella MA, Markowitz GS. Bisphosphonate nephrotoxicity. Kidney Int. 2008;74(11):1385–93.
5. Boonen S, Laan RF, Barton IP, Watts NB. Effect of osteoporosis treatments on risk of non-vertebral fractures: review and meta-analysis of intention-to-treat studies. Osteoporos Int. 2005;16(10):1291–8.
6. Bergner R, Dill K, Boerner D, Uppenkamp M. Elimination of intravenously administered ibandronate in patients on haemodialysis: a monocentre open study. Nephrol Dial Transplant. 2002;17(7):1281–5.
7. Bergner R, Henrich D, Hoffmann M, Schmidt-Gayk H, Lenz T, Upperkamp M. Treatment of reduced bone density with ibandronate in dialysis patients. J Nephrol. 2008;21(4):510–6.
8. Yamada S, Inaba M, Kurajoh M, Shidara K, Imanishi Y, Ishimura E, Nishizawa Y. Utility of serum tartrate-resistant acid phosphatase (TRACP5b) as a bone resorption marker in patients with chronic kidney disease: independence from renal dysfunction. Clin Endocrinol. 2008;69(2):189–96.
9. Nenonen A, Cheng S, Ivaska KK, Alatalo SL, Lehtimäki T, Schmidt-Gayk H, Uusi-Rasi K, Heinonen A, Kannus P, Sievänen H, Vuori I, Väänänen HK, Halleen JM. Serum TRACP 5b is a useful marker for monitoring alendronate treatment: comparison with other markers of bone turnover. J Bone Miner Res. 2005;20(10):1804–12.
10. Mehlhorn AT, Rechl H, Gradinger R, Stemberger A. Alendronate decreases TRACP 5b activity in osteoarthritic bone. Eur J Med Res. 2008;13(1):21–5.
11. Payne RB, Little AJ, Williams RB, Milner JR. Interpretation of serum calcium in patients with abnormal serum proteins. Br Med J. 1973;4(5893):643–6.
12. Seki M, Yabuno K, Miyawaki K, Miwa Y, Tomono K. Loading regimen required to rapidly achieve therapeutic trough plasma concentration of teicoplanin and evaluation of clinical features. Clin Pharmacol. 2012;4:71–5.
13. Clarke BL, Khosla S. Physiology of bone loss. Radiol Clin N Am. 2010; 48(3):483–95.
14. Melton LJ 3rd, Khosla S, Atkinson EJ, O'Fallon WM, Riggs BL. Relationship of bone turnover to bone density and fractures. J Bone Miner Res. 1997;12(7):1083–91.
15. Bauer DC, Garnero P, Hochberg MC, Santora A, Delmas P, Ewing SK, Black DM, Fracture Intervention Research Group. Pretreatment levels of bone turnover and the antifracture efficacy of alendronate: the fracture intervention trial. J Bone Miner Res. 2006;21(2):292–9.
16. Orwoll ES, Binkley NC, Lewiecki EM, Gruntmanis U, Fries MA, Dasic G. Efficacy and safety of monthly ibandronate in men with low bone density. Bone. 2010;46(4):970–6.
17. Hou Y, Gu K, Xu C, Ding H, Liu C, Tuoheti Y. Dose-effectiveness relationships determining the efficacy of ibandronate for management of osteoporosis: a meta-analysis. Medicine (Baltimore). 2015;94(26):e1007.
18. Leslie WD, Majumdar SR, Morin SN, Lix LM. Why does rate of bone density loss not predict fracture risk? J Clin Endocrinol Metab. 2015;100(2):679–83.
19. Liu WC, Yen JF, Lang CL, Yan MT, Lu KC. Bisphophonates in CKD patients with low bone mineral density. ScientificWorldJournal. 2013;2013:837573.
20. Ureña P, Hruby M, Ferreira A, Ang KS, de Vernejoul MC. Plasma total versus bone alkaline phosphatase as markers of bone turnover in hemodialysis patients. J Am Soc Nephrol. 1996;7(3):506–12.

7

Biocompatibility and small protein permeability of hydrophilic-coated membrane dialyzer (NV) in hemodialysis patients

Hirotoshi Kodama[1*], Akira Tsuji[2], Akihiro Fujinoki[1], Koujirou Ooshima[2], Kaori Ishizeki[2] and Tatsuo Inoue[1]

Abstract

Background: We evaluated the biocompatibility and small protein permeability of a newly developed hydrophilic-coated membrane dialyzer (NV) compared with conventional polysulfone dialyzer (APS) for hemodialysis (HD) therapy.

Methods: In a prospective crossover study, 11 maintenance HD patients (7 males; mean age 67.0 ± 10.2 years) received HD three times a week for 4 weeks with the NV membrane and then for another 4 weeks with the APS membrane. We evaluated the variation in several parameters including white blood cell (WBC) count and fibrinogen as indexes for biocompatibility. The plasma and dialysate concentrations of β_2-microglobulin (β_2-M), α_1-microglobulin (α_1-M), and albumin were measured at baseline and after 4 h of each study treatment in order to assess the removal of small proteins.

Results: Reductions in the WBC count were seen with APS compared with NV at 60 min (NV 5.65 ± 1.60, APS 5.17 ± 1.65 × 10^3/μL, $p < 0.05$) and 240 min (NV 5.28 ± 1.38, APS 4.63 ± 1.2 × 10^3/μL, $p < 0.005$) after the start of HD. With NV, we found significantly greater rates of variation of β_2-M (NV 45.5 ± 1.2, APS 40.1 ± 1.2%, $p < 0.0001$), α_1-M (NV 41.2 ± 9.9, APS 34.2 ± 18.5%, $p < 0.05$), and albumin (NV 31.6 ± 7.8, APS 18.1 ± 6.5%, $p < 0.0001$) during HD than with APS. However, there were no significant differences in the removal of β_2-M between the two dialyzers.

Conclusions: The clinical characteristics of NV may reveal an improved biocompatibility and a comparable efficiency in small protein removal as compared to those of APS.

Keywords: Hemodialysis, Polysulfone, Hydrophilic-coated membrane, Biocompatibility, Small protein permeability

Background

Biocompatibility and middle molecule clearance of hemodialysis (HD) membranes affect the survival, morbidity, and quality of life of uremic patients undergoing maintenance HD therapy. In particular, malnutrition [1] and dialysis-related amyloidosis due to the reference middle molecule β_2-microglobulin (β_2-M) [2] are the major long-term complications. A polysulfone (PS) dialyzer is the mainstay of HD treatment because of its high performance. However, TORAYLIGHT® NV dialyzer (NV; Toray Industries, Inc., Tokyo, Japan) is expected to have different characteristics from the conventional PS due to its newly developed hydrophilic-coated membrane [3]. We therefore designed this prospective, crossover study to evaluate the biocompatibility and low-molecular-weight protein permeability (small protein permeability) of NV compared with a conventional PS (APS; ASAHIKASEI Industries, Inc., Tokyo, Japan).

* Correspondence: hiro25@jcom.zaq.ne.jp
[1]Division of Blood Purification Center, Kamifukuoka General Hospital, 931 Fukuoka, Fujimino, Saitama 356-0011, Japan
Full list of author information is available at the end of the article

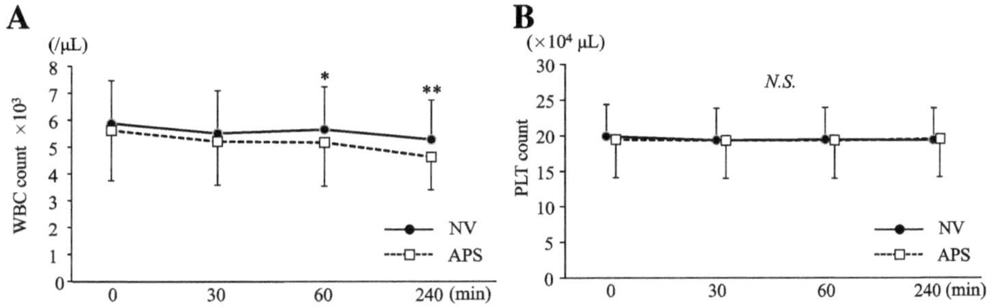

Fig 1 **a** WBC count and **b** PLT count. **a** Reduction in the white blood cell count were seen with the APS compared with the NV in 60 min (*$p < 0.05$) and 240 min (**$p < 0.005$) after the start of HD. **b** There were no significant differences between NV and APS

Methods

Eleven maintenance HD patients (7 males; mean age 67.0 ± 10.2 years) on regular thrice-weekly HD treatment for 4 h were enrolled in the study after they had given their written informed consent. The underlying renal diseases were diabetes mellitus ($N = 3$), glomerulonephritis ($N = 2$), and unknown ($N = 6$). The mean duration of dialysis treatment was 48.6 ± 45.0 (range 15 to 258) months. All of the patients underwent 12 consecutive HD treatments with NV-13U (1.3 m^2) and then switched with APS-13SA (1.3 m^2) as a control after a 2-week wash-out period.

Laboratory measurements

The platelet (PLT) count, white blood cell (WBC) count, and hematocrit (Hct) were measured at the beginning of dialysis and after 30, 60, and 240 min. To adjust for differences in the cell counts at the beginning of dialysis, we calculated the change ratio at each point using the following formula (1):

$$\text{Change ratio X min} = 100 + 100 \times \{(\text{Cell count} \times \text{min})/(\text{Cell count 0 min}) - 1\}$$

$$\text{Cell count 0 min: Cell count at the beginning of dialysis}$$

$$\text{Cell count X min: Cell count after X minutes from the beginning of dialysis} \quad (1)$$

We measured the urea nitrogen, serum creatinine, inorganic phosphorus, single-pool Kt/V [4], and hemoglobin levels; the removal rate of β_2-M; and the rate of variation of β_2-M, α_1-microglobulin (α_1-M), and albumin. We also measured the levels of platelet factor-4 (PF-4), β-thromboglobulin (β-TG), fibrinogen/fibrin degradation products (FDP), D-dimer, and fibrinogen (FIB).

Dialysate samples were collected at the final two dialysis sessions at a speed of 1.0 L/h using a fixed-quantity pump from the dialysate discharge line for 0–60, 60–180, and 180–240 min after the start of HD. On the assumption that each value measured before dialysis was 100%, the results were evaluated for variability.

This study was conducted in accordance with the guidelines of the Declaration of Helsinki and approved by the ethics committees of Kamifukuoka General Hospital and National Defense Medical College Hospital.

Statistical analyses

The continuous values of variables are expressed as the mean ± standard deviation or as the median (25th, 75th percentile). The comparative p values for continuous variables were calculated by an analysis of variance (ANOVA). All of the statistical analyses were carried out using the JMP Pro Version 11.2.0 software program (SAS Institute, Cary, NC, USA), setting the significance level at a p value of less than 0.05.

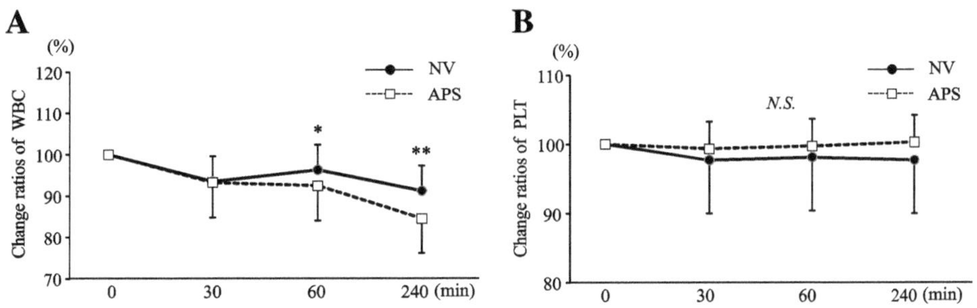

Fig 2 Change ratios of **a** WBC and **b** PLT. **a** The change ratios of the white blood cell count were significantly smaller with the NV than with the APS after 60 min (*$p < 0.01$) and 240 min (**$p < 0.05$). **b** There were no significant differences between NV and APS

Table 1 Clinical parameters of Hct, PF-4, β-TG, FDP, D-dimer, and change ratio of FIB

		0 (min)	30 (min)	60 (min)	240 (min)
Hct (%)	NV	32.2 ± 2.4	31.4 ± 2.7	32.1 ± 2.6	34.9 ± 3.3
	APS	32.0 ± 2.4	30.9 ± 2.3	31.5 ± 2.3	34.4 ± 2.8
PF-4 (ng/mL)	NV	7.45 ± 7.09	29.2 ± 13.5	16.9 ± 8.1	12.3 ± 7.4
	APS	6.77 ± 3.69	32.3 ± 21.5	17.3 ± 6.9	12.1 ± 5.8
β-TG (ng/mL)	NV	146 ± 41	128 ± 42	118 ± 36	104 ± 39
	APS	135 ± 33	125 ± 40	119 ± 36	101 ± 30
FDP (μg/mL)	NV	2.0(2.0, 2.0)	2.0(2.0, 2.0)	2.0(2.0, 2.0)	2.0(2.0, 3.0)
	APS	2.0(2.0, 2.0)	2.0(2.0, 2.0)	2.0(2.0, 3.0)	2.0(2.0, 2.0)
D-dimer (μg/mL)	NV	0.4(0.2, 0.5)	0.3(0.2, 0.5)	0.3(0.2, 0.5)	0.4(0.2, 0.5)
	APS	0.4(0.4, 0.5)	0.3(0.2, 0.5)	0.3(0.2, 0.5)	0.3(0.2, 0.5)
Change ratio of FIB (%)	NV	–	98.6 ± 2.8	102 ± 3	117 ± 8
	APS	–	97.8 ± 3.3	101 ± 4	116 ± 11

FDP and D-dimer are expressed as medians with 25th–75th percentiles
Hct hematocrit, *PF-4* platelet factor-4, *β-TG* thromboglobulin, *FDP* fibrinogen/fibrin degradation products, *FIB* fibrinogen

Results

Biocompatibility

Reductions in the WBC count were seen with APS compared with NV at 60 min (NV 5.65 ± 1.60, APS 5.17 ± 1.65 × 10^3/μL, $p < 0.05$) and 240 min (NV 5.28 ± 1.38, APS 4.63 ± 1.20 × 10^3/μL, $p < 0.005$) after the start of HD (Fig. 1). The PLT count was not markedly different between the two dialyzers. The change ratios of the WBC count were significantly smaller with NV than with APS after 60 min (NV 96.3 ± 2.3, APS 92.5 ± 7.5%, $p < 0.01$) and 240 min (NV 91.3 ± 2.3, APS 84.6 ± 11.3%, $p < 0.05$) (Fig. 2).

No significant differences were seen in the levels of Hct, PF-4, β-TG, FDP, or D-dimer or in the change ratio of FIB between NV and APS (Table 1). There were also no significant differences in the urea nitrogen, creatinine, inorganic phosphorus, single-pool Kt/V, or hemoglobin values between the two dialyzers (Table 2).

Small protein permeability

The intradialytic removal of α_1-M was greater with NV than with APS in the first hour (NV 15.7 ± 4.0, APS 10.7 ± 3.0 mg, $p < 0.001$) and last hour (NV 6.47 ± 2.35, APS 3.23 ± 0.74 mg, $p < 0.001$) as well as over the total HD session (NV 32.0 ± 11.3, APS 17.7 ± 6.3 mg, $p < 0.0001$) (Fig. 3). In addition, the removal of albumin was greater with NV than with APS in the first hour (NV 340 ± 125, APS 198 ± 59 mg, $p < 0.001$) and last hour (NV 109 ± 46, APS 32.0 ± 3.8 mg, $p < 0.001$) as well as over the total HD session (NV 693 ± 283, APS 249 ± 90 mg, $p < 0.001$) (Fig. 4). There were no significant differences in the removal of β_2-M between the two dialyzers (Fig. 5). However, the rates of variation during HD were greater with NV than with APS for β_2-M (NV 45.5 ± 1.2, APS 40.1 ± 1.2%, $p < 0.001$), α_1-M (NV 41.2 ± 9.9, APS 34.2 ± 18.5%, $p < 0.05$), and albumin (NV 31.6 ± 7.8, APS 18.1 ± 6.5%, $p < 0.001$).

Table 2 Clinical parameters

	NV	APS	*p*
Urea nitrogen (mg/dL)	61.1 ± 13.8	62.1 ± 11.7	N.S.
Creatinine (mg/dL)	9.98 ± 2.39	9.87 ± 2.23	N.S.
Phosphorus (mg/dL)	4.84 ± 1.31	4.95 ± 1.25	N.S.
Single-poor Kt/V	1.55 ± 0.22	1.63 ± 0.21	N.S.
Hemoglobin (g/dL)	10.5 ± 0.9	10.3 ± 0.7	N.S.

N.S. not significant

Discussion

The PS membrane has shown a very good biocompatibility due to its superior removal performance for small-molecule proteins such as β_2-M, high clearance of small-molecule solutes such as urea and creatinine [5], and low rate of complications such as leukopenia or disorders associated with the complement system [6]. Therefore, the PS membrane is widely used for HD treatment in Japan [7]. The NV membrane was developed as an alternative to PS. With NV, the mobility of water adjacent to the membrane surface is enhanced using a new hydrophilic polymer to reform the membrane surface. NV has antithrombotic activity and less platelet and leukocyte activation than PS, as well as the ability to sufficiently remove small solutes and low-molecular-weight proteins [3]. Further, NV induces less interleukin-6 activity, which may reduce the risk of erythropoiesis-stimulating agent hyporesponsiveness [8]. In this study, we evaluated the biocompatibility and protein permeability of NV compared with those of APS as a conventional PS.

The variation of several parameters such as the WBC, PLT, Hct and levels of PF-4, β-TG, FDP, D-dimer, and

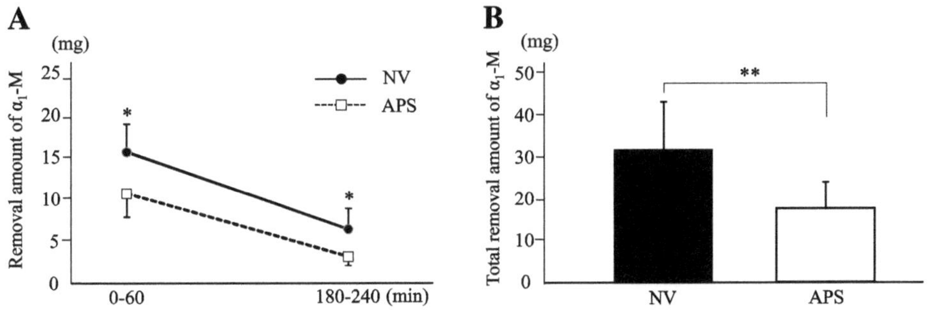

Fig 3 **a** Removal amount of α_1-M and **b** total removal amounts of α_1-M. Compared to APS. *$p < 0.001$ and **$p < 0.0001$ by paired *t* test. *α_1-M* α_1-microglobulin

FIB were compared to evaluate the biocompatibility of NV. PF4 and β-TG are substances contained within platelet α-granules, and changes in platelet PF4 or β-TG levels are useful indicators of platelet degranulation and activation during dialysis [9]. However, there were no significant changes observed in the coagulation factor values with either dialyzer. Although acute leukopenia is known to occur in all patients during the first 30 min of HD treatment [10], our study showed no reduction in the WBC during dialysis with either dialyzer. The platelet count usually decreases 5 to 15% at 15 to 30 min from the start of HD and recovers to the normal level by the end of the dialysis session [9, 11]. Oshihara [3] reported that the numbers of platelets adhering to the membrane surface were lower with NV than with the conventional PS (CX) membrane. In our results, the variations in the platelet counts with both membranes were stable, suggesting that both may prevent HD-associated thrombocytopenia.

It is known that WBC adhesion occurs with protein adsorption, and FIB adsorption promotes PLT adhesion on the dialysis membrane surface by blood exposure in HD treatment [12]. Platelet-derived microparticles are released from activated platelets during HD [13]. Although the biocompatibility of PS is generally regarded to be good, there are some reports that the PS dialyzer caused PLT depletion [14, 15]. On the other hand, the NV membrane has been reported that it not only inhibits the adhesion of blood components such as PLT and FIB but also acts as a highly biocompatible membrane to reduce blood cell stimulation because it is developed as a new hydrophilic polymer membrane [3]. With NV, the reduction rate of the WBC count was inhibited to a greater degree than with APS. However, the change ratio of FIB showed no significant difference between NV and APS. These results suggest that NV improves the biocompatibility compared with APS.

Dialysis-related amyloidosis is a major complication with long-term HD treatment and greatly affects patients' quality of life. The removal of β_2-M is therefore important to avoid this complication. However, there have been no reports of the small protein permeability of NV. We therefore designed this prospective crossover study to evaluate whether or not NV offers any advantages over APS. We found that the intradialytic removal of α_1-M and albumin but not β_2-M was significantly greater with NV than with APS. The rates of variation in the β_2-M and α_1-M levels during HD with NV were higher than with APS, but the differences were small. These results suggest that the removal performance of β_2-M with NV and APS should be almost equivalent.

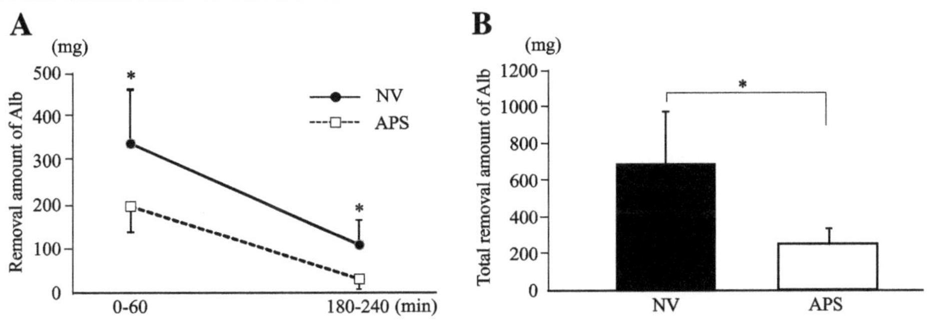

Fig 4 **a** Removal amount of Alb and **b** total removal amounts of Alb. Compared to APS. *$p < 0.0001$ by paired *t* test. *Alb* albumin

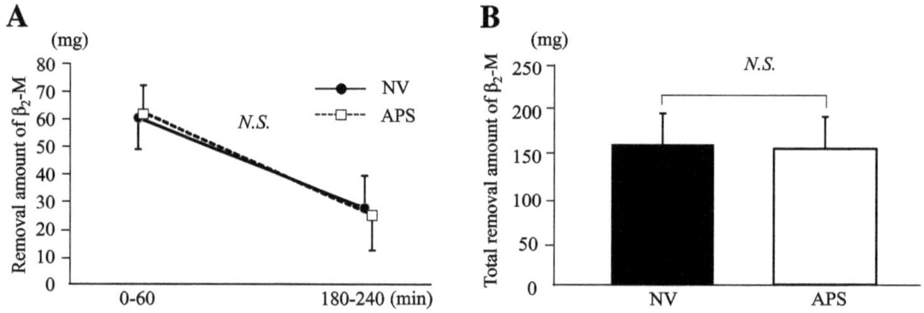

Fig 5 **a** Removal amount of β_2-M and **b** total removal amounts of β_2-M. There were no significant differences between NV and APS. *β_2-M* β_2-microglobulin

In addition, since the decrease in the serum albumin may cause low muscle mass [16], malnutrition [17], and mortality risk [18], it is important to select dialyzers with consideration of the laboratory data. NV removed significantly greater albumin than APS. Therefore, we should be cautious when using the NV membrane in elderly or malnourished patients, although the amount of albumin removed was less than 1 g (NV 693 ± 283, APS 249 ± 90 mg) in either dialyzer.

Because this was a short-term, prospective, crossover study involving only a few cases, large-scale and long-term future trials are necessary to corroborate our findings.

Conclusions

We designed this crossover study of the NV and APS membranes to evaluate the biocompatibility and small protein removal ability. The clinical characteristics of NV may reveal an improved biocompatibility and a comparable efficiency in small protein removal as compared to APS.

Abbreviations

Alb: Albumin; FDP: Fibrinogen/fibrin degradation products; FIB: Fibrinogen; Hct: Hematocrit; HD: Hemodialysis; PF-4: Platelet factor-4; PLT: Platelet; PS: Polysulfone; WBC: White blood cell; α_1-M: α_1-Microglobulin; β_2-M: β_2-Microglobulin; β-TG: β-Thromboglobulin

Acknowledgements

The authors thank all the staff members working at the Division of Blood Purification Center, Kamifukuoka General Hospital and Department of Blood Purification Therapy, National Defense Medical College Hospital.

Funding

This study has received research funds from the Foundation for Promotion of Defense Medicine.

Authors' contributions

HK designed the study, collected the clinical data, analyzed the data, and wrote the manuscript. AT designed the study and wrote the manuscript. AF collected the clinical data. KI, KO, and TI participated in its design and coordination. All authors read and approved the final manuscript.

Competing interests

The authors declare that they have no competing interests.

Author details

[1]Division of Blood Purification Center, Kamifukuoka General Hospital, 931 Fukuoka, Fujimino, Saitama 356-0011, Japan. [2]Department of Blood Purification, National Defense Medical College Hospital, 3-2 Namiki, Tokorozawa, Saitama 359-8513, Japan.

References

1. Kalantar-Zadeh K, Kopple JD, Block G, Humphreys MH. A malnutrition-inflammation score is correlated with morbidity and mortality in maintenance hemodialysis patients. Am J Kidney Dis. 2001;38:1251–63.
2. Gejyo F, Yamada T, Odani S, Nakagawa Y, Arakawa M, Kunitomo T, et al. A new form of amyloid protein associated with chronic hemodialysis was identified as beta 2-microgulobulin. Biophys Res Commun. 1985;129:701–6.
3. Oshihara W, Ueno Y, Fujieda H. A new polysulfone membrane dialyzer, NV, with low-founding and antithrombotic properties. Contrib Nephrol. 2017;189:222–9.
4. Shinzato T, Nakai S, Fujita Y, Takai I, Morita E, Nakane K, Maeda K. Determination of Kt/V and protein catabolic rate using pre- and postdialysis blood urea nitrogen concentrations. Nephron. 1994;67:280–90.
5. Fukuda M, Miyazaki M, Uezumi S, Yoshida M. Design and assessment of the new APS dialyzer (APS-SA series). J Artifs Organs. 2006;9:192–8.
6. Yamashita S, Mochizuki A, Nakazaki T, Seita Y, Sawamoto J, Endo F, et al. A new blood compatible and permselective hollow fiber membrane for hemodialysis. ASAIO J. 1996;42(6):1019–26.
7. Nakai S, Suzuki K, Masakane I, et al. Overview of regular dialysis treatment in Japan (as of 31 December 2009). Ther Apher Dial. 2010;14:505–40.
8. Kakuta T, Komaba H, Takagi N, Takahashi Y, Suzuki H, et al. A prospective multicenter randomized controlled study on interleukin-6 removal and induction by a new hemodialyzer with improved biocompatibility in hemodialysis patients: a pilot study. Ther Apher Dial. 2016;20(6):569–78.
9. Daugirdas JT, Bernardo AA. Hemodialysis effect on platelet count and function and hemodialysis-associated thrombocytoperia. Kidney Int. 2012;82:147–57.
10. Kaplow LS, Goffinet JA. Profound neutropenia during the early phase of hemodialysis. JAMA. 1968;203:1135–7.
11. Amato M, Salvadori M, Bergesio F, Messeri A, Filimberti E, Morfini M. Aspects of biocompatibility of two different dialysis membranes: cuprophane and polysulfone. Int J Artif Organs. 1988;11:175–80.
12. Reginald G. Mason, Hanson Y.K. chuang, S. Fazal Mohammad. Extracorporeal thrombogenesis: mechanisms and prevention. replacement of renal function by dialysis. 1983: 186-200.

13. Daniel L, Fakhouri F, Joly D, et al. Increase of circulating neutrophil and platelet microparticles during acute vasculitis and hemodialysis. Kidney Int. 2006;69:1416–23.
14. Kobari E, Terawaki H, Takahashi Y, et al. Dialyzer-related thrombocytopenia due to a polysulfone membrane. Intern Med. 2016;55:965–8.
15. Deprada L, Lee J, Gillespie A, Benjamin J. Thrombocytopenia associated with one type of polysulfone hemodialysis membrane: a report of 5 cases. Am J Kidney Dis. 2013;61:131–3.
16. Yasui S, Shirai Y, Tanimura M, Matsuura S, Saito Y, Miyata K. Prevalence of protein-energy wasting (PEW) and evaluation of diagnostic criteria in Japanese maintenance hemodialysis patients. Asia Pac J Clin Nutr. 2016;25(2):292–9.
17. Pifer TB, McCullough K, Port FK, Goodkin DA, Maroni BJ, Held PJ, et al. Mortality risk in hemodialysis patients and changes in nutritional indicators: DOPPS. Kidney Int. 2002;62:2338–245.
18. Dwyer JT, Larive B, Leung J, Rocco MV, Greene T, Burrowes J, et al. Are nutritional status indicators associated with mortality in hemodialysis (HEMO) study? Kidney Int. 2005;68:1766–76.

8

Determinants of difficulty in activities of daily living in ambulatory patients undergoing hemodialysis

Takaaki Watanabe[1], Toshiki Kutsuna[1,2], Kei Yoneki[1], Manae Harada[1], Takahiro Shimoda[1], Yusuke Matsunaga[3], Norio Murayama[4], Ryota Matsuzawa[5], Yasuo Takeuchi[6], Atsushi Yoshida[7] and Atsuhiko Matsunaga[1*]

Abstract

Background: Patients undergoing hemodialysis (HD) have difficulty performing activities of daily living (ADL) compared to healthy people. ADL difficulty is an early predictor of loss of independence and mortality in older community-living people. However, determinants of ADL difficulty in HD patients have not been clarified. This study aimed to identify factors associated with ADL difficulty in ambulatory HD patients.

Methods: Subjects were 216 Japanese outpatients (130 men, 86 women; mean age, 67 years) undergoing maintenance HD three times a week. Clinical characteristics, depressive symptoms, motor function (leg strength, balance, and walking speed), and ADL difficulty related to lower-limb function such as mobility issues were compared across three difficulty levels (higher, middle, and lower) as classified according to the percentages of patients with perceived difficulty. Multivariate logistic regression analysis was performed to examine whether clinical characteristics, depressive symptoms, and motor function could discriminate ADL difficulty at each level. Receiver operating characteristic curve analysis was performed to determine cut-off values of motor function for predicting ADL difficulty at each level.

Results: ADL difficulty was independently associated with age (odds ratio (OR) = 1.05, 95% confidence interval (CI) 1.00–1.10; $P = 0.039$), presence of depressive symptoms (OR = 4.24, 95%CI 1.13–15.95; $P = 0.033$), and usual walking speed (OR = 0.94, 95%CI 0.90–0.97; $P < 0.001$) for higher level difficulty; age (OR = 1.06, 95%CI 1.02–1.10; $P = 0.006$), maximum leg strength (OR = 0.97, 95%CI 0.94–1.00; $P = 0.043$), and usual walking speed (OR = 0.96, 95%CI 0.93–0.98; $P = 0.001$) for middle level difficulty; and age (OR = 1.06, 95%CI 1.02–1.10; $P = 0.006$) and usual walking speed (OR = 0.93, 95%CI 0.90–0.6; $P < 0.001$) for lower level difficulty. Cut-off values of usual walking speed for predicting ADL difficulty for higher, middle, and lower level difficulty were 83.7, 75.5, and 75.1 m/min, respectively.

Conclusions: A slow walking speed and old age were significantly and independently associated with ADL difficulty in ambulatory HD patients. Presence of depressive symptoms was significantly and independently associated with ADL difficulty at the higher level of difficulty in ambulatory HD patients. These findings provide useful data for planning effective therapeutic regimens to prevent ADL difficulty in ambulatory HD patients.

Keywords: Activities of daily living (ADL) difficulty, Depressive symptom, Walking speed, Hemodialysis patient

* Correspondence: atsuhikonet@gmail.com
[1]Department of Rehabilitation Sciences, Kitasato University Graduate School of Medical Sciences, 1-15-1 Kitasato, Sagamihara, Kanagawa 252-0373, Japan
Full list of author information is available at the end of the article

Background

Evaluation of physical functioning in maintenance hemodialysis (HD) patients is recommended by the Kidney Disease Outcomes Quality Initiative clinical practice guidelines [1] and European Renal Best Practice guidelines [2], as decreased physical functioning leads to a reduced quality of daily life and higher risk of mortality in this patient population [1–4]. These guidelines recommend assessment of physical functioning using both self-reported and open-field measures of physical performance [2, 5, 6]. In particular, self-reported measures of physical functioning have the advantage of being simple and easy to use [2].

In Japan, more than half of HD patients reportedly have the ability to perform basic activities of daily living (ADL) and instrumental ADL tasks without assistance [7]. However, even HD patients who can perform ADL tasks independently show high rates of ADL difficulty, i.e., difficulty carrying out routine self-care activities. Kutner et al. [8] reported that HD patients are more likely to have ADL difficulty compared to age-matched controls. Moreover, HD patients have been reported to show poor physical functioning (e.g., leg strength, standing balance, and walking ability), with high rates of depressive symptoms [9–13]. Recent studies have shown that poor standing balance, slow walking speed, presence of depression, and chronic kidney disease predict ADL difficulty in older community-living people [14–17]. Moreover, ADL difficulty has been shown to be an early predictor of loss of independence and mortality in older community-living people [18]. However, few studies have examined factors associated with ADL difficulty in HD patients. Therefore, this study aimed to identify factors associated with ADL difficulty in clinically stable ambulatory HD patients.

Methods

Study population

The study protocol was approved by the Ethics Committee of Kitasato University. Informed consent was obtained from each patient after providing a detailed explanation of the study protocol. From July 2007 to October 2016, clinically stable outpatients at the Sagami Circulatory Organ Clinic Hemodialysis Center were assessed for eligibility for inclusion in this cross-sectional study. Patients were undergoing maintenance HD therapy three times a week according to the Japanese Society for Dialysis Therapy guidelines. Patients were excluded if they fulfilled the following criteria: hospitalization ≤ 3 months prior to study enrollment; presence of uncontrolled cardiac arrhythmias, severe disdialysis syndrome (hypotension, nausea, and muscle spasm during hemodialysis), peripheral artery disease with apparent intermittent claudication or critical limb ischemia, chronic heart failure (New York Heart Association classes III to IV), or uncontrolled hypertension (blood pressure at rest > 180/110 mmHg); need for walking assistance; and presence of any other conditions that limited walking (e.g., dementia, low vision or blindness, paralysis due to stroke, and leg amputation).

Clinical characteristics

Information regarding age, sex, HD duration, body mass index (BMI), primary end-stage renal disease, and laboratory values (blood hemoglobin and serum albumin) was obtained from clinical records. BMI was calculated by dividing weight in kilograms by the square of height in meters. Blood hemoglobin and serum albumin concentrations were measured immediately before each hemodialysis session.

Presence of diabetes mellitus, cerebrovascular disease (stroke), and cardiac disease (angina pectoris, myocardial infarction, percutaneous coronary intervention, or coronary artery bypass grafting) was assessed based on clinical records. Moreover, to quantify comorbid illnesses, we used a comorbidity index developed for dialysis patients, which comprised the following primary causes of kidney disease: atherosclerotic heart disease, congestive heart failure, cerebrovascular accident/transient ischemic attack, peripheral vascular disease, dysrhythmia, and other cardiac diseases; chronic obstructive pulmonary disease; gastrointestinal bleeding; liver disease; cancer; and diabetes [19].

Depressive symptoms

A short, 10-item version of the Center for Epidemiological Studies Depression Screening Index (CES-D) was used to assess depressive symptoms in the last 7 days [13, 20, 21]. Each response item is rated on a scale ranging from 0 to 3. Total CES-D score was calculated as the sum of all item scores and ranged from 0 to 30. Higher scores indicated greater depressive symptoms, and the presence of depressive symptoms was defined as a score of ≥ 10 [21].

Motor function

Assessment of motor function included measurements of leg strength, standing balance, and walking ability. Leg strength was evaluated using a handheld dynamometer (μtas F-1; Anima, Tokyo, Japan). Patients were asked to sit on a bench with their hip and knee flexed at an angle of 90°, and then, the maximum voluntary isometric knee extensor strength was measured three times. Maximum leg strength was expressed as a percentage of body weight, i.e., the average of right and left maximum isometric leg strength divided by weight [22, 23].

Standing balance was evaluated by measuring one-leg standing time. The duration that patients could stand on one leg with their eyes open, while holding their hands at their waist without any aid or falling, was measured using a stopwatch [24]. The measurement was performed for up to 60 s and stopped if patients hopped, stepped, put the raised foot down on the other foot or on the floor, or released their hands from the waist. Patients underwent a second trial if they were unable to stand on one leg for 60 s in the first trial [25]. The maximum time of the two measurements was used for analysis.

Walking ability was evaluated by measuring usual walking speed along a 10-m walkway. Usual walking speed was defined as distance (10-m) divided by time (in minutes) from self-selected walking speed [22]. Usual walking speed was measured once and was expressed in meter per minutes.

ADL dependency

ADL dependency was assessed by the Functional Independence Measure (FIM). The FIM is widely used to measure patient functional status for performing ADL. In the USA, the FIM has been used as a primary outcome measure and, approximately, 60% of US hospitals used the FIM in 2002 [26]. The FIM comprises 13 motor items and five cognitive items, which are rated on a 7-point scale (1, complete assistance, to 7, complete independence) [27, 28]. In this study, only five motor items (transfer to bed, chair, or wheelchair; transfer to toilet; transfer to tub or shower; walking or wheelchair propulsion; and stair climbing) related to lower-limb function were used, with a total score of 7 to 35 points. Lower scores indicated greater ADL dependency.

ADL difficulty

ADL difficulty was assessed with a questionnaire developed for patients undergoing HD therapy to assess their perceived difficulty in performing ADL related to lower-limb function such as mobility. This questionnaire on perceived mobility difficulty for HD patients comprises 12 items divided into the following three categories, which were obtained by a factor analysis: "basic ADL," "ambulation," and "walking up or down stairs" [29, 30]. The reliability and validity of the questionnaire have been assessed in Japanese HD patients [29, 30]. The English version of this questionnaire was created through a process of repeated translation from Japanese to English by a bilingual physiotherapist (A.M.) and then back-translated by a bilingual translator.

Additional file 1: Table S1 shows the 12 items of the questionnaire. Patients were asked to rate their perceived difficulty in performing these items on a scale of 1 to 5 (1, not possible; 2, severe difficulty; 3, moderate difficulty; 4, mild difficulty; and 5, ease). ADL difficulty score was defined as the sum of all points and ranged from 12 to 60 points. Lower scores indicated greater ADL difficulty.

Statistical analysis

To compare score distribution, histograms of ADL dependency and difficulty scores from all patients were created at 5-point intervals. According to a method described previously [29], the 12 items of the ADL difficulty questionnaire were classified into three difficulty levels (higher, middle, and lower). Then, patients with a perceived difficulty score ≤ 3 for at least one item in each level were allocated into the difficulty group, and other patients (perceived difficulty score ≥ 4 for all items) were allocated into the non-difficulty group. Differences in clinical characteristics (age, sex, BMI, HD duration, primary cause of end-stage renal disease, hemoglobin, serum albumin, and comorbid conditions), depressive symptoms, motor function (maximum leg strength, one-leg standing time, and usual walking speed), and ADL dependency and difficulty scores between the two groups were assessed for significance using the non-paired t test and χ^2 test. Univariate and multivariate logistic regression analyses were performed to assess whether clinical characteristics and motor function could discriminate the presence of ADL difficulty for each level. Independent variables used for multivariate logistic regression analysis were age, sex, blood hemoglobin concentration, serum albumin concentration, comorbidity index, depression symptoms, maximum leg strength, one-leg standing time, and usual walking speed for each level. Receiver operating characteristic (ROC) curve analysis was performed to determine cut-off values of motor function for predicting ADL difficulty at each level. Cut-off values were determined according the maximum Youden index [31].

All analyses were performed using the Statistical Package for Social Sciences (IBM SPSS Statistics 24.0 for Windows; IBM Corp., Armonk, NY, USA). $P < 0.05$ was considered statistically significant.

Results

Patient characteristics, motor function, ADL dependency, and ADL difficulty

As shown in Fig. 1, 199 of 564 Japanese HD outpatients who were assessed for eligibility fell under the exclusion criteria, and 149 declined to participate. Consequently, 216 patients (130 men, 86 women) were included in this study.

Additional file 2: Table S2 shows the clinical characteristics, motor function, ADL dependency, and ADL difficulty of all 216 patients (mean age, 67.4 years; age range, 36–90 years). The most common underlying kidney disease was glomerulonephritis (35.2%), followed by diabetic nephropathy (31.9%). Mean ADL dependency and difficulty scores were 34.3 ± 0.9 and 43.6 ± 10.6 points, respectively.

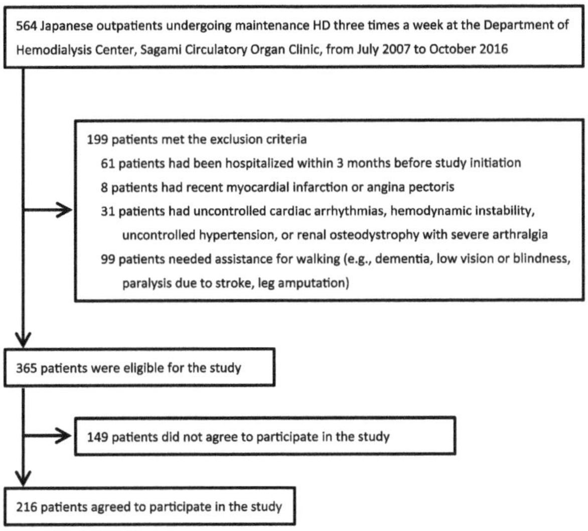

Fig. 1 Flow diagram of participant selection and exclusion

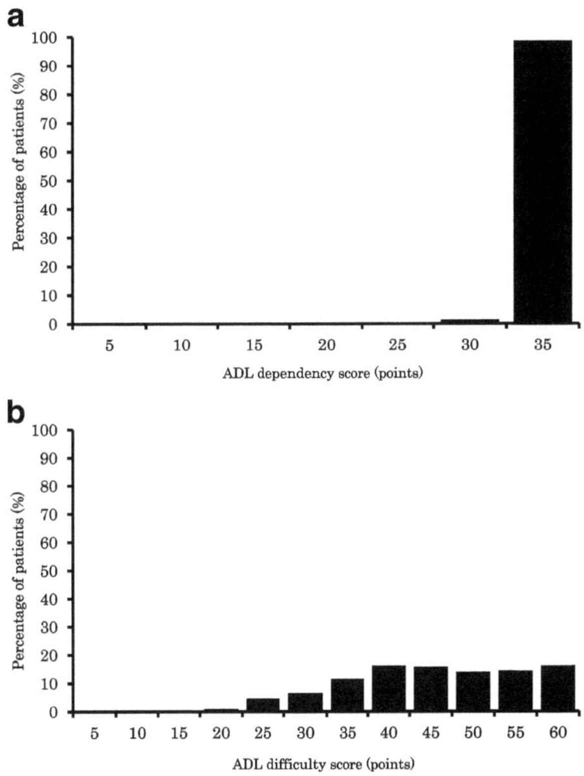

Fig. 2 Histogram of ADL dependency and ADL difficulty scores. **a** ADL dependency was assessed by the FIM. **b** ADL difficulty was assessed by the questionnaire on perceived mobility difficulty. ADL, activities of daily living; FIM, functional independence measure

Figure 2a shows the distribution of ADL dependency scores. Fifty-two percent (113 persons) scored full points. Figure 2b displays the distribution of ADL difficulty scores, showing wide variation. Four percent (nine persons) scored full points.

As shown in Fig. 3, patients found "walking up two flights of stairs" the most difficult of all 12 items, followed by "walking 1 km," "walking 600 m," "rising from the floor," "walking down two flights of stairs," "walking 300 m," "walking up one flight of stairs," "sitting down on the floor," "walking 20 m quickly," "walking down one flight of stairs," "walking 100 m," and "rising from a chair." Furthermore, based on the percentages of patients with a perceived difficulty score ≤ 3, "walking up two flights of stairs," "walking 1 km," "walking 600 m," and "rising from the floor" were classified as ADL items with higher level difficulty; "walking down two flights of stairs," "walking 300 m," "walking up one flight of stairs," and "sitting down on the floor" were classified as ADL items with middle level difficulty; and "walking 20 m quickly," "walking down one flight of stairs," "walking 100 m," and "rising from a chair" were classified as ADL items with lower level difficulty.

Differences in clinical characteristics, motor function, depressive symptoms, ADL dependency score, and ADL difficulty score between the difficulty and non-difficulty groups for each difficulty level are shown in Additional file 2: Table S2. For higher level difficulty, significant differences were observed between the two groups in age ($P < 0.001$), presence of depressive symptoms ($P = 0.002$), maximum leg strength ($P < 0.001$), one-leg standing time ($P < 0.001$), and usual walking speed ($P < 0.001$). For middle level difficulty, significant differences were observed in age ($P < 0.001$), presence of depressive symptoms ($P = 0.001$), maximum leg strength ($P < 0.001$), one-leg standing time ($P < 0.001$), and usual walking speed ($P < 0.001$). For lower level difficulty, significant differences were observed in age ($P < 0.001$), maximum leg strength ($P < 0.001$), one-leg standing time ($P < 0.001$), and usual walking speed ($P < 0.001$).

Univariate and multivariate logistic regression analyses on ADL difficulty

The results of univariate and multivariate logistic regression analyses on ADL difficulty are shown in Additional file 3: Table S3. As shown in Additional file 3: Table S3, the results of multivariate logistic regression analysis on ADL difficulty revealed that presence of depressive symptoms (odds ratio (OR) = 4.03, 95% confidence interval (CI) 1.12–14.50; $P = 0.033$) and usual walking speed (OR = 0.94, 95%CI 0.90–0.97; $P < 0.001$), after adjusting for age and sex (model 1), and presence of depressive symptoms (OR = 4.24, 95%CI 1.13–15.95; $P = 0.033$) and usual walking speed (OR = 0.94, 95%CI 0.90–0.97; $P < 0.001$), after adjusting for model 1 plus hemoglobin, serum albumin, and comorbidity index, were significantly associated with ADL difficulty at the higher level of difficulty. At the middle level of difficulty, maximum leg strength (OR = 0.97, 95%CI 0.94–1.00; $P = 0.043$) and usual walking speed (OR = 0.96, 95%CI

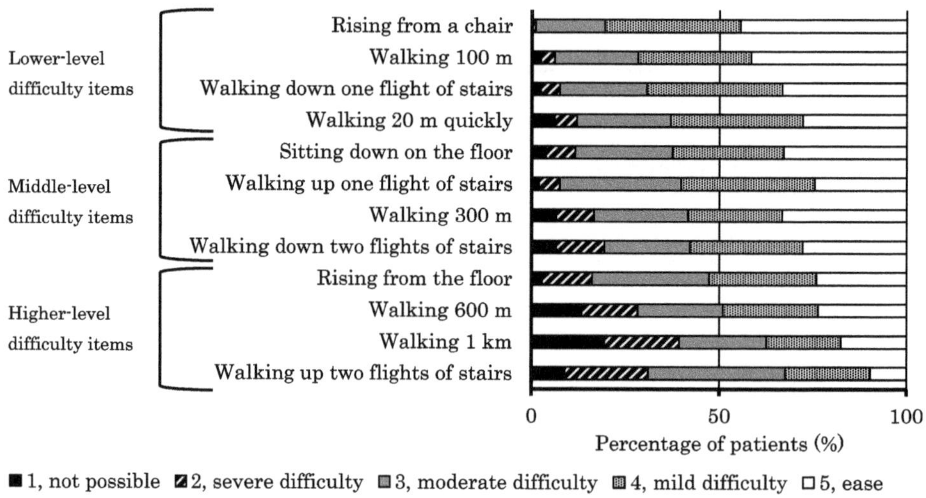

Fig. 3 Difficulty levels and distribution of 12 items of the questionnaire on perceived mobility difficulty

0.93–0.98; $P = 0.001$), in model 1, and maximum leg strength (OR = 0.97, 95%CI 0.94–1.00; $P = 0.043$) and usual walking speed (OR = 0.96, 95%CI 0.93–0.98; $P = 0.001$), in model 2, were significantly associated with ADL difficulty. At the lower level of difficulty, usual walking speed (OR = 0.93, 95%CI 0.90–0.96; $P < 0.001$), in model 1, and usual walking speed (OR = 0.93, 95%CI 0.90–0.96; P < 0.001), in model 2, were significantly associated with ADL difficulty.

ROC curves and cut-off values of usual walking speed for predicting ADL difficulty

Since usual walking speed was significantly associated with ADL difficulty across all three levels, ROC curves were generated for usual walking speed. Figures 4, 5, and 6 show the ROC curves of usual walking speed for predicting ADL difficulty at each level. The areas under the ROC curves of usual walking speed for predicting ADL difficulty at higher, middle, and lower levels were 0.82 ($P < 0.001$), 0.78 ($P < 0.001$), and 0.82 ($P < 0.001$), respectively. Cut-off values of usual walking speed for predicting ADL difficulty at higher, middle, and lower levels were 83.7, 75.5, and 75.1 m/min, respectively.

Discussion

In the present cross-sectional study, ADL difficulty scores varied widely among HD patients, whereas more than half of HD patients scored full points for ADL dependency. We classified the 12 items of the ADL difficulty questionnaire into three difficulty levels (higher, middle, and lower) based on the percentages of patients with a perceived difficulty score ≤ 3 in order to identify determinants of ADL difficulty. Multivariate logistic regression analysis revealed that common factors independently associated with ADL difficulty were old age and low usual walking speed for all difficulty levels, presence of depressive symptoms for higher level difficulty, and decreased maximum leg strength for middle level difficulty. Cut-off values of usual walking speed for predicting the presence of ADL difficulty for higher, middle, and lower level difficulty were 83.7, 75.5, and 75.1 m/min, respectively.

HD patients reportedly have a significantly higher ADL difficulty score compared to healthy controls [8]. Patients hospitalized due to heart failure have also been shown to have difficulty in walking (29.0%) and climbing stairs (45.9%) [32]. In the present study, 61 (28.2%) and 86 (39.8%) patients reported difficulty in walking 100 m

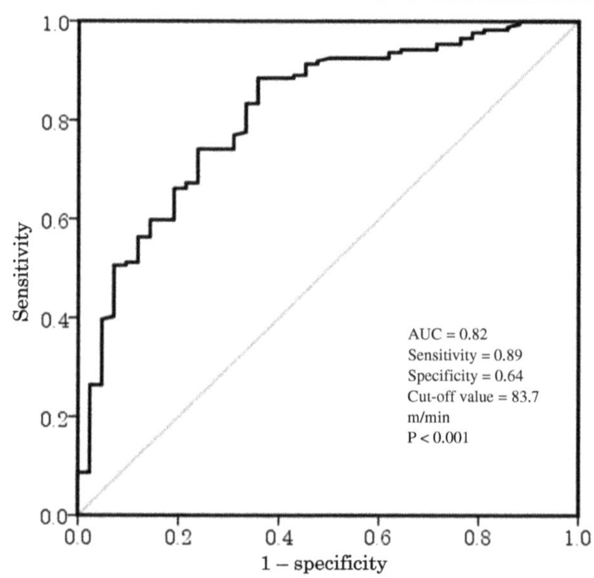

Fig. 4 ROC curve of usual walking speed for predicting ADL difficulty at higher level of difficulty. *ROC* receiver operating characteristic, *ADL* activities of daily living, *AUC* area under the curve

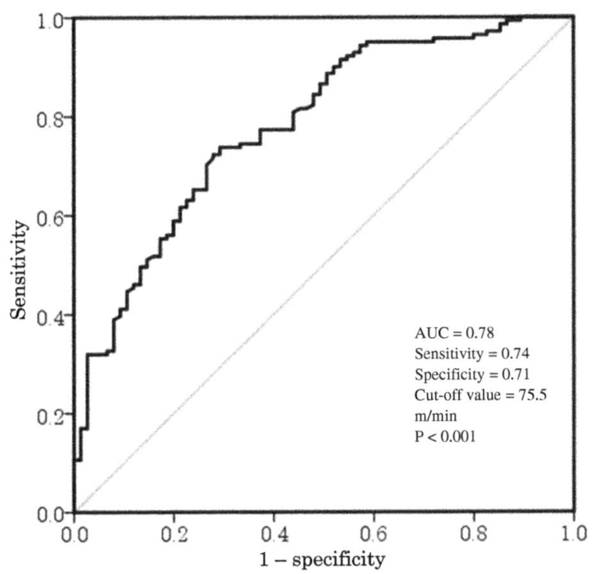

Fig. 5 ROC curve of usual walking speed for predicting ADL difficulty at middle level of difficulty. *ROC* receiver operating characteristic, *ADL* activities of daily living, *AUC* area under the curve

and walking up one flight of stairs, respectively, suggesting that prevalence rates of reported difficulty are similar between HD patients and hospitalized patients with heart failure.

In this study, usual walking speed was significantly associated with ADL difficulty at all three levels after adjustment for confounders. In a previous cross-sectional study, walking speed was associated with ADL difficulty in community-dwelling adults aged 65 and older [33]. Moreover, an 18-month prospective study reported that walking speed can predict the onset of ADL difficulty in older women aged 70–80 years [14]. Our findings are in line with these reports.

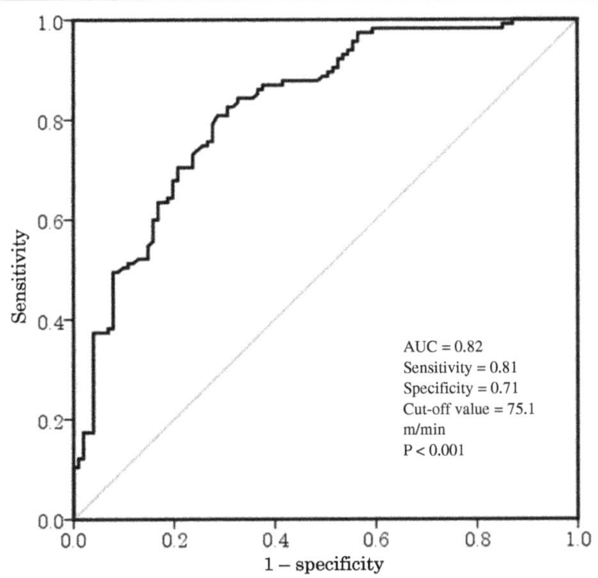

Fig. 6 ROC curve of usual walking speed for predicting ADL difficulty at lower level of difficulty. *ROC* receiver operating characteristic, *ADL* activities of daily living, *AUC* area under the curve

The presence of depressive symptoms was significantly associated with ADL difficulty at the higher level of difficulty. Depression has been attributed to disabilities in basic ADL (e.g., inability to bathe, eat, dress, transfer from a bed to a chair, use the toilet, or walk across a small room), mobility (e.g., unable to walk a short distance without help, or walking up and down stairs without help), and limited social activity (e.g., social withdrawal or social isolation) in older community-dwelling adults [34, 35]. Generally, collective social activity is defined as spending time and participating in activities together with other people, such as visiting cultural events, traveling, exercise, or participating in organizational activities. Therefore, social activity requires higher levels of mobility, e.g., more than that required to walk around at home. Moreover, the rate of onset of mobility disabilities after 6 years has been reported to be higher (67.1%) compared to that of basic ADL disabilities (36.1%) in patients with depression at baseline [34]. In our study, only a few participants had basic ADL disabilities. Therefore, depressive symptoms likely had a greater impact on high difficulty activities, such as walking long distances, than on easy activities in this study.

In this study, the cut-off values of usual walking speed for predicting ADL difficulty at higher, middle, and lower levels were 83.7, 75.5, and 75.1 m/min, respectively. These values were much higher compared to values reported previously, possibly because previous studies assessed ADL dependency in community populations. One study reported that usual walking speeds of 1.25 m/s (75.0 m/min) and 1.07 m/s (64.2 m/min) predict the onset of basic ADL dependency in men and women, respectively, among a Japanese community population aged 65 to 74 years with no ADL dependency [36]. In order to prevent ADL difficulty, higher physical functioning than that needed to prevent ADL dependency might be required. Therefore, the cut-off values obtained in this study might only be applicable to ambulatory HD outpatients.

Alavi et al. [37] reported that the ADL score is associated with age, gender, and education in hemodialysis and transplant patients. To the best of our knowledge, however, the present study is the first to examine determinants of ADL difficulty related to lower extremities after adjusting for confounders in HD patients. Walking speed and depressive symptoms, both predictors of ADL difficulty, have been reported to improve with adequate exercise training in HD patients [38, 39]. Thus, exercise training may help prevent the onset of ADL difficulty by improving walking speed and depressive symptoms.

This study has some limitations worth noting. First, our study might lack general applicability due to the small sample size and the single-center study design, which included only Japanese HD patients. Second, this study was a cross-sectional study, so a longitudinal study should be carried out in the future to investigate changes in ADL difficulty, physical functions, and depressive symptoms to examine further the determinants of ADL difficulty in HD patients. Third, only CES-D was used to evaluate depressive symptoms. More detailed evaluation including cognitive function will be necessary in the future.

Conclusions

This cross-sectional study revealed that a slow walking speed and old age are significantly and independently associated with ADL difficulty. The presence of depressive symptoms was significantly and independently associated with ADL difficulty at the higher level of difficulty in ambulatory HD patients. In addition, cut-off values of 83.7, 75.5, and 75.1 m/min for usual walking speed predicted the onset of ADL difficulty at higher, middle, and lower levels, respectively.

Additional files

Additional file 1: Table S1. Twelve items of the questionnaire on perceived mobility difficulty for HD patients. HD, hemodialysis.

Additional file 2: Table S2. Clinical characteristics, motor function, ADL dependency, and ADL difficulty of study subjects. Data are presented as mean ± standard deviation or number of subjects. *ADL items with higher level difficulty included "walking up two flights of stairs," "walking 1 km," "walking 600 m," and "rising from the floor." †ADL items with middle level difficulty included "walking down two flights of stairs," "walking 300 m," "walking up one flight of stairs," and "sitting down on the floor." ‡ADL items with lower level difficulty included "walking 20 m quickly," "walking down one flight of stairs," "walking 100 m," and "rising from a chair." BMI, body mass index: HD, hemodialysis; ADL, activities of daily living.

Additional file 3: Table S3. Univariate and multivariate logistic regression analyses on ADL difficulty. Univariate and multivariate logistic regression analyses were performed with ADL difficulty as a dependent variable and age, male sex, blood hemoglobin concentration, serum albumin concentration, comorbidity index, depression symptoms, maximum leg strength, one-leg standing time, and usual walking speed as independent variables for each level. *ADL items with higher level difficulty included "walking up two flights of stairs," "walking 1 km," "walking 600 m," and "rising from the floor." †ADL items with middle level difficulty included "walking down two flights of stairs," "walking 300 m," "walking up one flight of stairs," and "sitting down on the floor." ‡ADL items with lower level difficulty included "walking 20 m quickly," "walking down one flight of stairs," "walking 100 m," and "rising from a chair." ADL, activities of daily living; OR, odds ratio; CI, confidence interval.

Abbreviations

ADL: Activities of daily living; AUC: Area under the curve; BMI: Body mass index; CES-D: Center for Epidemiological Studies Depression Screening Index; CI: Confidence interval; FIM: Functional Independence Measure; HD: Hemodialysis; OR: Odds ratio; ROC: Receiver Operating Characteristic

Acknowledgements

The authors thank all patients who participated in this study. The authors also thank Drs. Shinya Nakajima, Yoriko Horiguchi, Tomoki Asai, and Sachiko Motohashi for performing the experiments, and the HD treatment staff at the Sagami Circulatory Organ Clinic for their contributions to this study.

Funding

This research was supported by JSPS KAKENHI Grant Numbers 23500614 and 26350631.

Authors' contributions

TW, TK, NM, YM, RM, YT, AY, and AM analyzed and interpreted the patient data regarding ADL difficulty and contributed significantly to the preparation of the manuscript. KY, MH, and TS performed measurements of motor function, depressive symptom, ADL dependency, and ADL difficulty. All authors read and approved the final manuscript.

Competing interests

The authors declare that they have no competing interests.

Author details

[1]Department of Rehabilitation Sciences, Kitasato University Graduate School of Medical Sciences, 1-15-1 Kitasato, Sagamihara, Kanagawa 252-0373, Japan. [2]Department of Physical Therapy, School of Health Sciences, Tokyo University of Technology, 5-23-22 Nishikamata, Ota-ku, Tokyo 144-8535, Japan. [3]Department of Sleep Medicine, Kitasato University Graduate School of Medical Sciences, 1-15-1 Kitasato, Sagamihara, Kanagawa 252-0373, Japan. [4]School of Allied Health Sciences, Kitasato University, 1-15-1 Kitasato, Sagamihara, Kanagawa 252-0373, Japan. [5]Department of Rehabilitation, Kitasato University Hospital, 1-15-1 Kitasato, Sagamihara, Kanagawa 252-0375, Japan. [6]Department of Nephrology in Internal Medicine, Kitasato University School of Medicine, 1-15-1 Kitasato, Sagamihara, Kanagawa 252-0373, Japan. [7]Department of Hemodialysis Center, Sagami Circulatory Organ Clinic, 4-21-15 Sonan, Sagamihara, Kanagawa 252-0312, Japan.

References

1. National Kidney Foundation. K/DOQI clinical practice guidelines: cardiovascular disease in dialysis patients. Am J Kidney Dis. 2005;45(4 Suppl 3) https://doi.org/10.1053/j.ajkd.2005.01.018.
2. Farrington K, Covic A, Aucella F, Clyne N, de Vos L, Findlay A, et al. Clinical practice guideline on management of older patients with chronic kidney disease stage 3b or higher (eGFR <45 mL/min/1.73 m2). Nephrol Dial Transplant. 2016;31(Suppl 2):ii1–ii66. https://doi.org/10.1093/ndt/gfw356.
3. Painter P, Marcus RL. Assessing physical function and physical activity in patients with CKD. Clin J Am Soc Nephrol. 2013;8(5):861–72. https://doi.org/10.2215/CJN.06590712.
4. Matsuzawa R, Matsunaga A, Wang G, Yamamoto S, Kutsuna T, Ishii A. Relationship between lower extremity muscle strength and all-cause mortality in Japanese patients undergoing dialysis. Phys Ther. 2014;94(7): 947–56. https://doi.org/10.2522/ptj.20130270.
5. Altintepe L, Levendoglu F, Okudan N, Guney I, Savas Cilli A, Ugurlu H, et al. Physical disability, psychological status, and health-related quality of life in older hemodialysis patients and age-matched controls. Hemodial Int. 2006; 10(3):260–6. https://doi.org/10.1111/j.1542-4758.2006.00106.x.

6. Kutner NG, Zhang R, Huang Y, Painter P. Gait speed and mortality, hospitalization, and functional status change among hemodialysis patients: a US renal data system special study. Am J Kidney Dis. 2015;66(2):297–304. https://doi.org/10.1053/j.ajkd.2015.01.024.
7. Jassal SV, Karaboyas A, Comment LA, Bieber BA, Morgenstern H, Sen A, et al. Functional Dependence and Mortality in the International Dialysis Outcomes and Practice Patterns Study (DOPPS). Am J Kidney Dis. 2016;67(2): 283–92. https://doi.org/10.1053/j.ajkd.2015.09.024.
8. Kutner NG, Brogan DJ. Assisted survival, aging, and rehabilitation needs: comparison of older dialysis patients and age-matched peers. Arch Phys Med Rehabil. 1992;73(4):309–15. https://doi.org/10.1016/0003-9993(92)90001-D.
9. Kaysen GA, Larive B, Painter P, Craig A, Lindsay RM, Rocco MV, et al. Baseline physical performance, health, and functioning of participants in the Frequent Hemodialysis Network (FHN) trial. Am J Kidney Dis. 2011;57(1): 101–12. https://doi.org/10.1053/j.ajkd.2010.08.021.
10. van den Ham EC, Kooman JP, Schols AM, Nieman FH, Does JD, Franssen FM, et al. Similarities in skeletal muscle strength and exercise capacity between renal transplant and hemodialysis patients. Am J Transplant. 2005; 5(8):1957–65. https://doi.org/10.1111/j.1600-6143.2005.00944.x.
11. Fahal IH, Bell GM, Bone JM, Edwards RH. Physiological abnormalities of skeletal muscle in dialysis patients. Nephrol Dial Transplant. 1997;12(1):119–27. https://doi.org/10.1093/ndt/12.1.119.
12. Painter P, Carlson L, Carey S, Paul SM, Myll J. Physical functioning and health-related quality-of-life changes with exercise training in hemodialysis patients. Am J Kidney Dis. 2000;35(3):482–92. https://doi.org/10.1016/S0272-6386(00)70202-2.
13. Lopes AA, Albert JM, Young EW, Satayathum S, Pisoni RL, Andreucci VE, et al. Screening for depression in hemodialysis patients: associations with diagnosis, treatment, and outcomes in the DOPPS. Kidney Int. 2004;66(5): 2047–53. https://doi.org/10.1111/j.1523-1755.2004.00977.x.
14. Chaves PH, Garrett ES, Fried LP. Predicting the risk of mobility difficulty in older women with screening nomograms: the Women's Health and Aging Study II. Arch Intern Med. 2000;160(16):2525–33. https://doi.org/10.1001/archinte.160.16.2525.
15. Fried LF, Lee JS, Shlipak M, Chertow GM, Green C, Ding J, et al. Chronic kidney disease and functional limitation in older people: health, aging and body composition study. J Am Geriatr Soc. 2006;54(5):750–6. https://doi.org/10.1111/j.1532-5415.2006.00727.x.
16. Connolly D, Garvey J, McKee G. Factors associated with ADL/IADL disability in community dwelling older adults in the Irish longitudinal study on ageing (TILDA). Disabil Rehabil. 2017;39(8):809–16. https://doi.org/10.3109/09638288.2016.1161848.
17. Tomita A, Burns JK. Depression, disability and functional status among community-dwelling older adults in South Africa: evidence from the first South African National Income Dynamics Study. Int J Geriatr Psychiatry. 2013;28(12):1270–9. https://doi.org/10.1002/gps.3954.
18. Hirvensalo M, Rantanen T, Heikkinen E. Mobility difficulties and physical activity as predictors of mortality and loss of independence in the community-living older population. J Am Geriatr Soc. 2000;48(5):493–8. https://doi.org/10.1111/j.1532-5415.2000.tb04994.x.
19. Liu J, Huang Z, Gilbertson DT, Foley RN, Collins AJ. An improved comorbidity index for outcome analyses among dialysis patients. Kidney Int. 2010;77(2):141–51. https://doi.org/10.1038/ki.2009.413.
20. Irwin M, Artin KH, Oxman MN. Screening for depression in the older adult: criterion validity of the 10-item Center for Epidemiological Studies Depression Scale (CES-D). Arch Intern Med. 1999;159(15):1701–4. https://doi.org/10.1001/archinte.159.15.1701.
21. Andresen EM, Malmgren JA, Carter WB, Patrick DL. Screening for depression in well older adults: evaluation of a short form of the CES-D (Center for Epidemiologic Studies Depression Scale). Am J Prev Med. 1994;10(2):77–84.
22. Kutsuna T, Matsunaga A, Matsumoto T, Ishii A, Yamamoto K, Hotta K, et al. Physical activity is necessary to prevent deterioration of the walking ability of patients undergoing maintenance hemodialysis. Ther Apher Dial. 2010; 14(2):193–200. https://doi.org/10.1111/j.1744-9987.2009.00750.x.
23. Bohannon RW. Comfortable and maximum walking speed of adults aged 20-79 years: reference values and determinants. Age Ageing. 1997;26(1):15–9. https://doi.org/10.1093/ageing/26.1.15.
24. Yamamoto S, Matsunaga A, Kamiya K, Miida K, Ebina Y, Hotta K, et al. Walking speed in patients with first acute myocardial infarction who participated in a supervised cardiac rehabilitation program after coronary intervention. Int Heart J. 2012;53(6):347–52. https://doi.org/10.1536/ihj.53.347.
25. Michikawa T, Nishiwaki Y, Takebayashi T, Toyama Y. One-leg standing test for elderly populations. J Orthop Sci. 2009;14(5):675–85. https://doi.org/10.1007/s00776-009-1371-6.
26. Hinkle JL. The use of the FIM™ instrument in the poststroke population. Top Stroke Rehabil. 2000;7(3):47–66. https://doi.org/10.1310/3LB6-CGVN-EAAU-0TEQ.
27. Granger CV, Hamilton BB, Keith RA, Zielezny M, Sherwin F. Advances in functional assessment for medical rehabilitation. Top Geriatr. 1986;1(3):59–74. https://doi.org/10.1097/00013614-198604000-00007.
28. Ottenbacher KJ, Hsu Y, Granger CV, Fiedler RC. The reliability of the functional independence measure: a quantitative review. Arch Phys Med Rehabil. 1966; 77(12):1226–32. https://doi.org/10.1016/S0003-9993(96)90184-7.
29. Ozawa T, Kutsuna T, Matsushima S, Kobayashi S, Henmi F, Matsuzawa R, et al. Development of a questionnaire for assessing perceived difficulty in performing activities of daily living related to lower-limb function in ambulatory hemodialysis patients (in Japanese). Phys Ther Jpn. 2010; 37(1):9–16.
30. Ozawa T, Matsunaga A, Kutsuna T, Matsushima S, Kobayashi S, Matsuzawa R, et al. Development of a questionnaire for assessing perceived difficulty in performing activities of daily living related to lower-limb function in ambulatory hemodialysis patients. Assessment of the responsiveness to exercise training (in Japanese). J Jpn Soc Dial Ther. 2010;43(6):515–22. https://doi.org/10.4009/jsdt.43.515.
31. Perkins NJ, Schisterman EF. The inconsistency of "optimal" cutpoints obtained using two criteria based on the receiver operating characteristic curve. Am J Epidemiol. 2006;163(7):670–5. https://doi.org/10.1093/aje/kwj063.
32. Dunlay SM, Manemann SM, Chamberlain AM, Cheville AL, Jiang R, Weston SA, et al. Activities of daily living and outcomes in heart failure. Circ Heart Fail. 2015;8(2):261–7. https://doi.org/10.1161/CIRCHEARTFAILURE.114.001542.
33. Capistrant BD, Glymour MM, Berkman LF. Assessing mobility difficulties for cross-national comparisons: results from the World Health Organization Study on Global AGEing and Adult Health. JAGS. 2014;62(2):329–35. https://doi.org/10.1111/jgs.12633.
34. Penninx BW, Leveille S, Ferrucci L, van Eijk JT, Guralnik JM. Exploring the effect of depression on physical disability: longitudinal evidence from the established populations for epidemiologic studies of the elderly. Am J Public Health. 1999;89(9):1346–52.
35. Djernes JK. Prevalence and predictors of depression in populations of elderly: a review. Acta Psychiatr Scand. 2006;113(5):372–87. https://doi.org/10.1111/j.1600-0447.2006.00770.x.
36. Shinkai S, Watanabe S, Kumagai S, Fujiwara Y, Amano H, Yoshida H, et al. Walking speed as a good predictor for the onset of functional dependence in a Japanese rural community population. Age Ageing. 2000;29(5):441-446. doi:doi.org/10.1093/ageing/29.5.441.
37. Alavi NM, Aliakbarzadeh Z, Sharifi K. Depression, anxiety, activities of daily living, and quality of life scores in patients undergoing renal replacement therapies. Transplant Proc. 2009;41(9):3693–6. https://doi.org/10.1016/j.transproceed.2009.06.217.
38. Headley S, Germain M, Mailloux P, Mulhern J, Ashworth B, Burris J, et al. Resistance training improves strength and functional measures in patients with end-stage renal disease. Am J Kidney Dis. 2002;40(2):355–64. https://doi.org/10.1053/ajkd.2002.34520.
39. Carney RM, Templeton B, Hong BA, Harter HR, Hagberg JM, Schechtman KB, et al. Exercise training reduces depression and increases the performance of pleasant activities in hemodialysis patients. Nephron. 1987;47(3):194–8. https://doi.org/10.1159/000184490.

9

Influence of continuous erythropoietin receptor activator (CERA) administration intervals on erythropoietic effect in hemodialysis patients

Shoichiro Daimon[1*], Hiromi Nuka[2], Kinya Kitada[2], Yasunori Suzuki[2], Fae Kim[2] and Mitsuhiro Kawano[2]

Abstract

Background: Erythropoietin deficiency is the major cause of anemia in hemodialysis patients. Although continuous erythropoietin receptor activator (CERA) has a long half-life and once-monthly administration is recommended, the optimal interval to achieve the greatest efficacy is not known.

Methods: In 44 hemodialysis patients, CERA was administered at an interval of once every 2 weeks (Q2W) and 4 weeks (Q4W) consecutively and reticulocyte counts and hemoglobin levels were compared prospectively. In six patients with CERA 100 μg/4 weeks, CERA intervals were further changed to 1 week (Q1W).

Results: Mean reticulocyte counts were higher during Q2W than Q4W (41.5 ± 10.7 and $36.4 \pm 8.8 \times 10^3/\mu L$, respectively, $p < 0.0001$), and hemoglobin levels decreased during Q4W. These results were irrespective of the CERA dose (50, 100, and 150 μg/4 weeks). In six patients with CERA 100 μg/4 weeks, although not significant, reticulocyte counts were higher during Q2W and Q1W than Q4W and hemoglobin levels were highest during Q1W ($p < 0.05$).

Conclusions: In our hemodialysis patients, an interval of CERA shorter than 4 weeks appeared to be more effective for the treatment of anemia.

Keywords: CERA, Interval, Reticulocyte, Hemoglobin

Background

Anemia is common in patients with chronic renal failure. Its causes include erythropoietin (EPO) deficiency, iron deficiency, inflammation, hyperparathyroidism, and in hemodialysis patients, blood loss related to the hemodialysis procedure. Although all these factors contribute to the anemia of hemodialysis patients, EPO deficiency is thought to be the major one. Anemia is associated with poorer patient survival [1, 2] and quality of life [3]. After the introduction of erythropoietin-stimulating agents (ESAs), the management of renal anemia has improved and has been associated with improved survival of hemodialysis patients [4].

Traditional ESAs have relatively short intravenous half-lives (epoetin alfa and beta, 7–9 h) [5] and require frequent administration. Continuous erythropoietin receptor activator (CERA) has a long half-life (134 and 139 h following intravenous and subcutaneous administration, respectively) [6] and is administered at wider intervals than epoetin or darbepoetin alfa for renal anemia in patients with chronic kidney disease. Although conversion to CERA with intervals of once every 2 weeks (Q2W) or 4 weeks (Q4W) from other ESAs is achieved safely in hemodialysis patients and once-monthly administration is recommended in Japan, the optimal interval of CERA administration is not known. Recently, it is reported that more continuous erythropoiesis was achieved with a Q2W administration of CERA than Q4W [7], and Q2W administration of CERA is more effective than Q4W to achieve target hemoglobin (Hb) levels [8]. Although we also reported more effective

* Correspondence: dai-clinic@m2.spacelan.ne.jp
[1]Department of Nephrology, Daimon Clinic for Internal Medicine, Nephrology and Dialysis, Oshino 1-400, Nonoichi, Ishikawa-pref 921-8802, Japan
Full list of author information is available at the end of the article

erythropoiesis of CERA by Q2W than Q4W, the fluctuation of Hb levels during Q4W is greater than that during Q2W [9], which makes it difficult to compare the true effect of the interval of CERA administration on Hb levels.

Usually the responsiveness to ESAs in hemodialysis patients is defined by the ESA dose and Hb levels [10], with low Hb levels at the same dose of ESAs meaning hypo-responsiveness to ESAs. This "responsiveness" is not equal to "red blood cell (RBC) production". In the absence of considerable blood loss, Hb levels are affected not only by the RBC production rate but also by the death rate, which means RBC lifespan. In hemodialysis patients, shortened and high interindividual variability of RBC lifespan is reported [11] and may have a substantial impact on Hb levels, which has been largely neglected.

For these reasons, Hb levels alone are not suitable to evaluate the erythropoietic effect of CERA according to administration interval, which prompted us to compare also reticulocyte counts during 4-, 2-, and 1-week intervals of CERA administration.

Methods

This prospective study focused on 44 hemodialysis patients in Daimon Clinic for Internal Medicine, Nephrology and Dialysis, whose Hb levels were controlled between 9 and 12 g/dL without changes in the CERA dose administered by Q2W for more than 3 months. Table 1 shows patient characteristics at baseline. Hb was controlled within a narrow range (10.9 ± 0.8 g/dL) under the same dosage of CERA administered by Q2W (50 µg per 4 weeks, $N = 25$; 100 µg, $N = 13$; and 150 µg, $N = 6$). Serum levels of hepcidin-25 were measured using a liquid chromatography-tandem mass spectrometric method [12]. Reticulocyte counts and Hb levels were evaluated every week for 4 weeks, and then CERA administration intervals were changed to 4 weeks (same dosage per 4 weeks). After the 4-week wash-out period, weekly reticulocyte counts and Hb levels were evaluated again for 4 weeks. To compare the erythropoietic effect of CERA by Q2W and Q4W, we evaluated the mean reticulocyte counts of the first hemodialysis session of the week during the 4 weeks of the evaluation period.

In 6 of 13 patients, 100 µg of CERA was administered every 4 weeks and Hb levels were between 9 and 12 g/dL at the end of the above study, after which CERA intervals were further changed to 1 week (Q1W) (25 µg of CERA every week) and reticulocyte counts and Hb levels were evaluated prospectively for a further 8 weeks (Fig. 1).

As a rule, iron has been administered orally in our clinic, with intravenous iron not administered during the study period. In 28 of the 44 patients, oral iron had been prescribed every day at least 3 months before the study (sodium ferrous citrate, $N = 21$; ferric citrate, $N = 7$, respectively) and did not change during the study period.

This study was approved by the local ethics committee (issue 2014-A1 at Daimon Clinic for Internal Medicine, Nephrology and Dialysis), and written informed consent was obtained from all patients.

Statistical analyses

Data were expressed as the mean ± SD. Paired and unpaired t tests and chi square test were used to compare the data. Statistical significance is defined as p less than 0.05.

Results

Figure 2 shows the weekly changes of reticulocyte counts during CERA administration by Q2W and Q4W. Three groups by CERA dose (50, 100, and 150 µg/4W) showed a similar pattern of reticulocyte count changes. As shown in Table 2, mean reticulocyte counts were higher during Q2W than during Q4W irrespective of CERA dose ($p < 0.005$, $p < 0.05$, and $p < 0.05$ for CERA 50, 100, and 150 µg/4W, respectively). Although Hb levels were stable during the period of CERA by Q2W, after the switch to Q4W, Hb levels showed a tendency to decrease (Fig. 3).

In six patients with CERA 100 µg per 4 weeks who were switched to Q1W further, as shown in Fig. 4, reticulocyte counts were maximal ($50–56 \times 10^3/\mu L$) around 2 weeks after the switch to Q1W and Hb increased gradually and reached a plateau 6 weeks after the switch to Q1W. Mean reticulocyte counts during the evaluation periods of Q4W, Q2W, and Q1W were 34.6 ± 22.3, 41.9 ± 19.9, and 38.3 ± 10.8 × $10^3/\mu L$, respectively (p = n.s.). Mean Hb levels were 11.1 ± 0.9, 11.2 ± 1.3, and 12.0 ± 2.2 g/dL, respectively ($p < 0.05$ Q1W vs. Q2W and Q1W vs. Q4W). Serum iron and ferritin levels at the switch to Q1W were 105.3 ± 42.5 µg/dL and 145.3 ± 81.5 ng/mL, and 8 weeks later, 75.3 ± 40.9 µg/dL (p = n.s.) and 91.6 ± 109.6 ng/mL ($p < 0.05$), respectively.

Discussion

EPO deficiency is the major cause of anemia in patients with chronic renal failure. ESAs correct anemia by binding to erythropoietin receptors expressed on progenitor cells in the bone marrow which leads to inhibition of cell apoptosis and enhancement of proliferation and differentiation [13]. The stimulated progenitor cells differentiate to erythroblasts, then mature to reticulocytes and finally to RBCs. Hematopoiesis by ESA administration influences iron metabolism. Although the precise mechanisms are not clear, in hemodialysis patients, ESA administration exerts a biphasic pattern of serum hepcidin-25 levels; early upregulation followed by late downregulation [14], and low serum hepcidin levels

Table 1 Patient characteristics at baseline

CERA dosage (μg/4 weeks)	Male (%)	Age (years)	Diabetes (%)	HD vintage (months)	BUN (mg/dL)	Cr (mg/dL)	TP (g/dL)	Alb (g/dL)	Hb (g/dL)	CRP (mg/dL)	Fe (μg/dL)	Ferritin (ng/mL)	Hepcidin-25 (ng/mL)
50 (*N* = 25)	16 (64.0)	70.0 ± 11.3 (35–87)	13 (52.0)	105.5 ± 90.6	62.6 ± 13.6	10.7 ± 2.1	6.5 ± 0.5	3.8 ± 0.3	10.9 ± 0.8	0.35 ± 0.53	79.7 ± 26.0 (36–123)	143.2 ± 155.0 (16.1–824)	74.2 ± 41.9 (0.4–175.9)
100 (*N* = 13)	9 (69.2)	70.6 ± 7.7 (53–85)	4 (30.8)	67.4 ± 66.4	67.5 ± 14.2	10.4 ± 1.9	6.7 ± 0.3	3.7 ± 0.3	11.0 ± 0.7	0.25 ± 0.52	82.1 ± 31.7 (32–145)	89.1 ± 70.4 (25.1–233)	38.9 ± 33.6 (0.2–122)
150 (*N* = 6)	5 (83.3)	69.0 ± 9.3 (51–75)	5 (83.3)	88.5 ± 45.4	57.9 ± 23.2	9.1 ± 4.0	6.6 ± 0.4	3.3 ± 0.2	10.4 ± 1.0	2.46 ± 3.17	44.8 ± 15.8 (26–68)	128.6 ± 89.6 (54.6–263)	90.2 ± 29.3 (55.7–137.1)
All (*N* = 44)	30 (68.2)	70.0 ± 9.9 (35–87)	22 (50.0)	91.9 ± 79.6	63.4 ± 15.2	10.4 ± 2.4	6.6 ± 0.4	3.7 ± 0.3	10.9 ± 0.8	0.61 ± 1.40	75.6 ± 29.0 (26–145)	125.2 ± 127.7 (16.1–824)	66.0 ± 41.7 (0.2–175.9)

Variables are represented as mean ± standard deviation

HD hemodialysis, *BUN* blood urea nitrogen, *Cr* creatinine, *TP* total protein, *Alb* albumin, *Hb* hemoglobin, *CRP* C-reactive protein, *Fe* iron

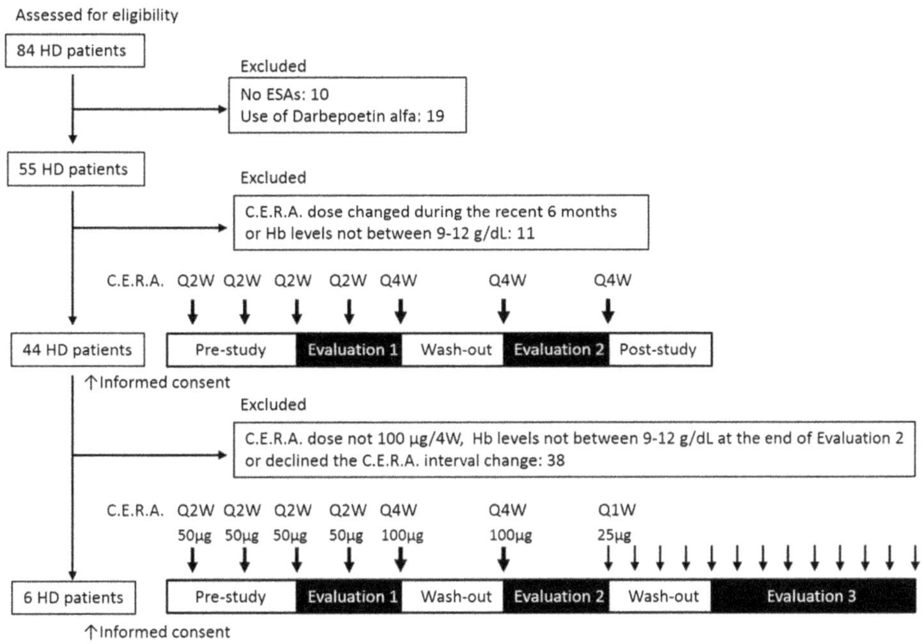

Fig. 1 Study design schema

facilitate iron utilization, which results in a decrease of serum ferritin levels. The degree of iron utilization and recruitment to the hematopoietic system seems to differ according to the type of ESAs [14–16] and interval of dosing [7, 8]. Transient reduction of serum hepcidin and ferritin levels induced by CERA administration reach a maximum around 1 week after dosing and return to pre-administration levels by 4 weeks, with this being the rationale of the once-monthly administration of CERA. These transient changes of serum ferritin and hepcidin levels induced by CERA are considered to be due to sustained stimulation of erythropoiesis by CERA which lasts

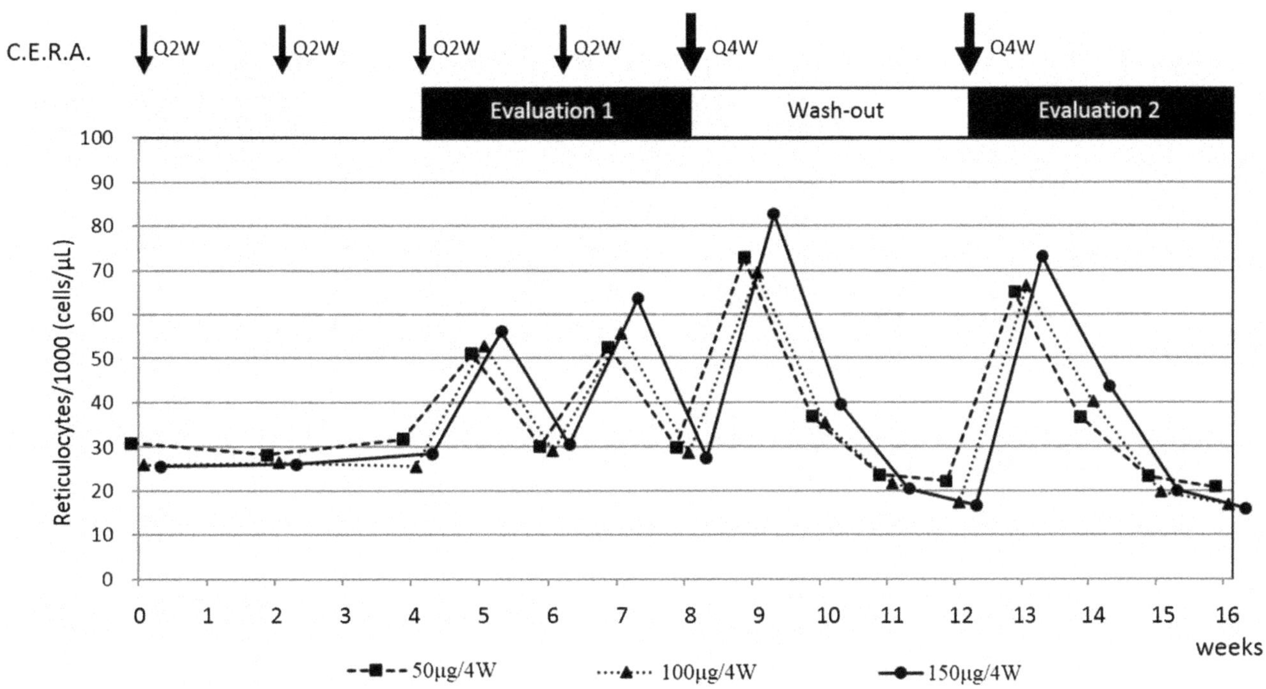

Fig. 2 Reticulocyte counts according to the dosage of CERA

Table 2 Mean reticulocyte counts during the administration of CERA by Q2W and Q4W

CERA dosage (μg/4 weeks)	Q2W/1000 (cells/μL)	Q4W/1000 (cells/μL)	*p* value
50 (*N* = 25)	40.7 ± 10.0	36.2 ± 9.9	<0.005
100 (*N* = 13)	41.6 ± 12.5	35.8 ± 7.8	<0.05
150 (*N* = 6)	44.7 ± 10.8	38.4 ± 7.0	<0.05
All (*N* = 44)	41.5 ± 10.7	36.4 ± 8.8	<0.0001

Variables are represented as mean ± standard deviation

much longer than that induced by epoetin. Although CERA has a long half-life, and once-monthly administration of CERA is safe and reported to save up to 144 injections per hemodialysis patient per year compared with three times weekly dosing [17], it is reported that Q2W administration of CERA is more effective than Q4W to achieve target Hb levels [7, 8, 17], which made us wonder what would be the optimal interval of CERA administration from the standpoint of efficacy.

As shown in Table 2, our study demonstrated higher mean reticulocyte counts in patients with CERA administered at Q2W than Q4W. In six patients, we further evaluated Hb levels and reticulocyte counts after CERA was administered by Q2W, Q4W, and Q1W sequentially (Fig. 4). During Q1W, Hb increased gradually and reached a higher level than that during Q2W and Q4W. Reticulocyte counts were highest in the first 2–4 weeks during the period of Q1W and persisted around the same levels as those of Q2W. Although timing effect of CERA administration on serum iron and ferritin levels must be taken into consideration, decrease of serum iron and ferritin levels during Q1W may indicate more effective iron recruitment for erythropoiesis than Q4W. Although the number of patients on Q1W was very small, this result suggests that not only Q2W but also Q1W administration of CERA has a greater erythropoietic effect than Q4W, and Q1W may have more potential to increase Hb levels than Q2W.

For the production of RBCs, erythropoietin is mandatory, since otherwise erythroid progenitor cells are rapidly lost to apoptosis [18]. Although CERA has a longer half-life than traditional ESAs, our results suggest that 4 weeks as a CERA administration interval is too long to achieve sustained erythropoiesis, and it is anticipated that the longer the interval of CERA administration is, the more erythroid progenitor cells might be lost to apoptosis, resulting in a decrease in the RBC production rate.

We evaluated the erythropoietic effect of CERA administered at different intervals by comparing reticulocyte counts and Hb levels. For this purpose, the CERA dose had to be kept stable during the study period. But it is sometimes difficult to maintain Hb levels within the target ranges without changing the dose of CERA for a substantial period, which meant that the study period had to be rather short. Especially when the CERA interval changes, Hb levels become unstable, and so as the wash-out period of

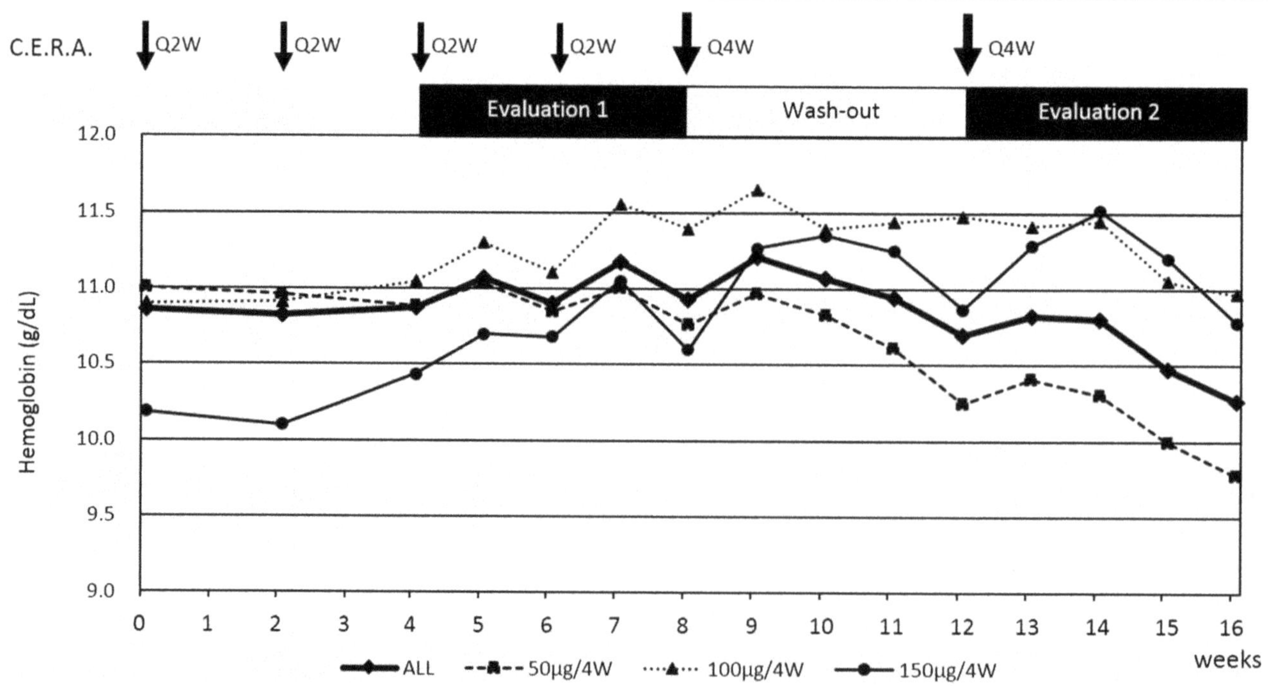

Fig. 3 Hemoglobin levels according to the dosage of CERA

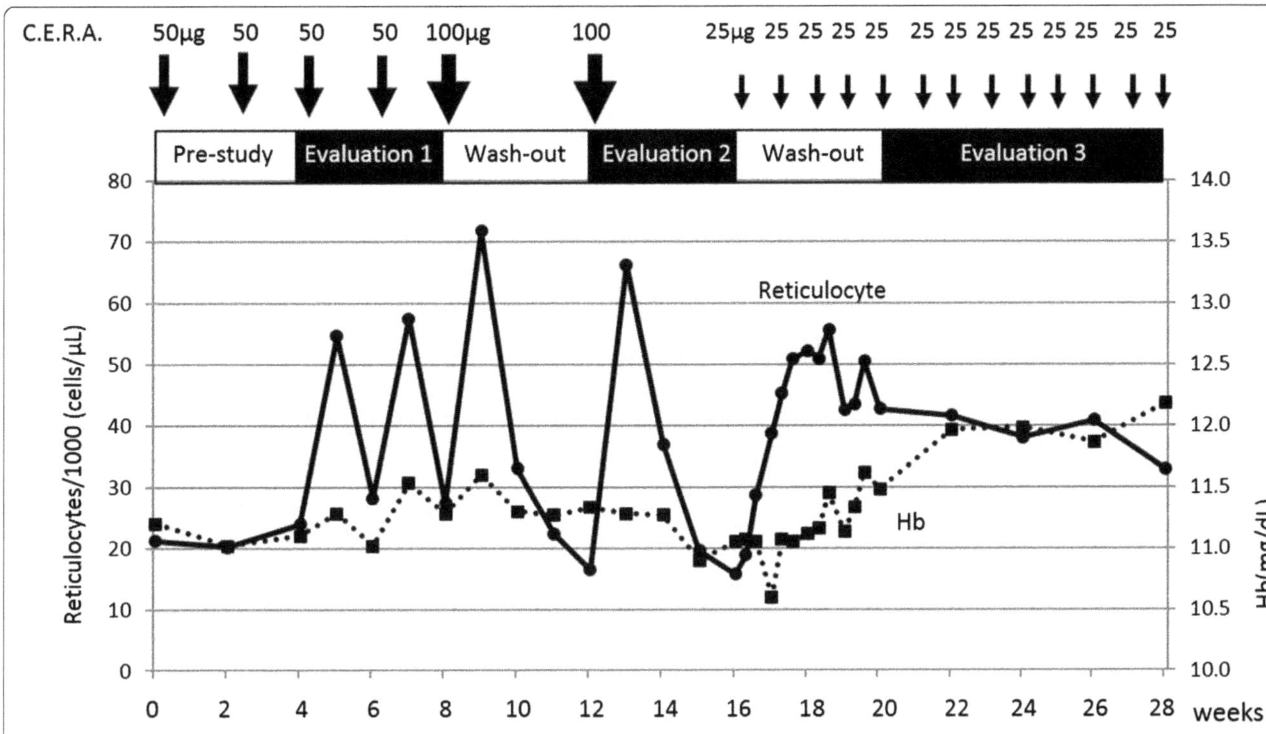

Fig. 4 Reticulocyte counts and hemoglobin levels when 100 μg of CERA per 4 weeks was administered by Q2W, Q4W, and Q1W

evaluation of CERA administration, we adopted only 4 weeks provisionally. As shown in Fig. 5, which illustrates the changes of reticulocyte counts and Hb levels during 100 μg of CERA, as Q4W was missed (this patient was excluded from evaluation in this study), reticulocyte counts decreased to minimal values at 4 weeks after the administration of CERA and persisted at the same level until the next administration of CERA. Although this is just a single observational datum, this example suggests that the

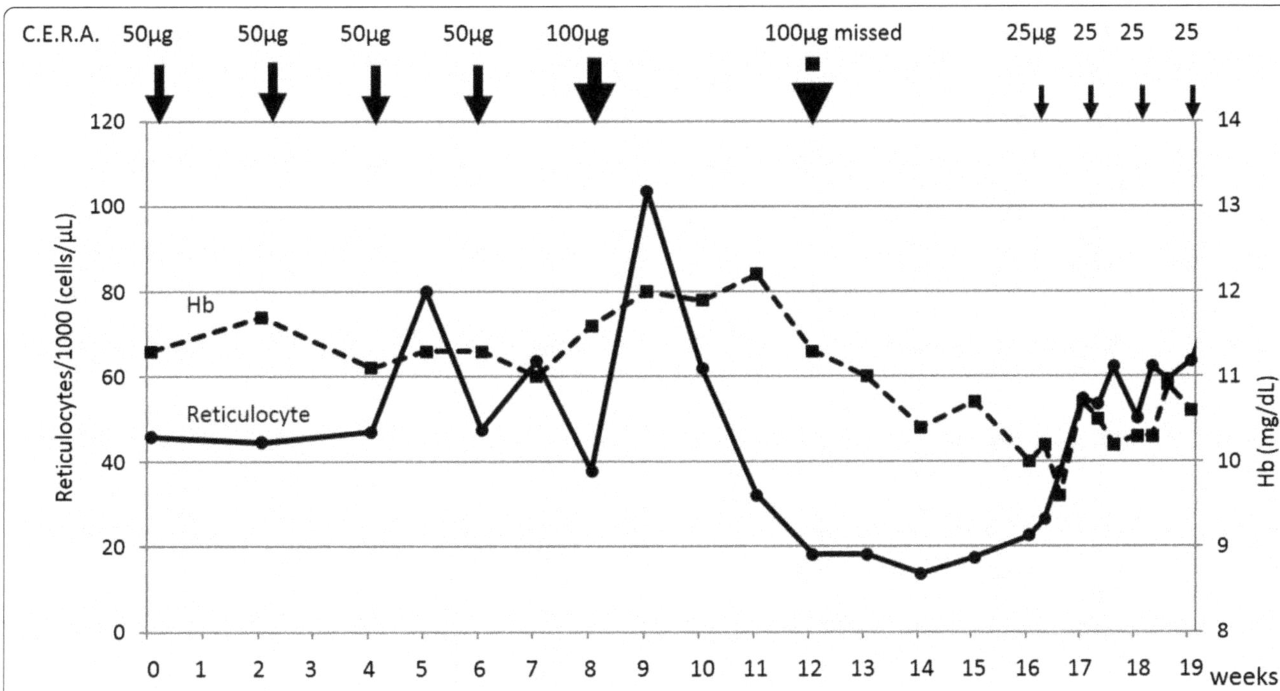

Fig. 5 Reticulocyte count and hemoglobin levels in a patient in whom CERA administration was missed

erythropoietic effect of CERA is not sustained for more than 4 weeks. This is in accordance with the reports of reticulocyte dynamics in hemodialysis patients treated with CERA [15, 19].

To compare the Hb levels of hemodialysis patients with CERA administered by different intervals, as we reported elsewhere [9], we need to consider the fluctuation patterns of Hb levels, which differ according to the CERA interval. Reticulocyte counts were maximal at 7–10 days of CERA administration and returned to the same levels by the next monthly CERA administration [15, 19], which influenced Hb levels. As a result, not only reticulocyte counts but also Hb levels differ according to the timing of the CERA administration and bloodwork, with the timing effect more prominent when CERA administration intervals are longer. This is also the case when we evaluate the serum iron, ferritin, or hepcidin levels which change in a mirror-image manner to the reticulocyte counts [7, 9, 15, 19].

In this study, Hb levels in the three groups of patients with CERA at doses of 50, 100, and 150 μg per 4 weeks were the same, which means that as a whole patients in the group with smaller dose of CERA have a higher responsiveness to CERA than patients in the group with a larger dose. But this "responsiveness" to ESAs is not equivalent to the "RBC production rate" by ESAs. The anemia of hemodialysis patients is not exclusively attributable to hypoproduction of RBCs. In the absence of considerable blood loss due to hemorrhage or the hemodialysis procedure itself, Hb levels of hemodialysis patients are affected by a shortened RBC lifespan. In healthy adults, the RBC lifespan is about 120 days within a narrow distribution. On the other hand, it is reported that in hemodialysis patients, the mean RBC lifespan is 89 days with high interindividual variability [11]. Although the influence of RBC lifespan on Hb levels in hemodialysis patients is substantial, this factor has been largely neglected [20]. In hemodialysis patients, RBC lifespan is influenced by the uremic state [21, 22], ESA administration [19, 23], and/or inflammation. The higher levels of CRP and hepcidin and lower levels of iron in patients receiving CERA 150 μg/4W than in those receiving 100 or 50 μg/4W may indicate the bluntness of iron recruitment for erythropoiesis but may also indicate a shorter RBC lifespan in patients requiring higher doses of CERA. Also, the highest level of Hb seen during evaluation 3 as compared to that during evaluation 1 and 2 with the same reticulocyte counts may suggest a longer RBC lifespan during Q1W of CERA than that during Q2W and Q4W.

For the effective treatment of anemia in hemodialysis patients, we need to consider multiple factors such as iron deficiency, inflammation, hyperparathyroidism, and dialysis dose and adjust them whenever possible. Also our study suggests that by changing the interval of CERA, the CERA dose can be reduced without exacerbating Hb control. Moreover, it is anticipated that the more sustained erythropoiesis and RBC production associated with a shorter interval of CERA can prevent the occurrence of Hb overshoot or Hb cycling. Although any effects of such factors on the mortality of hemodialysis patients have not been well documented [24], a shorter interval of CERA administration has advantages in stabilizing Hb levels, reducing the cost of ESAs, and reducing the workload associated with frequent changes of the ESA dose.

Conclusions

In hemodialysis patients, a shorter interval of CERA administration can produce more RBC and increase Hb levels. To achieve efficient and sustained RBC production and maintenance of Hb levels within the narrow target range, shorter than a 4-week interval of CERA administration appears preferable.

Abbreviations

CERA: Continuous erythropoietin receptor activator; EPO: Erythropoietin; ESA: Erythropoietin-stimulating agent; Q2W: Once every 2 weeks; Hb: Hemoglobin; RBC: Red blood cell

Acknowledgements

The authors thank all staff members working at Daimon Clinic for Internal Medicine, Nephrology and Dialysis.

Funding

This study was not supported by any grants or funding.

Authors' contributions

HN, KK, YS, and FK participated in the design of the study. MK conceived of the study and participated in its design. SD was responsible for the research idea and study. All authors read and approved the final manuscript.

Competing interests

The authors declare that they have no competing interests.

Author details

[1]Department of Nephrology, Daimon Clinic for Internal Medicine, Nephrology and Dialysis, Oshino 1-400, Nonoichi, Ishikawa-pref 921-8802, Japan. [2]Division of Rheumatology, Department of Internal Medicine, Kanazawa University Graduate School of Medicine, Kanazawa, Japan.

References

1. Ma JZ, Ebben J, Xia H, Xia H, Collins AJ. Hematocrit level and associated mortality in hemodialysis patients. J Am Soc Nephrol. 1999;10:610–9.

2. Foley RN, Parfrey PS, Morgan J, et al. Effect of hemoglobin in hemodialysis patients with asymptomatic cardiomyopathy. Kidney Int. 2000;58:1325–35.
3. Perlman RL, Finkelstein FO, Liu L, et al. Quality of life in chronic kidney disease (CKD): a cross-sectional analysis in the Renal Research Institute-CKD study. Am J Kidney Dis. 2005;45:658–66.
4. Regidor DL, Kopple JD, Kovesdy CP, et al. Association between changes in hemoglobin and administered erythropoietin-stimulating agent and survival in hemodialysis patients. J Am Soc Nephrol. 2006;17:1181–91.
5. Halstenson CE, Macres M, Katz SA, et al. Comparative pharmacokinetics and pharmacodynamics of epoetin alfa and epoetin beta. Clin Pharmacol Ther. 1991;50:702–12.
6. Macdougal IC, Robson R, Opatrna S, et al. Pharmacokinetics and pharmacodynamics of intravenous and subcutaneous continuous erythropoietin receptor activator (CERA) in patients with chronic kidney disease. Clin J Am Soc Nephrol. 2006;1:1211–5.
7. Morikami Y, Fujimori A, Okada S, Kumei M, Mizobuchi N, Sakai M. Comparison of 2-week versus 4-week dosing intervals of epoetin beta pegol on erythropoiesis and iron metabolism in hemodialysis patients. Ther Apher Dial. 2014;18:414–20.
8. Toida T, Sato Y, Shibata N, Kitamura K, Fujimoto S. A randomized control study on the procedure for switching epoetin beta (EPO) to epoetin beta pegol (CERA) in the treatment of renal anemia in maintenance hemodialysis patients. Blood Purif. 2014;38:174–9.
9. Daimon S. Comparison of the effect of the same dose of a 4-weekly continuous erythropoietin receptor activator administered once every 2 or 4 weeks in hemodialysis patients. Ther Apher Dial. 2014;18:518–21.
10. Fukuma S, Yamaguchi T, Hashimoto S, et al. Erythropoiesis-stimulating agent responsiveness and mortality in hemodialysis patients: results from a cohort study from the dialysis registry in Japan. Am J Kidney Dis. 2012;59:108–16.
11. Sato Y, Mizuguchi T, Shigenaga S, et al. Shortened red blood cell lifespan is related to the dose of erythropoiesis-stimulating agents requirement in patients on hemodialysis. Ther Apher Dial. 2012;16:522–8.
12. Itkonen O, Parkkinen J, Stenman UH, Hämäläinen E. Preanalytical factors and reference intervals for serum hepcidin LC-MS/MS method. Clin Chim Acta. 2012;413:696–701.
13. Fisher JW. Erythropoietin: physiology and pharmacology update. Exp Biol Med. 2003;228:1–14.
14. Takasawa K, Tomosugi N, Takaeda C, Maeda T, Ueda N. Regulation of hepcidin-25 by short and long-acting rhEPO may be dependent on ferritin and predict the response to rhEPO in hemodialysis patients. Nephron Extra. 2014;4:55–63.
15. Jonckheere S, Dierick J, Vanhouteghem H, Devieeschouwer M, Stove V. Erythrocyte indices in the assessment of iron states in dialysis-dependent patients with end-stage renal disease on continuous erythropoietin receptor activator versus epoetin β therapy. Acta Haematol. 2010;124:27–33.
16. Kakimoto-Shino M, Toya Y, Kuji T, Fujikawa T, Umemura S. Changes in hepcidin and reticulocyte levels in response to continuous erythropoietin receptor activator administration in hemodialysis patients: a randomized study. Ther Apher Dial. 2014;18:421–6.
17. Sulowicz W, Locatelli F, Ryckelynck JP, et al. Once-monthly subcutaneous C.E.R.A. maintains stable hemoglobin control in patients directly from epoetin one to three times weekly. Clin J Am Soc Nephrol. 2007;2:637–46.
18. Polenakovic M, Sikole A. Is erythropoietin a survival factor for red blood cells? J Am Soc Nephrol. 1996;7:1178–82.
19. Forni V, Bianchi G, Ogna A, et al. Reticulocyte dynamic and hemoglobin variability in hemodialysis patients treated with Darbepoetin alfa and C.E.R.A.: a randomized controlled trial. BMC Nephrol. 2013;14:157–66.
20. Kalicki RM, Uehlinger DE. Red cell survival in relation to changes in the hematocrit: more important than you think. Blood Purif. 2008;26:355–60.
21. Erslev AJ, Besarab A. The rate and control of baseline red cell production in hematologically stable patients with uremia. J Lab Clin Med. 1995;126:283–6.
22. Hocken AG. Haemolysis in chronic renal failure. Nephron. 1982;32:28–31.
23. Schwartz AB, Kahn SB, Kelch B, Kim KE, Pequignot E. RBC improved survival due to recombinant human erythropoietin explains effectiveness of less frequent, low dose subcutaneous therapy. Clin Nephrol. 1992;38:283–9.
24. Singh AK, Milford E, Fishbane S, Keithi-Reddy SR. Managing anemia in dialysis patients: hemoglobin cycling and overshoot. Kidney Int. 2008;74: 679–83.

10

Improvement of the fraction of human mercaptalbumin on hemodialysis treatment using hydrogen-dissolved hemodialysis fluid

Kenji Maeda[1*], Shigehito Yoshizaki[2], Toshiro Iida[1], Tomoyoshi Terada[3], Seiichi Era[3], Keiichiro Sakashita[4] and Hajime Arikawa[5]

Abstract

Background: Oxidative stress (OS) is said to increase in hemodialysis therapy, so that the electrolyzed water-hemodialysis (EW-HD) dissolving hydrogen in hemodialysis fluid has been tried for the reduction of OS. It is reported that the risk of cardiovascular disease events increased if the fraction of reduced albumin (human mercaptalbumin (f(HMA))) was low and that the f(HMA) rose at the dialyzer outlet on EW-HD. Therefore, we studied whether the f(HMA) of hemodialysis patients was improved when they received long-term EW-HD treatment.

Methods: We produced hydrogen-dissolved hemodialysis fluid with EW-C81-HD and carried out EW-HD treatment for 12 patients. The serum albumin redox states of pre- and post-HD were measured in the summer of 2014 (EWHD2014) and in the winter of 2015 (EWHD2015) after 6 months by high-performance liquid chromatography using Shodex-Asahipak ES-502N 7C column. For comparison, 38 conventional hemodialysis (C-HD) patients and 24 healthy subjects were selected.

Results: The f(HMA) of EWHD2015 significantly increased from EWHD2014 on both pre- and post-HD (pre, 51.32 ± 5.63 % → 58.03 ± 7.43 %; post, 72.04 ± 5.73 % → 76.42 ± 4.67 %). The f(HMA) of C-HD at pre- and post-HD were 51.07 ± 9.07 and 70.53 ± 8.05 %, respectively. The f(HMA) of healthy subjects was 79.11 ± 5.46 %. The f(HMA) of EWHD2014 at pre-HD evidenced no significant difference with that of C-HD at pre-HD, but the f(HMA) of EWHD2015 at pre-HD was significantly higher than that of C-HD at pre-HD. The f(HMA) of C-HD at post-HD was significantly lower than that of both EWHD2015 at post-HD and healthy subjects, but the f(HMA) of EWHD2015 at post-HD showed no significant difference with that of healthy subjects.

Conclusions: Our data suggest that the f(HMA) may be raised with long-term hemodialysis treatment using hydrogen-dissolved hemodialysis fluid.

Keywords: Hemodialysis, Hydrogen-dissolved hemodialysis fluid, Electrolyzed water-hemodialysis, Human mercaptalbumin, Human nonmercaptalbumin, Albumin redox, Oxidative stress

* Correspondence: daikoupaper@gmail.com
[1]Daiko Sunadabashi Clinic, Nagoya, Japan
Full list of author information is available at the end of the article

Background

The dialysis patient population in Japan was 310,007 at the end of 2012. The characteristics of the dialysis patients include the long dialysis vintage, aging, and increased rate of diabetic nephropathy on primary disease. The patient population surviving over 25 years of dialysis was 12,307 (4.1 %). Their mean age was 66.9 years, and the percentage over 75 years of age was 29.6 %. On the primary disease, the percentage of diabetic nephropathy was 37.1 % and that of chronic glomerulonephritis was 33.6 % [1]. The life convalescence of a dialysis patient is far worse than that of the general population [2], and one of the main causes is considered to be oxidative stress (OS) related with hemodialysis therapy [3, 4]. One of the OS markers was the albumin oxidation-reduction ratio [5]. The reduced form of albumin decreases from a point of chronic kidney disease before the dialysis therapy [6], and that is lower in hemodialysis and peritoneal dialysis patients. The cardiovascular event and death risk are as high as the reduced form of albumin is low [7, 8].

In present dialysis therapy, various kinds of treatments are carried out to reduce the risk of mortality and the frequency of complications. The hydrogen molecules remove a hydroxyl radical and reduce the OS [9], so its effects are expected on the hemodialysis therapy.

The electrolyzed water-hemodialysis (EW-HD) dissolving hydrogen in hemodialysis fluid is one of the various kinds of treatments to reduce OS. The EW-HD treatment was first reported by Huang et al. [10]. In Japan, the clinical application of EW-HD was carried out by Nakayama et al. [11]. Its effects such as anemia improvement, blood pressure control, and the reduction of the OS were then reported [12, 13].

We began the EW-HD treatment from January 2014 in Daiko Sunadabashi Branch Clinic, too, and began examining clinical effects of EW-HD from July. One previous report showed that EW-HD might improve OS more effectively than conventional HD (C-HD) session. In this report, the authors adapted the redox state of human serum albumin (HSA-redox) as a marker of OS: they found that a fraction of reduced albumin (human mercaptalbumin (f(HMA))) rose at the dialyzer outlet only on EW-HD treatment [14]. However, there is still no long-term study regarding the long-term effect of EW-HD on HSA-redox profile. Therefore, we studied whether the f(HMA) of HD patients increased when they received long-term EW-HD treatment. This is why we report here this interesting f(HMA) increase with long-term EW-HD treatment.

Methods

Subject

Twelve patients (male/female; 6/6) received EW-HD, 38 (male/female; 24/14) received C-HD, and 24 people were healthy subjects (male/female; 11/13). The age and/or other parameters are shown in Table 1. No patient who took a drug had a reduction action.

Primary disease, age, and sex were not required for the condition of the subjects, but the patients having cirrhosis or a malignant tumor were excluded.

Production of the hydrogen-dissolved hemodialysis fluid

The reverse osmosis water dissolving hydrogen (H2-RO water) that was produced by the Reverse Osmosis Purified Water Production System for EW-HD; EW-C81-HD (Trim Medical Institute Co., Ltd. Sendai, Japan) was used for the product water. The hydrogen-dissolved hemodialysis fluid was produced by the Multiple Patient Dialysis Fluid Supply System; DAB-20NX (NIKKISO Co., Ltd. Tokyo, Japan). The concentrated liquid for hemodialysis fluid was produced by Dialysis Powder Mixing Device; DAD-50 (NIKKISO Co., Ltd. Tokyo, Japan) using H2-RO water and Dialysis Powder; D DRY®-2.5S/3.0S (NIKKISO Co., Ltd. Tokyo, Japan). (Fig. 1).

Table 1 Profile of subjects

	Median (min – max)		
	EW-HD[a]	C-HD	Healthy subjects
Gender (M/F)	6/6	24/14	11/13
Age (years old)	70 (57–83)	73 (37–89)	39 (21–54)
Primary disease (DM/non-DM)	6/6	14/24	–
Body weight at post-HD (kg)	48.7(43.7–64.7)	53.3 (33.3–87.5)	–
HD treatment time (hours)	4.0 (3.5–4.0)	4.0 (3.0–5.0)	–
HD vintage (months)	8 (1–150)	22 (2–128)	–
EW-HD vintage (days)	75 (19–210)	–	–

There was no significant difference between EW-HD and C-HD
[a]At 2014

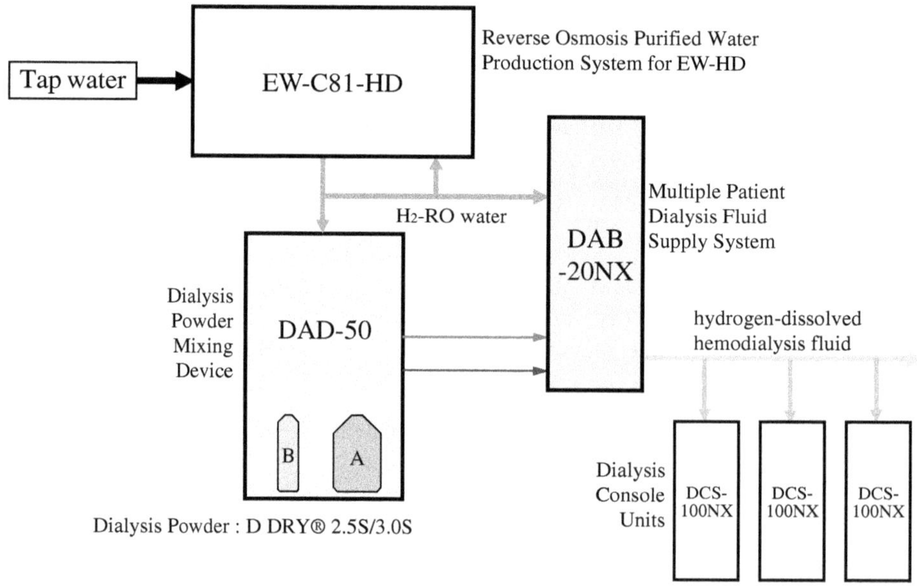

Fig. 1 Schema of production process of hydrogen-dissolved hemodialysis fluid

Dialysis conditions

The dialysis conditions for the hemodialysis patients are shown in Table 2. All patients did not receive hemodiafiltration treatment. There were no differences in treatment time, hemodialysis frequency, dialyzer type and membrane material, membrane area, quantity of blood flow (Q_B), or dialysis dose between EW-HD and C-HD. The quantity of hemodialysis fluid flow (Q_D) was 500 mL/min in all patients. The dialysis powder of C-HD was Kindaly 4E (Fuso Pharmaceutical Industries, Ltd., Osaka, Japan). The compositions of hemodialysis fluid in C-HD are almost the same as those in EW-HD.

Table 2 Dialysis condition

	EW-HD (n = 12) EWHD2014 → EWHD015	C-HD (n = 38)	Notes
Treatment mode	Hemodialysis	Hemodialysis	
Treatment time (hour/session)	3.92 ± 0.19 → 3.96 ± 0.14	3.95 ± 0.48	Mean ± SD ns
Hemodialysis frequency	3 times/week	3 times/week	
Dialyzer type/membrane material	V/PS: 6; IV/CTA: 6 → V/PS: 7; IV/CTA: 5	V/PS: 14; IV/PS: 8, CTA: 16	Polysulfone (PS), cellulose triacetate (CTA)
Dialyzer membrane area (m^2)	1.5 (1.3–2.1) → 1.7 (1.5–2.1)	1.8 (1.3–2.5)	Median (min–max) ns
Q_B (mL/min)	200 (180–230) → 200 (200–230)	200 (150–250)	Median (min–max) ns
Q_D (mL/min)	500	500	
Dialysis dose: KT/V for urea	1.45 ± 0.15 → 1.55 ± 0.19	1.45 ± 0.24	Mean ± SD ns
Body weight pre-HD (kg)	52.9 ± 6.4 → 54.3 ± 6.3	56.6 ± 11.5	Mean ± SD ns
post-HD (kg)	50.7 ± 6.4 → 51.9 ± 6.5	54.1 ± 10.9	Mean ± SD ns
Dialysis powder	D DRY®-2.5S/3.0S	Kindaly 4E	
Compositions of hemodialysis fluid			
Na^+ (mEq/L)	140.0	140.0	
K^+ (mEq/L)	2.0	2.0	
Ca^{2+} (mEq/L)	2.75	2.75	
Mg^{2+} (mEq/L)	1.0	1.0	
Cl^- (mEq/L)	112.25	112.25	
HCO_3^- (mEq/L)	25.0	27.5	
CH_3COO^- (mEq/L)	10.0	8.0	
$C_6H_{12}O_6$ (mg/dL)	100.0	125.0	

ns no significant difference between EW-HD and C-HD

Measurements

HMA and HNA (human nonmercaptalbumin) were measured by high-performance liquid chromatography (HPLC) as reported in the previous paper [14]. Briefly, the HPLC system consisted of an AS-8010 auto-sampler (Tosoh, Tokyo, Japan; 2 μL injection volume) and a CCPM double-plunger pump (Tosoh) in conjunction with a CO-8011 system controller (Tosoh). Chromatographs were obtained using a UV6000LP photodiode alley detector (detection area, 200–600 nm with 1 nm step; Thermo Electron, Waltham, MA, USA). A Shodex-Asahipak ES-502 N 7C column (10 × 0.76 cm I.D., DEAE form for ion-exchange HPLC; Showa Denko, Tokyo, Japan; column temperature, 35 ± 0.5 °C) was used in this study.

The f(HMA) was calculated with the following equation, f(HMA) = [HMA/(HMA + HNA)] × 100 (%).

The serum samples were collected from EW-HD patients in August/September 2014 (EWHD2014) and February/March 2015 (EWHD2015), from C-HD patients in August 2014 ~ February 2015, from healthy subjects in September/October 2014. The samples were frozen at −80 °C until measurement. The sampling from the patients was carried out at the pre- and post-HD at the beginning of the week.

The hydrogen concentration in hemodialysis fluid was measured by Portable Dissolved Hydrogen Meter; DH-35A (DKK-TOA CO., LTD. Tokyo, Japan).

Data analysis

The data were shown in mean ± standard deviation. The Stat View 5.0 (Hulinks Inc., Tokyo, Japan) software was used for statistical tests. The differences of EWHD2014 and EWHD2015 were compared by paired *t* test. The multiple comparison procedure was carried out for statistical analysis among EW-HD, C-HD, and healthy subjects. We assumed less than 5 % of levels of significance as a statistical significance standard.

Results

The f(HMA) of pre- and post-HD were 51.32 ± 5.63 and 72.04 ± 5.73 % at EWHD2014, respectively. The f(HMA) of pre- and post-HD were 58.03 ± 7.43 and 76.42 ± 4.67 % at EWHD2015, respectively. The f(HMA) of pre- and post-HD on C-HD were 51.07 ± 9.07 and 70.53 ± 8.05 %, respectively. The f(HMA) of healthy subjects was 79.11 ± 5.46 % (Table 3).

Table 4 shows the blood data of the patients at the time of sampling.

On the EW-HD, the f(HMA) at 2015 significantly increased from 2014 on both pre- and post-HD (Fig. 2).

On comparison with C-HD at pre-HD, the f(HMA) of EWHD2014 showed no significant difference with that of C-HD, but the f(HMA) of EWHD2015 was significantly higher than that of C-HD (Fig. 3).

In the relationship between the HD vintage and f(HMA) at pre-HD, there were no correlation both in C-HD and EWHD2014(Fig. 4).

On comparison among EWHD2015, C-HD and healthy subjects, the f(HMA) of C-HD at post-HD were significantly lower than those of EWHD2015 at post-HD and healthy subjects, but the f(HMA) of EWHD2015 at post-HD showed no significant difference with that of healthy subjects (Fig. 5).

The concentration of hydrogen in hemodialysis fluid was measured several times after the beginning of EW-HD, and ranged 47~196 ppb (Table 5).

Discussion

Albumin is the main antioxidant in plasma [5], and we paid attention to HSA-redox and examined it. As for the human albumin, the free thiol of 34-cysteine is reduced albumin (HMA), and the disulfide bond of 34-cysteine is oxidative albumin (HNA). HMA plays an important role in the antioxidant mechanism in extracellular fluid [5]. The f(HMA) in serum decreases with aging, but that in cerebrospinal fluid does not change [15]. The control mechanism of albumin redox has not fully been examined, but Matsuyama et al. reported that human astrocytes and aortic endothelial cells are actively converted to HMA from HNA [15]. The f(HMA) decreases with a renal dysfunction [6], so the kidney may do some kind of participation in albumin redox. In the hemodialysis patients who have almost no renal function, it is thought that the albumin redox adjustment function is lowered during non-hemodialysis treatment. In the albumin redox of hemodialysis patients, the f(HMA) increased to nearly normal levels post-HD when hemodialysis treatment was performed, but decreased afterward , and was

Table 3 Albumin redox of patients and healthy subjects

(%) mean ± SD

	EWHD2014 (*n* = 12)		EWHD2015 (*n* = 12)		C-HD (*n* = 38)		Healthy subjects (*n* = 24)
	Pre-HD	Post-HD	Pre-HD	Post-HD	Pre-HD	Post-HD	
f(HMA)	51.32 ± 5.63	72.04 ± 5.73	58.03 ± 7.43	76.42 ± 4.67	51.07 ± 9.07	70.53 ± 8.05	79.11 ± 5.46
f(HNA)	48.68 ± 5.63	27.96 ± 5.73	41.97 ± 7.43	23.58 ± 4.67	48.93 ± 9.07	29.47 ± 8.05	20.89 ± 5.46

f(HMA) fraction of human mercaptalbumin, *f(HNA)* fraction of human nonmercaptalbumin
f(HNA) = 100 − f(HMA)

Table 4 Data of blood and physical situation in patients

	Mean ± SD		
	EWHD2014 ($n = 12$)	EWHD2015 ($n = 12$)	C-HD ($n = 38$)
BUN (mg/dL)	56.05 ± 11.25	56.53 ± 13.39	62.27 ± 12.73
Cr (mg/dL)	8.98 ± 2.32	9.20 ± 1.78	10.05 ± 2.4
UA (mg/dL)	6.99 ± 1.21	6.98 ± 1.12	6.84 ± 1.29
Hb (g/dL)	10.91 ± 1.033	10.98 ± 0.73	11.26 ± 1.20
WBC (/μL)	6121 ± 2493	6605 ± 2039	5827 ± 2046
CRP (mg/dL)	0.552 ± 1.015[a]	0.542 ± 0.747	0.234 ± 0.492[b]
Alb (g/dL)	3.49 ± 0.20	3.65 ± 0.24*	3.53 ± 0.23
GOT (U/L)	13.3 ± 2.4	14.1 ± 2.3	31.4 ± 105.0
GPT (U/L)	9.2 ± 2.8	10.3 ± 5.0	25.5 ± 88.1
T-Cho (mg/dL)	154 ± 39	165 ± 47	146 ± 24
nPCR (g/kg/day)	0.81 ± 0.13	0.83 ± 0.16	0.87 ± 0.15
%CGR (%)	93.2 ± 32	98.2 ± 27	99.0 ± 25.4
BMI (kg/m^2)	20.1 ± 2.9	20.6 ± 3.2*	21.5 ± 3.3
GNRI (−)	89.2 ± 5.0	92.1 ± 6.3**	91.3 ± 5.1

*$p < 0.05$ (paired t-test vs EWHD2014); **$p < 0.01$ (paired t-test vs EWHD2014)
Other data were no significant difference
[a] $n = 10$
[b] $n = 13$

lower than for healthy persons before hemodialysis treatment [16]. The data of our study indicated similar results but the significant difference with healthy subjects was not only the f(HMA) of post-HD in EWHD2015, but the low numerical value.

As to previous study regarding the relationship between HSA-redox and EW-HD, Terawaki et al. [14] reported the beneficial effect of single EW-HD session on HSA-redox [14]. Our present study, however, deals with the long-term (201~392 days) effect of EW-HD treatment on HSA-redox profile. In our study, data were collected at only one point in C-HD; however, it was thought that there was little possibility of the change by HD vintage (Fig. 4). It is suggested that the f(HMA) of hemodialysis patients improves with long-term EW-HD treatment.

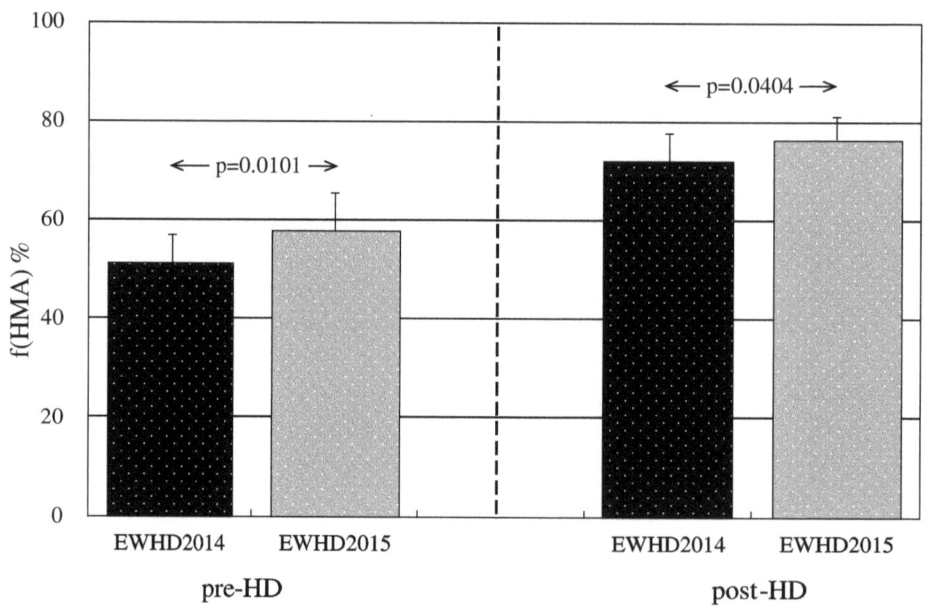

Fig. 2 Comparison of the f(HMA) on EWHD2014 vs EWHD2015. $n = 12$: both at pre- and post-HD

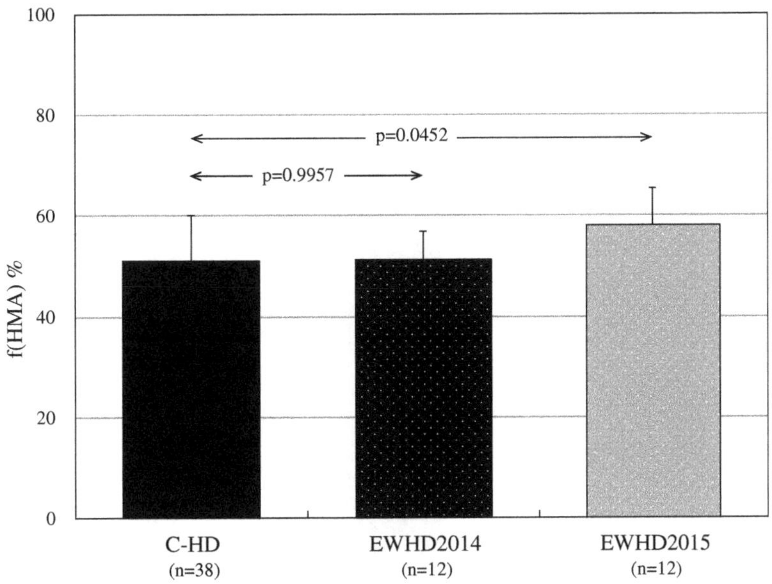

Fig. 3 Comparison of the f(HMA) in pre-HD

Terawaki et al. reported that the risk of cardiovascular disease (CVD) events and mortality were very high at pre-HD f(HMA) <40 % or post-HD f(HMA) <60 %; in particular, the odds ratios of CVD incidence and mortality in the post-HD f(HMA) < 60 % were 20.6 and 25.6 times by those in the post-HD f(HMA) ≥60 %, respectively [7]. In our study, the C-HD treatment patients who were f(HMA) <40 % at pre-HD were 4 (10.5 %) and, those of the f(HMA) < 60 % at post-HD were 3 (7.9 %), but no EW-HD treatment patient corresponded to those conditions.

The pre-HD albumin levels at EWHD2015 were significantly increased compared with those at EWHD2014, to 3.65 from 3.49 g/dL, likewise BMI and GNRI were significantly increased (Table 4). If all the rising values were HMA, the f(HMA) increased only to 53.45 from 51.32 %. And, the dialyzer and/or the reduction of body weight that influence on albumin leakage during hemodialysis were no different between EWHD2014 and EWHD2015 (Table 2). Therefore, EW-HD is more likely to contribute to the rise of HMA. Long-term EW-HD treatment presumably resulted in the rise of HMA by the

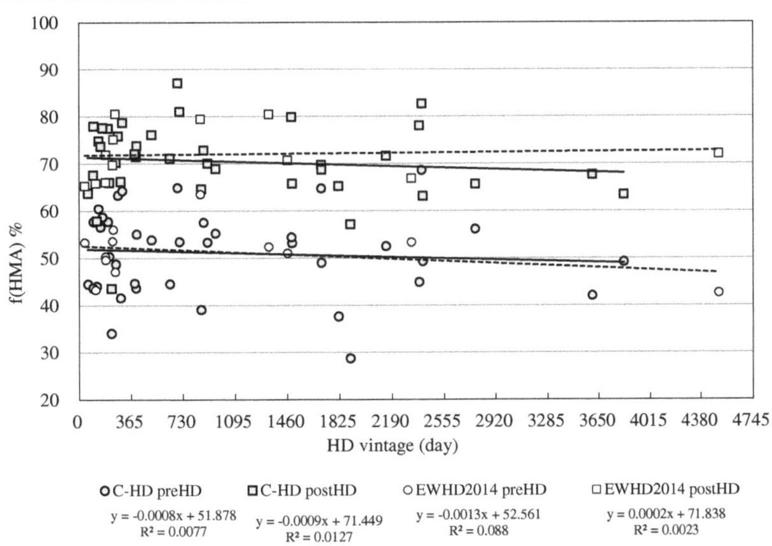

Fig. 4 Relationship of the HD vintage and f(HMA)

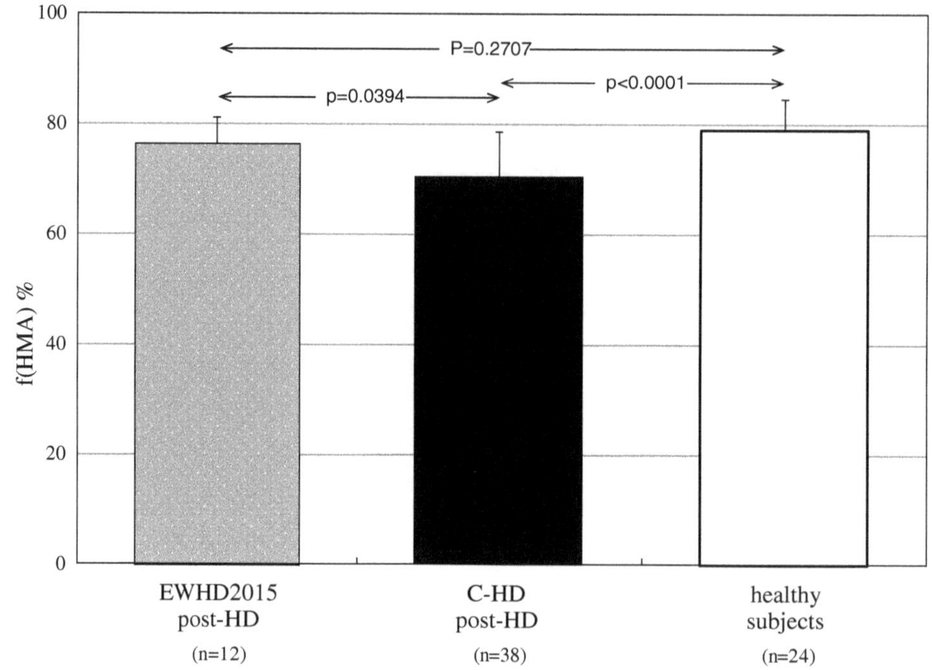

Fig. 5 Comparison of the f(HMA) in post-HD and healthy subjects

accumulation of albumin reduction effect in the dialyzer [14] and/or the improvement of blood vessel wall function [15]. In a comparison of EWHD2014 and EW2015, the pre-HD f(HMA) values increased and the difference in the f(HMA) value between pre- and post-HD decreased. It is thought that the latter contribution is greater, and the possible effectiveness of the prevention of CVD events by long-term EW-HD treatment was suggested.

Nakayama et al. reported that EW-HD ameliorated inflammatory reactions and offered a novel therapeutic option for control of uremia [17]. Huang et al. reported that 1-year treatment improved T cell damage [18]. MIA syndrome has been proposed as one of the disease states influencing the vital prognosis of hemodialysis patients. MIA syndrome is a syndrome that occurs in relation to malnutrition, inflammation and atherosclerosis, of which inflammation is considered to take a central role [19]. The inflammatory reaction and the oxidation LDL generation may be decrease directly or indirectly by the reduction action of hydrogen, so we expect that longer-term EW-HD treatment will show clinical usefulness such as a lower frequency of complications and/or improvement of vital prognosis.

Table 5 Hydrogen concentration of the EW-HD fluid

Measurement day	Minimum	Maximum
2014/04/17	47	107
2014/06/18	62	122
2014/08/04	50	111
2014/11/10	67	161
2015/02/02	84	196

Concentration unit is ppb

Study limitations

There are several limitations in this study. The number of EW-HD subjects is small, and the observation period in EW-HD treatment is not sufficient to detect any clinical outcome. It will therefore be necessary to evaluate albumin redox in more patients with longer-term EW-HD treatment.

Conclusions

Our data suggest that the f(HMA) may be raised with long-term hemodialysis treatment using hydrogen-dissolved hemodialysis fluid.

Acknowledgements

This study was supported by Kiyomi Inada, Ritsuko Ando, Izumi Tamai, Chie Shirakawa, and Syunsuke Nakashima of the Daiko Sunadabashi Clinic and Yukie Hirabayashi, Yayoi Kondo, and Hirochika Kato of the Daiko Sunadabashi Branch Clinic.

Authors' contributions

KM and KS conceived of the study and participated in its design and coordination. HY and TI participated in the design of the study. KM, HY, and TI carried out the selections of patients. TT and SE carried out the measurements of the samples. HA, KS, and ES performed the statistical analysis. KS and SE helped to draft the manuscript. KM organized the study project and drafted the final manuscript. All authors read and approved the final manuscript.

Authors' information

KM is the director of the Daiko Sunadabashi Clinic, the representative director of the Japanese Academy of Home Care Physicians, the chairman of the Public Interest Incorporated Foundation Aichi Kidney Foundation, and the professor emeritus of Nagoya University. HY is the director of the Daiko Sunadabashi Branch Clinic. TI is the physician of the Daiko Sunadabashi Clinic. SE is the professor of the Gifu University Graduate School of Medicine. TT is the lecturer of the Gifu University Graduate School of Medicine. KS is the head of the Laboratory of Dialysis Medical Care and Technology. HA is the associate professor of the Chubu Gakuin College.

Competing interests

The authors declare that they have no competing interests.

Author details

[1]Daiko Sunadabashi Clinic, Nagoya, Japan. [2]Daiko Sunadabashi Branch Clinic, Nagoya, Japan. [3]Department of Physiology and Biophysics, Graduate School of Medicine, Gifu University, Gifu, Japan. [4]Laboratory of Dialysis Medical Care and Technology, Nagoya, Japan. [5]Department of Early Childhood Education, Chubu Gakuin College, Seki, Gifu, Japan.

References

1. Nakai S, Hanafusa N, Masakane I, Taniguchi M, Hamano T, Shoji T, et al. An overview of regular dialysis treatment in Japan (as of 31 December 2012). Ther Apher Dial. 2014;18:535–602.
2. Nakai S, Masakane I, Akiba T, Iseki K, Watanabe Y, Itami N, et al. Overview of regular dialysis treatment in Japan (as of 31 December 2005). Ther Apher Dial. 2007;11:411–41.
3. Locatelli F, Canaud B, Eckardt KU, Stenvinkel P, Wanner C, Zoccali C. Oxidative stress in end-stage renal disease: an emerging threat to patient outcome. Nephrol Dial Transplant. 2003;18:1272–80.
4. Morena M, Delbosc S, Dupuy AM, Canaud B, Cristol JP. Overproduction of reactive oxygen species in end-stage renal disease patients: a potential component of hemodialysis-associated inflammation. Hemodial Int. 2005;9:37–46.
5. Anraku M, Chuang VT, Maruyama T, Otagiri M. Redox properties of serum albumin. Biochim Biophys Acta. 1830;2013:5465–72.
6. Terawaki H, Yoshimura K, Hasegawa T, Nakayama M, Hosoya T, Era S, et al. Oxidative stress is enhanced in correlation with renal dysfunction: examination with the redox state of albumin. Kidney Int. 2004;66:1988–93.
7. Terawaki H, Takada Y, Era S, Funakoshi Y, Nakayama K, Nakayama M, et al. The redox state of albumin and serious cardiovascular incidence in hemodialysis patients. Ther Apher Dial. 2010;14:465–71.
8. Terawaki H, Matsuyama Y, Matsuo N, Terada T, Era S, Hosoya T, et al. A lower level of reduced albumin induces serious cardiovascular incidence among peritoneal dialysis patients. Clin Exp Nephrol. 2012;16:629–35.
9. Ohsawa I, Ishikawa M, Takahashi K, Watanabe M, Nishimaki K, Yamagata K, et al. Hydrogen acts as a therapeutic antioxidant by selectively reducing cytotoxic oxygen radicals. Nat Med. 2007;13:688–94.
10. Huang KC, Yang CC, Lee KT, Chiang-Ting Chien CT. Reduced hemodialysis-induced oxidative stress in end-stage renal disease patients by electrolyzed reduced water. Kidney Int. 2003;64:704–14.
11. Nakayama M, Kabayama S, Terawaki H, Nakayama K, Kato K, Sato T, et al. Less-oxidative hemodialysis solution rendered by cathode-side application of electrolyzed water. Hemodial Int. 2007;11:322–7.
12. Huang KC, Yang CC, Hsu SP, Lee KT, Liu HW, Morisawa S, et al. Electrolyzed-reduced water reduced hemodialysis-induced erythrocyte impairment in end-stage renal disease patients. Kidney Int. 2006;70:391–8.
13. Nakayama M, Kabayama S, Nakano H, Zhu WJ, Terawaki H, Nakayama K, et al. Biological effects of electrolyzed water in hemodialysis. Nephron Clin Pract. 2009;112:c9–c15.
14. Terawaki H, Zhu WJ, Matsuyama Y, Terada T, Takahashi Y, Sakurai K, et al. Effect of a hydrogen (H_2)-enriched solution on the albumin redox of hemodialysis patients. Hemodial Int. 2014;18:459–66.
15. Matsuyama Y, Hayashi T, Terawaki H, Negawa T, Terada T, Okano Y, et al. Human astrocytes and aortic endothelial cells actively convert the oxidized form of albumin to the reduced form: reduced albumin might participate in redox regulation of nerve and blood vessel systems. J Physiol Sci. 2009;59:207–15.
16. Soejima A, Matsuzawa N, Hayashi T, Kimura T, Ootsuka R, Fukuoka K, et al. Alteration of redox state of human serum albumin before and after hemodialysis. Blood Purif. 2004;22:525–9.
17. Nakayama M, Nakano H, Hamada H, Itami N, Nakazawa R, Ito S. A novel bioactive haemodialysis system using dissolved dihydrogen (H2) produced by water electrolysis: a clinical trial. Nephrol Dial Transplant. 2010;25:3026–33.
18. Huang KC, Hsu SP, Yang CC, Ou-Yang P, Lee KT, Morisawa S, et al. Electrolysed-reduced water dialysate improves T-cell damage in end-stage renal disease patients with chronic haemodialysis. Nephrol Dial Transplant. 2010;5:2730–7.
19. Stenvinkel P, Heimbürger O, Lindholm B, Kaysen GA, Bergström J. Are there two types of malnutrition in chronic renal failure? Evidence for relationships between malnutrition, inflammation and atherosclerosis (MIA syndrome). Nephrol Dial Transplant. 2000;15:953–60.

11

Clinical evaluation of a newly developed automated hemodialysis system as a clinical trial

Takashi Shigematsu[1*], Jun Minakuchi[2], Satoshi Funakoshi[3], Junichiro Hashiguchi[4], Hiroshi Yoshimoto[5], Kyoko Ito[6], Takuya Ban[7] and Tetsunosuke Kunitomo[7]

Abstract

Background: To cope with the increasing number of patients on long-term hemodialysis (HD), especially those with diabetic nephropathy, we designed a fully automated HD system to decrease staff workload and hence human errors related to HD treatment. In this study, we evaluated this new system as a clinical trial.

Methods: Based on a dialysis machine combined with a central dialysate delivery system (CDDS), the new system is characterized by the use of back ultrafiltrated dialysate (BUD) as a substitute fluid for priming, bonus shot and blood return, and the attachment of double endotoxin retentive filters (ETRFs).

Results: The subjects comprised 61 patients from five HD facilities enrolled in a randomized, open-labeled crossover study after giving written informed consent.
A total of 348 HD treatments for 58 of the 61 patients were studied under a protocol designed in accordance with good clinical practice (GCP) guidelines and approved by the respective institutional review boards. No severe adverse effects were observed with either the test or control systems. The incidence of clinical events, including blood pressure decline, residual blood, and error in fluid removal, was not statistically significant in either group. Neither endotoxins nor bacteria were detected in the dialysate passing through the double filters.

Conclusions: This study confirmed the safety and effectiveness of an automated HD system based on CDDS. (This Clinical Trial No. is 21500BZZ00045000)

Keywords: Hemodialysis, Automated system, Clinical trial, Ultrafiltrated dialysate, Endotoxin retentive filter

Background

More than 95% of patients on maintenance dialysis for end-stage renal disease (ESRD) in Japan undergo hemodialysis (HD). At the end of 2014, the number of such patients exceeded 320,000. The following two points are of particular importance:

1. The proportion of dialysis patients with diabetic nephropathy has been increasing steadily, reaching nearly 45% of patients commencing dialysis and 36.6% of existing patients.

2. The population of dialysis patients is aging rapidly. For both men and women, many patients commencing dialysis are between 80 and 84 years old, representing more than 15 and 17% of those commencing dialysis, respectively, with the median age at commencement of initiating dialysis now 69.1 years [1, 2].

Although those trends seen in Japan are also observed worldwide, the following problems such as an increase in the number of patients requiring various

* Correspondence: taki@wakayama-med.ac.jp
[1]Department of Nephrology, Wakayama Medical University, Wakayama 641-8509, Japan
Full list of author information is available at the end of the article

medical cares including considerable extra support from the staffs have become more prominent in the current setting of maintenance HD in Japan.

Thus, in Japan, the dialysis staffs' shortages have become evident. The advantage of the central dialysate delivery system (CDDS) is its ability to deliver dialysis fluid to multiple patients at the same time, but full automation of the device has been required in order to decrease the number of operations, especially during the beginning and end of dialysis when multiple tasks converge.

Hemodialysis treatment is especially suitable for full automation because it involves multiple repetitions of similar operations. By implementing full automation with safety devices and fail-safe systems in place, we can achieve both the pursuit of a decrease in operational burden and an increase in efficiency, as well as safety from human error.

With the purification of dialysis fluid [3], fully automated devices actively utilizing back ultrafiltration dialysate (BUD) came into use [4]. Blood return to the arterial side is usually performed by reversing the rotation of the blood pump in a similar manner to automatic devices using physiological saline.

We developed a dialysis console using BUD, and special features of this device are that rotation of the blood pump is not reversed during blood return to the arterial side and the blood return speed can be controlled while blood return pressure is monitored. We evaluated the safety and effectiveness of this novel fully automatic dialysis machine in a clinical trial, and present the results here.

Methods

Newly developed machine

Figure 1 shows the flow scheme of a newly developed machine (TR-3000MA) as well as that of the conventional basic machine (TR-3000M) used as a control one in this study. To develop this new automated machine (TR-3000MA) based upon the conventional machine (TR-3000M), the following five features were additively designed: (1) automatic priming, (2) automatic blood removal, (3) fast fluid replacement, (4) automatic blood return, and (5) manual solution sending. To realize these function, it is noted to apply two major manipulations:

1. Non-reversed rotation of blood pump during blood return to the patient
2. Assurance of quality of back ultrafiltrated dialysate (BUD). Contrasting strikingly with the preceding machine [5], non-reversed rotation of blood pump was materialized by the device shown in Fig. 2, where blood return speed is controlled based upon the blood return pressure monitored. To control the quality of BUD, a double endotoxin (ET) retentive filter (ETRF) was placed immediately before the dialyzer on the dialysis unit side, and furthermore, the following were devised: (1) auto-flushing of the ETRF, (2) leakage test of ETRF, (3) countermeasure to failure of a single ETRF, and (4) monitoring of ETRF use duration.

Study protocol

Prior to the clinical trial, the study plan including the inclusion and exclusion criteria of patients as shown below

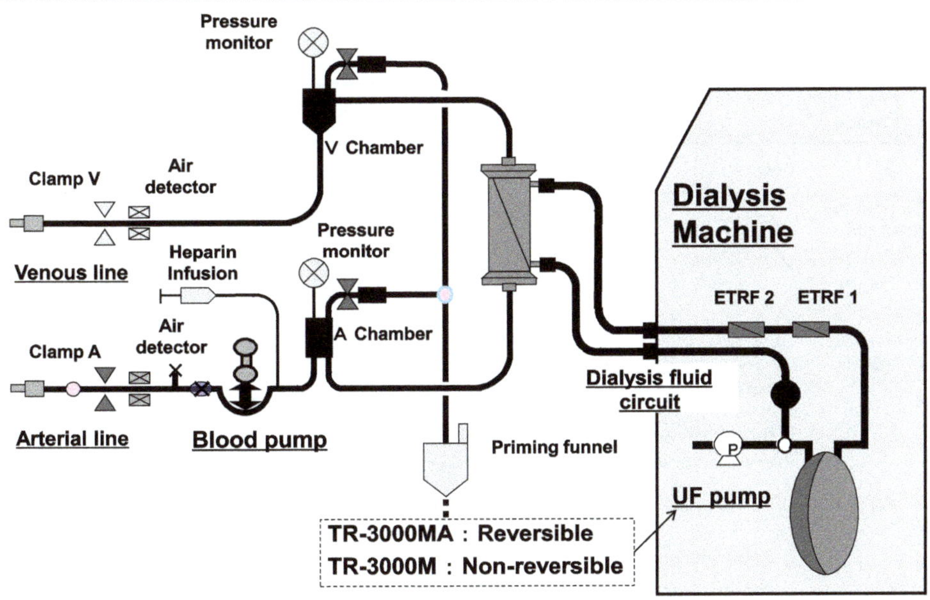

Fig. 1 Schematic illustration of the whole system

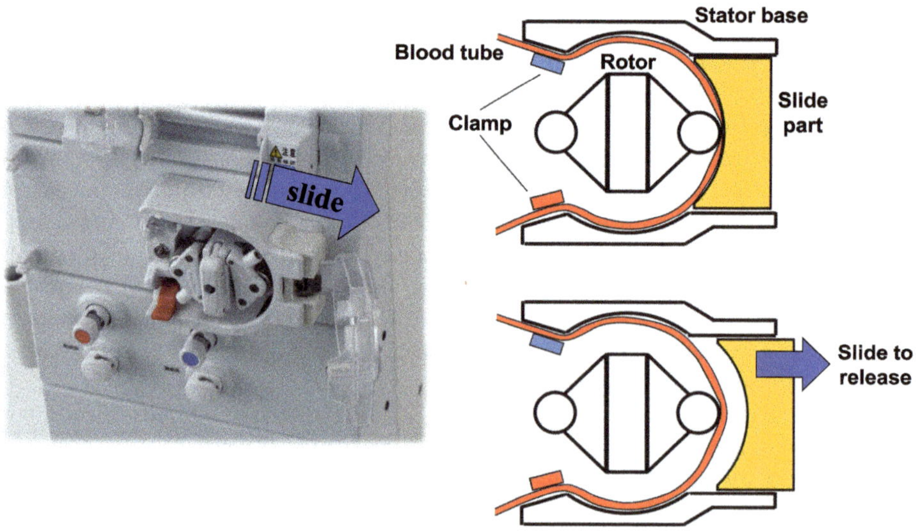

Fig. 2 A releasable blood pump. When the blood pump cover is opened, the casing slides to release the pumping unit

was reviewed by the institutional review board of each participating institution.

Inclusion criteria:

1. Duration of HD—more than 6 months
2. Age—more than 20 and less than 75
3. Treatment schedule—basically 3 to 5 h per treatment and three times a week
4. Physical condition—stable outpatient receiving HD as scheduled

Exclusion criteria:

1. Patients to whom kidney transplantation is planned
2. Patients to whom the shift from HD to other modalities such as HDF, CAPD, and so on is investigated
3. Patients who suffer from acute myocardial infarction, unstable angina, and cardiac insufficiency (NYHA; more than III)
4. Patients whose values of hepatic markers (AST, ALT) are higher than normal more than by two times
5. Patients who suffer from severe anemia (hematocrit; less than 20%)
6. Patients who suffer from malignant tumors

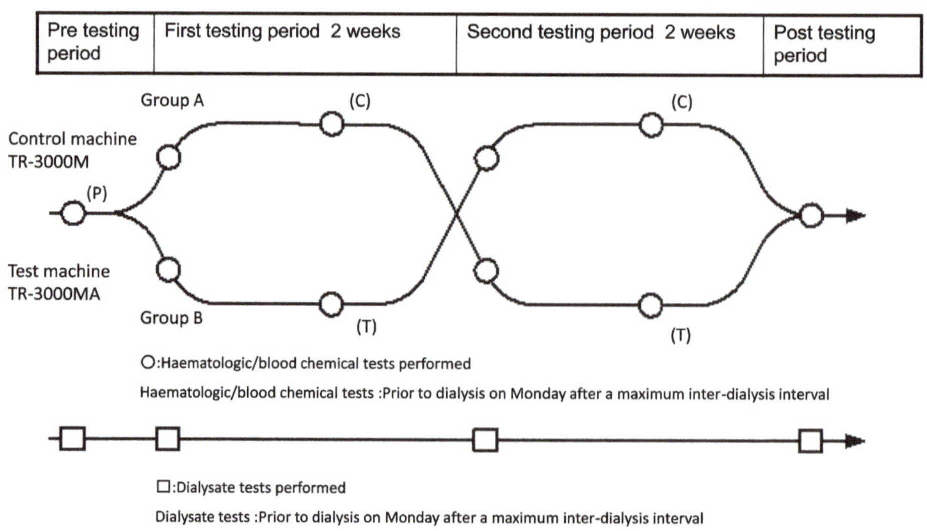

Fig. 3 Crossover diagram in this study. "T" expresses the test machine (TR-3000MA). "C" expresses the control machine (TR-3000M)

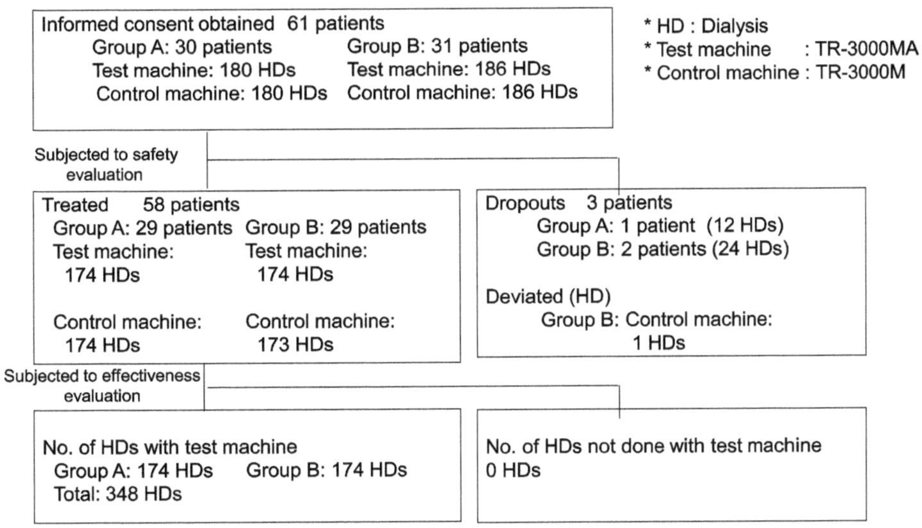

Fig. 4 Disposition of patients

7. Patients who suffer from uncontrollable hypertension or hypotension
8. Patients who are pregnant or are suspected to be pregnant
9. Patients from whom more than 150 mL/min of extracorporeal blood volume cannot be obtained

Subjects were given an explanation of the clinical trial using the informed consent form and written information, and informed consent was given in writing by each subject. The clinical trial was conducted with due ethical considerations, such as maintaining subject confidentiality.

Basic frame of protocol

This clinical trial was an open-label, controlled crossover, non-inferiority test of TR-3000MA to the conventional machine (TR-3000M) combined CDDS. Figure 3 depicts the frame of the protocol, where long-term dialysis patients enrolled in five institutions were assigned to group A or B. Total of 60 patients were planned to be enrolled. Patients classified in group A were treated with dialysis with TR-3000M six times for 2 weeks and then switched to that with TR-3000MA six times for next 2 weeks, and those of group B were vice versa. Hematologic/blood chemical tests and biological dialysate tests were carried out at the timing shown in Fig. 3. Basically, data were compared between the phase of TR-3000MA and that of TR-3000M and analyzed mainly using the chi-square test, while patient-dependent biomarkers were analyzed using paired *t* test.

Assessment of the safety and the effectiveness

The safety (i.e., of devices/machine and of entry of BUD into the body) and effectiveness (i.e., performance of auxiliary functions as intended) of the study test

Table 1 Background characteristics of the hemodialysis patients

		Group A[*1]	Group B[*1]	Significant difference
Sex	Male	25	22	NS[*2]
	Female	4	7	
Age (years)	Mean	62.8	59.9	NS[*3]
	SD	8.06	8.99	
Dialysis duration (years)	Mean	10.05	9.00	NS[*3]
	SD	8.95	7.91	
Height (cm)	Mean	162.21	161.17	NS[*3]
	SD	8.41	7.43	
Dry weight (kg)	Mean	55.86	59.28	NS[*3]
	SD	8.99	13.23	

[*1]Refer to Fig. 2
[*2]Chi-square test
[*3]Paired *t* test

Table 2 Hematological and laboratory results of hemodialysis patients

	Units	Pretesting(P)*1	Control machine (C)*1	Test machine (T)*1	Significant difference (paired *t* test)		
					(P)-(C)	(C)-(T)	(P)-(T)
Leucocyte count (WBC)	/μL	6048.3 ± 1950.10	5974.1 ± 1931.60	6051.7 ± 2070.96	NS	NS	NS
Urea nitrogen	mg/dL	72.3 ± 14.01	70.7 ± 14.50	71.2 ± 14.49	NS	NS	NS
Creatinine	mg/dL	11.6 ± 2.46	11.5 ± 2.43	11.5 ± 2.41	NS	NS	NS
hsCRP*1 (pre-dialysis)	mg/L	2114.8 ± 3817.68	2312.7 ± 4485.56	1360.1 ± 1810.18	NS	NS	NS
hsCRP*1 (post-dialysis)	mg/L	2453.9 ± 4815.46	2415.4 ± 4807.21	1533.0 ± 2115.53	NS	NS	NS

*1 *hsCRP* high-sensitivity C-reactive protein

machine were assessed in comparison with a control one (TR-3000M) in stable-phase chronic dialysis patients for the purpose of confirming its acceptability for a plurality of operators at multiple institutions.

Safety endpoints comprised (1) occurrence of adverse events, (2) failure of the study machine, and (3) comparison of high-sensitivity C-reactive protein (CRP) values pre- and post-dialysis as a bioreactive marker to the quality of BUD infused into patients.

For adverse events for which the occurrence was foreseeable during the use of the study machine, a set of criteria was devised in advance at a clinical trial research meeting and used as the observation parameters in the clinical trial.

1) Decrease in blood pressure—fall in systolic blood pressure by ≥ 20%
2) Residual blood corresponding in volume to approximately two thirds of the hollow fibers
3) Water removal error ≤ 400 g

Failure of the study machine denoted either premature discontinuation of dialysis or completion of dialysis delayed by 1 h or longer related to the machine, as agreed upon at the clinical trial research meeting.

An effectiveness endpoint consisted of checking and evaluating whether the test machine had performed auxiliary functions as intended. The evaluation was made not for each patient but for each session of dialysis.

Results

The disposition of the enrolled patients and their background characteristics are shown in Fig. 4 and Table 1, respectively. There were no significant intergroup differences in respect of distribution by sex, age, dialysis duration, height, and dry weight (Table 1). As for underlying diseases, patients with chronic glomerulonephritis (33 patients, 54.1%) tended to be more frequent and patients with diabetic nephropathy (15 patients, 24.6%) fewer than the national mean percentages at the end of 2009 in a report of the statistical investigation.

Of the 61 patients who gave informed consent, there were 3 who withdrew consent before pre-testing, and there was a protocol deviation in one session of dialysis in group B (control machine). Consequently, 58 treated patients were subjected to the safety evaluation. For the effectiveness evaluation, 174 dialyses with the test machine in group A and 174 dialyses with the control one in group B were subjected to the assessment.

Results of the safety evaluation are summarized in Tables 2 and 3. There was no significant difference in high-sensitivity CRP values because there was no significant elevation in this parameter. It was also judged that there were 57 events judged to be adversely associated with 348 dialyses using the test machine and 61 adverse events associated with 347 dialyses using the control one. There was no significant difference in the number of adverse events between the machines as a result of statistical tests of the incidence with due consideration to the number of dialyses performed. As none of the events came under the definition of failure framed in advance in association with the use of the study systems, it was judged that there was no significant difference in this respect between the test and control machines. Collectively, it was concluded that there was no difference in safety between the test and control machines.

Data especially concerning the events agreed upon at the clinical trial research meeting, among other adverse events, are presented in Table 4.

Table 3 Results of the safety evaluation (test and control machines)

Endpoints	No. of adverse events		Statistical test		Significant difference
	Test machine	Control machine	χ^2	*P* value	
Adverse event occurrence	57*1	61*1	0.285	0.593	NS
Study machine failure status	0*1	0*1			NS
Highly sensitive CRP	0*2	0*2			NS

*1 No. of dialyses are 348 (test machine) and 347 (control machine)
*2 No. of tests performed are 116 (test machine) and 114 (control machine)

Table 4 Occurrence of adverse events (AE) agreed upon at the clinical trial research meeting and results of statistical analysis

	Test/control machine[*1]	No. of events	Incidence (%)	No. patients with AE	Statistical test	Significant difference
Decrease in blood pressure	Test	24	6.897	12	$\chi^2 = 0.165$ $P = 0.684$	NS
	Control	26	7.493	14		
Residual blood	Test	3	0.862	1	$\chi^2 = 3.004$ $P = 0.125$	NS
	Control	0	0.000	0		
Water removal error	Test	6	1.724	6	$\chi^2 = 2.295$ $P = 0.130$	NS
	Control	11	3.170	7		

[*1]No. of dialyses are 348 (test machine) and 347 (control machine)

Decrease in blood pressure

A fall in blood pressure occurred during 24 dialyses with the test machine in 12 patients and during 26 dialyses with the control one in 14 patients. Of these patients, eight were common to both test and control machines. As for the circumstances in which a fall in blood pressure occurred, the event was peculiar to the study subjects, and it was found that the event occurred concomitantly with changes in water removal volume and dry weight on the day, according to the case report forms and findings by the responsible investigator. Therefore, we judged that there was no causal relationship of a decrease in blood pressure with the study machine.

Residual blood

There were three events of residual blood occurring in one patient on the test machine and no event with the control one. The events were confined to this one patient and were judged to be peculiar to this subject.

Water removal error

Water removal error occurred at 6 dialyses with the test machine in six patients and at 11 dialyses with the control one in seven patients. The results showed a significantly lower incidence for the test machine. However, the measurement of the UF pump capacity (i.e., determination of water removal precision) performed at the relevant institution on the occasion the error occurred showed no error in water removal volume, and the determination of water removal precision made after retrieval of the study machines also failed to demonstrate any error in water removal volume. As a result of the deliberation with the responsible investigators based on these considerations, the errors were thought to be attributable to errors in pre-dialysis measurement of body weight and subjects' diet adjustment. The responsible investigators and the sponsor thus judged that there was no problem with the water removal precision of the study machine.

As shown in Table 5, there were a total of 16 cases of interruption of the automatic blood return function (8 cases of air abnormality, 3 of inadequate blood pump stop position, 2 of venous pressure elevation, and 3 of arterial pressure elevation [needle tip, thrombus]). The inadequate blood pump stop position was caused by automatic blood return being started when the blood pump segment had not been fully opened. In all these events, nevertheless, the machine stopped automatically as the safety monitor functioned, and the staff manually completed blood return.

Figure 5 shows the results of water quality tests of water and dialysate samples taken at the following sites: (1) outlet of reverse osmosis (RO) equipment, (2) outlet of CDDS, (3) inlet of the dialysis machine, and (4) inlet of the dialyzer. The apparatus used at the five institutions included 7 RO equipment, 7 CDDS, and 23 dialysis machines, and the data shown represent the measurements performed four times for each site. Clinical trials were conducted after the confirmation that water/dialysate met the specified water quality standards [6, 7].

Discussion

As noted by the Japan Society for Dialysis Therapy [1], both the number of dialysis patients (304,592) and dialysis machines (121,835) showed a tendency to increase as of December 31, 2014. The status quo of the number of nurses is only being maintained. The increases in both the patient population and the patients requiring nursing care are likely to be related to the progressive increase in reported medical incidents in dialysis rooms [8, 9], with 2905 events in 2009 compared with 1946 events in 2005.

In view of the above factors, dialysis operations have been partially automated in order to prevent manipulative errors related to the increased burden on nurses, as well as to realize the practicability of concurrent care of several patients. With an automated machine, the nurse can concentrate on patient care because the dialysis

Table 5 Results of the effectiveness evaluation

Auxiliary function	No. of completed operations/ no. of operations	Operation completion rate (%)
Priming	348/348	100.0
Bonus shot	25/25	100.0
Blood return	329/345	95.4

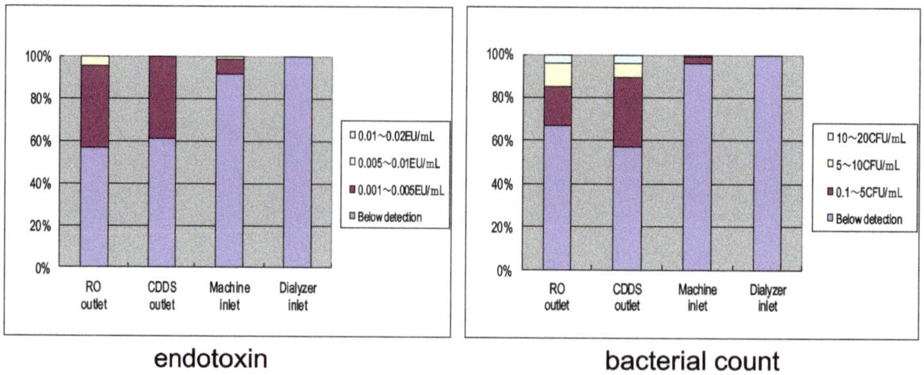

Fig. 5 Water quality of product water and dialysate

machine should perform safety monitoring of the intra-circuit pressure, air bubbling, etc. after the nurse has programmed the machine.

The use of BUD instead of saline leads to cost reductions, as does automation of those operations that place an increased burden on staff—starting dialysis, when blood pressure falls in a patient and completion of dialysis. The lessening of workload is particularly conspicuous when CDDS is used because one staff member can prepare and initiate dialysis to several patients simultaneously. We also confirmed that the system readily fulfills the water quality control standards required for the use of BUD, and the CDDS has been judged a suitable system for producing sufficiently purified dialysate (Fig. 5).

By the way, the first clinical use of BUD was tried as "Pull and Push Therapy" by Drs. T. Shinzato and K. Maeda [10] in 1982. Although the filtration through not a dialyzer but a special filter was used, use of the filtered dialysate was approved as the substitution fluid for hemodiafiltration as Gambro's AK-100Ultra machine in 1998 [4]. As mentioned above, TR-3000MA machine was the first automated machine without the reversed rotation of blood pump during blood return, which is noted to decrease the operation risk as compared to the reversing rotation system of blood pump.

Through this clinical trial, the safety of this system was proved and later was approved by the Japanese Government. Since then, the quantitative effectiveness of this system including the labor-saving effect is being confirmed.

Conclusions

We confirmed the availability of fully automated dialysis machine by the clinical trial study.

Acknowledgements

Transparency declarations: none to declare.

I (TS) thank Ms. Yoko Doi and Midori Matsudaira for giving fine secretarial works.

Funding

This study was performed as the phase III clinical trial funded by Toray Medical Co. Ltd. Tokyo, Japan. The role of the funding body was a reward to the data collection of investigators in each chronic hemodialysis institution.

Authors' contributions

The corresponding author (TS) planned the study, searched the literature, assessed the studies, extracted the data, analyzed the data, and prepared the article. JM, SF, JH, HY, and KI assisted in the data collection and article preparation. TB and TK gave the detail of the study protocol from phase III clinical trial detail. All authors read and approved the final manuscript.

Competing interests

The corresponding author (TS) has received an honorarium from Toray Medical Co. Ltd., Tokyo, Japan. TB is an employee of Toray Medical Co., Ltd., Japan. TK is a scientific advisory board in Toray Medical Co., Ltd., Japan. However, this involvement does not raise the question of bias in the work reported, or in the conclusions, implications, or opinions stated.

Author details

[1]Department of Nephrology, Wakayama Medical University, Wakayama 641-8509, Japan. [2]Department of Nephrology and Blood Purification, Kawashima Hospital, Tokushima, Japan. [3]Department of Nephrology and Blood Purification, Nagasaki Jin Hospital, Nagasaki, Japan. [4]Department of Blood Purification, Nagasaki Jin Clinic, Nagasaki, Japan. [5]Division of Nephrology and Dialysis, Department of Medicine, Social Insurance Chuo General Hospital, Tokyo, Japan. [6]Department of Blood Purification, Heisei Hidaka Clinic, Takasaki, Japan. [7]Toray Medical Co., Ltd., Tokyo, Japan.

References

1. Masakane I, Nakai S, Ogata S, Kimata N, Hanafusa N, Hamano T, Wakai K, Wada A, Nitta K. Annual Dialysis Data Report 2014, JSDT Renal Data Registry (JRDR). Renal Replacement Ther. 2017;3:18. https://doi.org/10.1186/s41100-017-0097-8.
2. Hanafusa N, Nakai S, Iseki K, Tsubakihara Y. Japanese society for dialysis therapy renal data registry—a window through which we can view the details of Japanese dialysis population. Kidney Int Suppl (2011). 2015;5(1):15–22.

3. Koda Y, Mineshima M. Advances and advantages in recent central dialysis fluid delivery system. Blood Purif. 2009;27(Suppl 1):23–7.
4. Kawanishi H, Akiba T, Masakane I, Tomo T, Mineshima M, Kawasaki T, Hirakata H, Akizawa T. Standard on microbiological management of fluids for hemodialysis and related therapies by the Japanese Society for Dialysis Therapy. Ther Aphresis Dial. 2008;13:161–6.
5. Tsuchiya S, Moriishi M, Takahashi N, Watanabe H, Kawanishi H, KimS-T MK. Experience with the JMS fully automated dialysis machine. ASAIO J. 2003;49:547–53.
6. Kawanishi H, Moriishi M, Takahashi N, Tsuchiya S. The central dialysis fluid delivery system (CDDS): is it specialty in Japan? Renal Replace Therap. 2016;2:1. https://doi.org/10.1186/s41100-016-0016-4.
7. Tomo T, Shinoda T. Standardization of water purification in the central dialysis fluid delivery system: validation and parametric method. Blood Purif. 2009;27(Suppl 1):36–40.
8. Japanese Council for Quality Health Care. Annual Report on Medical Malpractice/Errors Information Gathering Project 2005: JCQHC. https://jcqhc.or.jp/en/.
9. Japanese Council for Quality Health Care. Annual Report on Medical Malpractice/Errors Information Gathering Project 2009 JCQHC. https://jcqhc.or.jp/en/.
10. Usuda M, Shinzato T, Sezaki R, Kawanishi A, Maeda K, Kawaguchi S, Shibata M, Toyoda T, Asakura Y, Ohbayashi S. New simultaneous HF and HD with no infuse fluid. Trans Am Soc Artif Organs. 1982;28:24–7.

12

Effectiveness case of Jidabokuippo (traditional Japanese Kampo medicine) on pain, venous thrombosis, and subcutaneous hematoma after percutaneous femoral catheterization in a hemodialysis patient

Kentaro Wada[1*], Haruhito A. Uchida[2] and Yuko Wada[3]

Abstract

Background: The authors herein report a case of pain, femoral vein thrombosis, and inguinal subcutaneous hematoma caused by percutaneous femoral vascular catheterization in a hemodialysis (HD) patient complicated with vascular access occlusion. The pain was well-controlled without using analgesics such as non-steroidal anti-inflammatory drugs (NSAIDs). The thrombosis and hematoma increased in size and was also treated by conservative treatment using traditional Japanese Kampo medicine (jidabokuippo: JDI) to resolve *oketsu*: a sign of microcirculating disorder. JDI improves the blood circulation in the affected lesion and alleviates contusion-induced blood flow and repairs blood flow without forming thrombosis. These catheter-related complications were successfully treated by JDI.

Case presentation: A 41-year-old man under HD was admitted because of permanent vascular access failure. He had a history of side effects of gastrointestinal bleeding associated with use of NSAIDs and accompanied with femoral vein thrombosis and inguinal subcutaneous hematoma caused by percutaneous femoral vascular catheterization. The hematoma increased in size and was treated using JDI. In the present case, pain, venous thrombosis, and subcutaneous hematoma surprisingly improved with use of JDI in addition to combination therapy with anticoagulant (warfarin potassium) and antibiotic (meropenem hydrate), without using analgesics such as NSAIDs.

Conclusions: The present case indicated as follows: JDI controls the pain associated with hematoma without analgesics such as NSAIDs; JDI also has an effect of improving the complications associated with venous thrombosis and subcutaneous hematoma caused by catheterization in HD patients safely. JDI, one of Kampo drugs, has few side effects and can be used as needed.

Keywords: Pain, Thrombosis, Hematoma, Catheterization, Hemodialysis, Jidabokuippo

* Correspondence: kyw620@hotmail.co.jp
[1]Division of Nephrology and Dialysis, Department of Internal Medicine, Nippon Kokan Fukuyama Hospital, 1844, Tsunoshita, Daimon-cho, Fukuyama City, Hiroshima 721-0927, Japan
Full list of author information is available at the end of the article

Background

Percutaneous femoral catheterization is considered a quick and an easy access for emergency case under hemodialysis (HD) patient complicated with vascular access occlusion. However, it may cause severe and fatal complications such as infection, hematoma, deep vein thrombosis, and vessel perforation [1].

Conservative treatment of hematoma is acceptable if no hemodynamic dysfunction is present; no compartment syndrome is present; pain control is well-managed by analgesic drugs such as non-steroidal anti-inflammatory drugs (NSAIDs); and the hematoma does not increase in size.

The authors herein report a case of pain, femoral vein thrombosis, and inguinal subcutaneous hematoma caused by percutaneous femoral vascular catheterization. The thrombosis and hematoma increased in size and was successfully treated by conservative treatment using traditional Japanese Kampo medicine (jidabokuippo: JDI) to resolve *oketsu*: a sign of microcirculating disorder. The pain was also well-controlled without using analgesics. To our knowledge, no reports are available concerning the effectiveness of JDI for catheter-related complications in patients under HD.

Case presentation

A 41-year-old man (Japanese) under HD attributable to lupus nephritis for approximately 16 years with a history of vascular access trouble several times was admitted to our hospital because of permanent vascular access failure (day 1). Ultrasonography revealed that thrombosis obstructed the vascular access almost completely from the anastomosis of the brachial artery and artificial vessel toward the anastomosis of the brachial vein and artificial vessel. He had a risk factor of thrombosis with history of systemic lupus erythematosus (SLE) for 20 years. However, the laboratory data findings showed that anti-double strand DNA IgG antibody and anticardiolipine antibody remained negative, and 50% hemolytic unit factor (CH50), C3, and C4 remained within normal range for recent 15 years. Thrombocytopenia was not observed. These data indicated that immunological activity of SLE was in remission.

The authors concluded the patient had no indication of thrombectomy nor percutaneous angioplasty. Percutaneous femoral vascular catheter was inserted (left) under ultrasonography guidance using the Seldinger technique because the patient had a history of carotid vein damage and subclavian vein stenosis. Since maintaining the appropriate blood flow rate was difficult, femoral vascular catheter was inserted again in the opposite (right) side. After the first HD session of catheterization, he complained of pain in the left groin; a hard, smooth, painful mass was palpable; and subcutaneous hemorrhage was also observed. The left groin was compressed with an elastic bandage.

On day 3, laboratory data findings showed elevation of d-dimer level (13.2 μg/mL) without any abnormality in blood coagulopathy, but no progression in the decrease of hemoglobin level. The patient also showed shivering and spiking fever (39 °C) and complained of continuous pain in the groin; therefore, the catheter was immediately removed. Contrast-enhanced computed tomography (CECT) revealed a thrombosis in the right side of the external iliac vein (Fig. 1, left panel) and a soft-tissue mass in the left side of the groin (Fig. 1, right panel), but revealed no pulmonary embolism.

Warfarin potassium was administered to maintain prothrombin time-international normalized ratio with the range from 1.5 to 2.5 (2.0 mg/day). On the other hand, blood culture test was positive (*Staphylococcus aureus*), and laboratory data findings showed elevation of both white blood cell count (12,400/μL) and C-reactive protein (CRP) (8.6 mg/dL). Meropenem hydrate (0.5 g/day) was also administered for infectious disease.

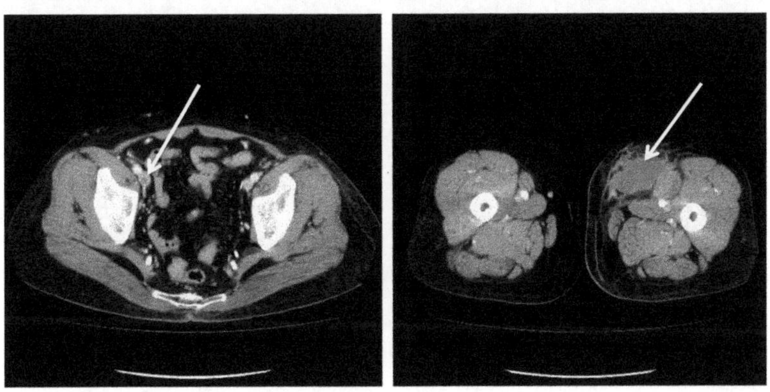

Fig. 1 A contrast-enhanced computed tomography scan revealed (*left panel*) venous thrombosis in the external iliac vein (*arrow*) and (*right panel*) hematoma inside the sartorius muscle and rectus femoris muscle (*arrow*) (day 3)

The authors did not place an inferior vena cava filter to protect from new onset of pulmonary embolism attributable to the findings as follows: ultrasonic echocardiography showed no abnormality, and the possibility remained concerning risk of exacerbation of infections by catheterization.

Based on these findings, the patient was diagnosed as *oketsu* (blood stasis syndrome). Traditional Japanese Kampo medicine, JDI (7.5 g/day: Tsumura, Tokyo, Japan), was administered to improve the symptoms.

Visual analogue scale (VAS) scale in the groin reduced from 85 (day 1) to 33 mm (day 7), thereafter, 12 mm (day 12). The subcutaneous hemorrhage disappeared completely on day 16. The firm mass in the left groin gradually reduced in size and was not palpable on day 19.

Because laboratory data showed improvement in CRP concentration of less than 0.01 mg/dL, blood culture test remained negative, and clinical symptoms dramatically improved, meropenem hydrate administration was terminated on day 14. A d-dimer concentration also reduced from 13.2 to 0.4 μg/mL on day 14. The patient underwent successful arteriovenous graft formation in the right forearm on day 15.

The CECT on day 21 revealed that venous thrombosis in the right external iliac vein reduced (Fig. 2, left panel), and hematoma inside the left sartorius muscle and rectus femorius also reduced (Fig. 2, right panel); therefore, the patient was discharged on day 22. The patient did not use analgesic drugs such as NSAIDs throughout the hospitalization.

JDI administration was terminated because no symptoms were observed on day 21. No adverse reactions to the JDI treatment were observed.

Neither pulmonary embolism nor recurrence of venous thrombosis occurred until 6 months after discharge, thereby, terminating warfarin potassium administration.

At present, the patient is clinically well, showing no signs of exacerbation or relapse of venous thrombosis and subcutaneous hematoma.

Discussion

The authors found out two important clinical issues in this case. JDI controls the pain associated with subcutaneous hematoma without using analgesics such as NSAIDs. JDI also has an effect of improving the complications associated with venous thrombosis and subcutaneous hematoma caused by percutaneous catheterization in HD patients.

First, the pain was well-controlled by conservative treatment using traditional Japanese Kampo medicine JDI without using analgesics. Several reports in the literature describe the randomized controlled trial comparing the effects on rib fracture between JDI and NSAIDs showing that the treatment period was shorter in JDI than NSAIDs; thereby, JDI is an excellent analgesic from the viewpoint of medical economics [2].

The prescription JDI has been developed by Shuan Kagawa (herbalist), who lived in the eighteenth century, Edo era, Japan [3]. JDI is an herbal mixture that improves the blood circulation in the affected lesion and alleviates contusion-induced swelling and pain. JDI also has been reported to undo the stagnant blood flow and repair blood flow without forming thrombosis. JDI is composed of seven herbs as follows: cinamon bark, cnidium rhizome, nuphar rhizome, quercus bark, glycyrrhiza root, rhubarb rhizome, and clove floral bud [4]. Cnidium rhizome exerts anti-inflammatory and analgesic actions. Nuphar rhizome promotes the resorption of the internal hemorrhage, thereby repairing damaged tissue. Quercus bark has analgesic, anti-inflammatory, detoxyfying, and hemostatic properties. Rhubarb rhizome and clove floral bud improve microcirculation [4]. Several

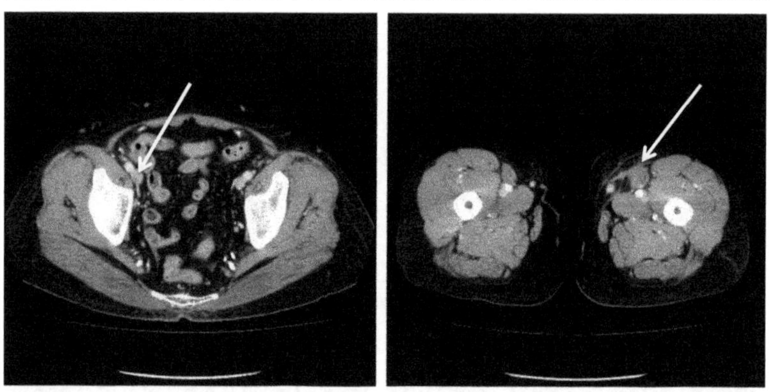

Fig. 2 A contrast-enhanced computed tomography scan revealed that (*left panel*) venous thrombosis in the external iliac vein reduced compared with day 3 (*arrow*) and (*right panel*) hematoma inside the sartorius muscle and rectus femoris muscle also reduced compared with day 3 (*arrow*) (day 21)

reports in the literature describe that JDI includes herbs with established antioxidant activity, which may act synergistically when administered as a combination [5–7]. Antioxidant activity has been reported to be involved in the improvement of swelling and pain associated with trauma [8]; therefore, JDI has mainly been used for bruises and sprains in Japan [4]. Nevertheless, no reports were available concerning the effectiveness of JDI in HD patients. The current report indicates the possibility that the pharmacological effect of JDI could be useful for HD patients with catheter-related complications such as pain, thrombosis, and hematoma. Moreover, in this case, JDI was firstly administered as analgesic and was surprisingly effective to resolve thrombosis and subcutaneous hematoma, probably in part, attributable to the effect of cnidium rhizome and quercus bark [4]. It still remains unclear whether JDI administration under the specific condition with renal dysfunction affected the improvement of these catheter-related complications. However, treatment by JDI should be considered as an option for catheter-related complications among all patients with history of side effects caused by NSAIDs.

In the pathological state, *ketsu* (blood and its metabolic products that circulate throughout the body) manifests *stagnation* known as *oketsu* according to the diagnostic criteria [9]. The major formulations against *oketsu* for the similar symptoms are as follows: (1) tsudosan, (2) tokakujyokitou, (3) keishibukuryogan, and (4) JDI. To distinguish JDI from other three formulations when prescribing, abdominal symptoms type of *sho* based on Japanese Kampo medicine show the characteristics as follows: (1) tsudosan, complaint of having stuck sensations in the region beneath the heart; (2) tokakujyokitou, lower abdominal strain appearing accompanied by severe sharp pain on gentle rubbing by fingertip; and (3) keishibukuryogan, pain at side of navel on palpitation. The pain produced at either side of the navel on palpitation is an important abdominal symptom of *ketsu* congestion. *Ketsu*-improving agent such as keishibukuryogan may clear up this condition. The present case did not show such abdominal symptoms. No specific abdominal symptoms (type of *sho* by Kampo diagnosis) exist in the use of JDI [4]; therefore, JDI has been widely used and classified as one of the major drugs improving the pathological state called *oketsu* in Japanese Kampo medicine.

According to the theory of Japanese Kampo medicine, venous thrombosis and subcutaneous hematoma caused by catheterization are considered as an *oketsu* condition: a sign of microcirculating disorder. In the present case, pain, thrombosis, and subcutaneous hematoma surprisingly improved with use of JDI in addition to combination therapy with anticoagulant and antibiotic. This could be attributable to that *oketsu* condition was improved by JDI. The result that the patient had no complication such as thrombosis or coagulation inside the HD circuit also indicates that JDI unlikely inhibits the action of warfarin and heparin. For the treatment of more severe pain, thrombosis, and hematoma by catheterization, it remains unclear which is better either JDI alone therapy or combination therapy with other Kampo *oketsu*-improving agents such as tsudosan, tokakujyokitou, and keishibukuryogan in addition to JDI. This issue remains to be solved in the future.

Second, femoral vein thrombosis and inguinal hematoma were caused by percutaneous femoral catheterization. The hematoma increased in size and was successfully treated by conservative treatment using traditional Japanese Kampo medicine JDI to resolve *oketsu*. The venous thrombosis decreased in size after combination therapy with JDI and warfarin potassium.

Because anticoagulants such as heparin are regularly administered in HD treatment, HD patients frequently have complications associated with bleeding. The present case also had a history of side-effects of gastrointestinal bleeding associated with use of NSAIDs, therefore, he was administered JDI. JDI can thus be used safely and economically in HD patients with history of gastrointestinal bleeding caused by NSAIDs.

According to the clinical guidance for the evaluation and the treatment of cardiovascular complications in HD patients by Japanese Society for Dialysis Therapy [10], they state that warfarin potassium for HD patients should be strictly monitored attributable to high risk of bleeding complications such as cerebral hemorrhage in the population [11, 12]. Warfarin potassium significantly increases the risk for bleeding as creatinine clearance. Non-vitamin K-dependent oral anticoagulant agents (NOACs) are currently recommended for patients with atrial fibrillation at risk for stroke instead of warfarin potassium, however, all NOACs are dependent on kidney function for elimination therefore contraindicated in HD population [13]. Anticoagulant therapy for HD patients is difficult accordingly.

If the patient was administered only warfarin potassium as an anticoagulant therapy and meropenem hydrate without JDI, the possibility remains that the pain control might be more difficult, and it might take longer to diminish venous thrombosis and hematoma. Therefore, the quality of life of the patient might be reduced attributable to extension of hospitalization or medication period.

Because JDI contains rhubarb rhizome (laxative) [4], the associated side effects of digestive symptoms such as epigastralgia and diarrhea could be caused. In the present case, the patient did not complain of such symptoms. While taking JDI, the frequency of his bowel movements improved regularly approximately once daily. HD patients overall require water restriction, thereby complicating constipation frequently. Laxative effect of rhubarb rhizome may be rather favorable for bowel movement in HD patients.

The favorable indication of JDI in HD patients could be characterized as follows: (1) pain with history of NSAIDs-related gastrointestinal bleeding, (2) complications associated with venous thrombosis or subcutaneous hematoma caused by catheterization, and (3) under treatment with anticoagulants (bleeding tendency). On the other hand, unfavorable indication of JDI in HD patients could be characterized as follows: patients who cannot follow water restriction. Because herbal medicines are generally in granule forms and bitter taste, it requires a certain amount of drinking water at the time of medication. They are more difficult to take than a tablet form; therefore, JDI in capsules or tablets should be desirable in the future. Because the patient accompanied with shivering and high fever, he was administered JDI with use of a jelly specialized for Kampo drugs without drinking water (Rakuraku fukuyaku jelly for Kampo medicine, Ryukakusan, Tokyo, Japan) [14].

JDI can be not only safely used for HD patients with fewer side-effects but also a cheap medicine from the viewpoint of medical economics. Traditional Japanese Kampo and modern medical approaches should be incorporated into the future medical system to exploit the advantage of both medicine. A large number of cases using JDI should be accumulated to maximize the benefits and confirm the excellent effectiveness of JDI in the future.

Conclusions

The present case indicated as follows: JDI controls the pain associated with hematoma without analgesics such as NSAIDs; JDI also has an effect of improving the complications associated with venous thrombosis and subcutaneous hematoma caused by catheterization in HD patients safely. JDI, one of Kampo drugs, has few side effects and can be used as needed.

Abbreviations

CECT: Contrast-enhanced computed tomography; CH50: 50% hemolytic unit factor; CRP: C-reactive protein; HD: Hemodialysis; JDI: Jidabokuippo; NOACs: Non-vitamin K-dependent oral anticoagulant agents; NSAIDs: Non-steroidal anti-inflammatory drugs; SLE: Systemic lupus erythematosus; VAS: Visual analogue scale

Acknowledgements

The authors would like to express our sincere thanks to the medical staffs of Nippon Kokan Fukuyama Hospital, Hiroshima, Japan, for collecting samples of the patient and analyzing the samples.

Funding

Not applicable. Our manuscript does not contain funding.

Authors' contributions

KW is responsible for the manuscript. KW and YW performed the acquisition and interpretation of data and drafted and revised the manuscript. HAU helped to draft the manuscript. All authors read and approved the final manuscript.

Authors' information

KW is a Director of the Division of Nephrology and Dialysis, Department of Internal Medicine, Nippon Kokan Fukuyama Hospital, Hiroshima, Japan.
HAU is the associate professor of the Department of Chronic Kidney Disease and Cardiovascular Disease, Okayama University Graduate School of Medicine, Dentistry and Pharmaceutical Sciences, Okayama, Japan.
YW is a Director of the Division of Nephrology and Dialysis, Department of Internal Medicine, Central Hospital, Hiroshima, Japan.

Competing interests

The authors declare that they have no competing interests.

Author details

[1]Division of Nephrology and Dialysis, Department of Internal Medicine, Nippon Kokan Fukuyama Hospital, 1844, Tsunoshita, Daimon-cho, Fukuyama City, Hiroshima 721-0927, Japan. [2]Department of Chronic Kidney Disease and Cardiovascular Disease, Okayama University Graduate School of Medicine, Dentistry and Pharmaceutical Sciences, Okayama, Japan. [3]Division of Nephrology and Dialysis, Department of Internal Medicine, Central Hospital, Hiroshima, Japan.

References

1. Oliver MJ. Acute dialysis catheters. Semin Dial. 2001;14:432–5.
2. Nakae H, Yokoi A, Kodama H, Horikawa A. Evid Based Complement Alternat Med. 2012;2012:837–958.
3. Asada S. Futsugo-yakushitsu-hokan-kuketsu. Tokyo: Futsugo-yakushitsu 20; 1878 [in Japanese].
4. The Japan Society for Oriental Medicine. Introduction to KAMPO: Japanese traditional medicine. Tokyo: Elsevier Japan K.K; 2005.
5. Nakae H, Hebiguchi M, Okuyama M. Jidabokuippo use in patients with fractures of the extremities. Pers Med Univers. 2015;4:66–9.
6. Nakae H. Clinical evaluation of oxidative stress after taking jidabokuippo. Kampo Med. 2010;61:847–52 [in Japanese].
7. Nakae H. Determination of the total antioxidant capacity for comparing different types of suspensions of Kampo extract. Int J Integr Med. 2011;3:62–6 [in Japanese].
8. Povlishock JT, Kontos HA. The role of oxigen radicals in the pathobiology of traumatic brain injury. Hum Cell. 1992;5:345–53.
9. Terasawa K, Shinoda H, Imadaya A, et al. The presentation of diagnositic criteria for "oketsu" syndrome. Kampo Med. 1983;34:1–17 [in Japanese].
10. Japanese Society for Dialysis Therapy. Clinical guidance for the evaluation and the treatment of cardiovascular complications in hemodialysis patients. J Jpn Soc Dial Ther. 2011;44:337–425 [in Japanese].
11. Bleyer AJ, Russell GB, Satko SG. Sudden and cardiac death rates in hemodialysis patients. Kidney Int. 1999;55:1553–9.
12. Reiter MJ, Reiffel JA. Importance of beta blockade in the therapy of serious ventricular arrhythmias. Am J Cardiol. 1991;82:91–191.
13. Chan KE, Giugliano RP, Patel MR, et al. Nonvitamin K anticoagulant agents in patients with advanced chronic kidney disease or on dialysis with AF. J Am Coll Cardiol. 2016;67:2888–99.
14. Wada K. Kampo medicine for dialysis patients. Tokyo: Nakayama Shoten Co., Ltd.; 2005 [in Japanese].

13

Effects, safety, and plasma levels of topiroxostat and its metabolites in patients receiving hemodialysis

Satoko Oyama[1*], Chihiro Hirose[1], Kenichiro Hori[1], Katsuhiro Sugano[1], Jie Zhang[1], Miyuki Tamura[2] and Kimio Tomita[1]

Abstract

Background: Serum uric acid concentrations have been associated with mortality in patients receiving hemodialysis. Treatment options are sometimes limited because of the accumulation of a drug and/or its metabolites. The aim of the present study is to investigate the efficacy, safety, and plasma levels of topiroxostat, a selective xanthine oxidase inhibitor, and its metabolites in patients receiving hemodialysis.

Methods: This was a 52-week open study. The plasma concentrations of topiroxostat and its metabolites were measured. The endpoints selected were effects on serum uric acid concentrations and the safety and tolerability of topiroxostat. A statistical analysis was performed using a paired t test with Bonferroni corrections.

Results: Nineteen participants were followed for 52 weeks without significant adverse effects. Serum uric acid concentrations decreased from 527 ± 49 to 325 ± 62, 297 ± 99, 297 ± 68, and 296 ± 83 μmol/L (weeks 4, 12, 26, and 52; $p < 0.001$, respectively). The dosage of topiroxostat was 20 mg twice per day in all patients. The clearances of topiroxostat and its metabolites by a dialyzer by use of an arterio-venous method were 55.9 ± 31.1 mL/min (topiroxostat), 143.9 ± 37.0 mL/min (*N*-oxide), 179.0 ± 41.1 mL/min (N_1-glucuronide), and 192.9 ± 37.0 mL/min (N_2-glucuronide). Plasma concentrations of topiroxostat did not increase during the 52-week study period. The concentrations of the metabolites of topiroxostat (N_1-glucuronide and N_2-glucuronide) slightly increased at the 0-h point on week 4 and remained at similar levels for 52 weeks.

Conclusions: Topiroxostat effectively reduced serum uric acid concentrations in patients receiving hemodialysis. Topiroxostat and its metabolites were partly cleared during hemodialysis and were sufficiently low to allow for the continued administration of the drug for 52 weeks.

Keywords: Dialysis, Drug clearance, Selective xanthine oxidase inhibitor, Topiroxostat, Uric acid

Background

Epidemiological studies have suggested that increased serum uric acid levels are a risk factor for cardiovascular mortality. All-cause mortality in 5 years was previously reported to be significantly higher in hyperuricemic than in normouricemic men and women [1]. Hyperuricemia has been strongly associated with the relative risks of death from all causes, coronary heart disease, stroke, hepatic disease, and renal failure, and serum uric acid may be a significant risk factor for reduced life expectancy in 49,413 Japanese male workers [2]. Although uric acid has been identified as a strong risk factor for myocardial infarction, stroke, and chronic kidney disease progression [3], other studies have not reported a significant relationship between uric acid concentrations and mortality [4]. High serum uric acid concentrations appear to be associated with mortality in patients with renal disease receiving hemodialysis [5]. On the other hand, higher uric acid concentrations have been associated with a lower risk of all-cause and cardiovascular mortalities in the hemodialysis population when six countries affiliated with the Dialysis Outcomes and

* Correspondence: satokomonchi@gmail.com
[1]The Chronic Kidney Disease Research Center, Tomei Atsugi Hospital, 232, Funako, Atsugi City, Kanagawa 243-8571, Japan
Full list of author information is available at the end of the article

Practice Patterns Study (DOPPS) were analyzed [6]. Therefore, the extent to which serum uric acid is associated with mortality in patients with chronic kidney disease receiving hemodialysis remains controversial.

Intervention studies have suggested beneficial effects of allopurinol on cardiovascular events in patients receiving hemodialysis [7]. Febuxostat has also been shown to improve endothelial dysfunction and reduce serum uric acid concentrations and oxidative stress in hyperuricemic patients receiving hemodialysis [8]. A recent study suggested that the administration of topiroxostat, a xanthine oxidase inhibitor, at a dose of 160 mg effectively reduced serum uric acid concentrations in hyperuricemic stage 3 chronic kidney disease patients with or without gout [9]. Most of these intervention studies have suggested the benefit of lowering uric acid concentrations. However, the effects of topiroxostat on dialysis patients have not yet been examined in detail.

The excessive accumulation of the active form and metabolites of a drug may eventually induce serious adverse effects, particularly in patients with end-stage renal failure. A recent study proposed the extra-renal pathway of uric acid [10]. In addition, the levels of the uric acid transporter ABCG2 (ATP-binding cassette subfamily G member 2) were found to be increased in the intestine of a 5/6 nephrectomy rat model of chronic kidney disease [11]. Uric acid metabolism may also be affected by end-stage renal failure.

Topiroxostat is inactivated through the liver and is almost cleared from blood even in patients with moderate renal dysfunction [12]. The metabolites of topiroxostat are excreted into feces and urine. The main metabolites of topiroxostat, *N*-oxide, N_1-gluculonide, and N_2-gluculonide, are excreted into urine about 4.8, 43.3, and 16.1 % of the dose, respectively [13]. Therefore, the concentrations of these metabolites could increase in patients with severe renal dysfunction. The metabolites of topiroxostat have a negligible low activity (*N*-oxide, 1/188; N_1-gluculonide and N_2-gluculonide, less than 1/1449 compared with topiroxostat); however, the effects of these metabolites on patients with unexpectedly high concentration are not known. There are no reports concerning the safety, the concentration of topiroxostat and its metabolites, and its clearance during hemodialysis in patients receiving hemodialysis.

The aim of the present study is to investigate the efficacy and safety of topiroxostat in patients receiving hemodialysis for 52 weeks.

Methods

The protocol and informed consent form were approved by the Review Board of Tomei Atsugi Hospital (approved on October 3, 2013, and June 10, 2016). This study complied with the Declaration of Helsinki and the Ethical Guidelines for Clinical Studies by the Ministry of Health, Labour and Welfare, Japan. Participants were all recruited from Tomei Atsugi Hospital and Aikawa Clinic in Kanagawa, Japan, between November 2013 and July 2016. Twenty patients older than 20 years old were enrolled in this study after providing written informed consent. An explanation of the present study included the study hypothesis, benefits of this study, and the risks of adverse effects associated with topiroxostat such as gouty arthritis, liver dysfunction, and skin rash.

Study design

Participants were followed up for 52 weeks. The endpoints analyzed were as follows: (1) change from the baseline serum uric acid concentration, the achievement rate of the target serum uric acid concentration (≤357 μmol/L) according to the guidelines of the Japanese Society of Gout and Nucleic Acid Metabolism; (2) the safety and tolerability of topiroxostat; (3) plasma concentrations of topiroxostat and its metabolites following the administration of topiroxostat; (4) clearances of topiroxostat and its metabolites by a dialyzer using an arterio-venous method; and (5) plasma concentrations of topiroxostat and its metabolites for 52 weeks.

Eligible patients were those whose serum uric acid concentration was more than 476 μmol/L at least 8 weeks before the study, receiving steady hemodialysis over 5 months. None of the participants had been treated with uric acid-lowering drugs at least 12 weeks before the initiation of the study. The exclusion criteria were hyperuricemia possibly secondary to a malignant tumor and genetic diseases, hypothyroidism, polycystic kidney disease, hepatic dysfunction (AST or ALT over 100 IU/L), cancer, pregnancy, breastfeeding, serious hepatic disease, serious heart disease, allergy to topiroxostat, and any other significant medical conditions.

Chronic hemodialysis patients with a serum uric acid concentration of more than 476 μmol/L were treated with topiroxostat for 52 weeks. Topiroxostat was orally administered at 20 mg twice per day at the start of the study, followed by a stepwise increase to a maximal dose of 60 mg twice per day according to the clinical condition of each patient. Drugs other than topiroxostat that may influence the serum concentration of uric acid were discontinued during the study. Serum biochemical tests were performed once a month during the study. Patient samples were tested for blood urea nitrogen, creatinine, total protein, albumin, AST, ALT, alkaline phosphatase, total bilirubin, LDH, total cholesterol, triglycerides, HDL cholesterol, and LDL cholesterol.

Topiroxostat was prescribed in the morning and late evening. Patients who received dialysis in a morning session were administered the morning dose of the drug at the time of dialysis. Patients who received dialysis in an afternoon session were administered the morning dose of the drug early in the morning and at dialysis. This means the concentrations of topiroxostat and its metabolites were measured 8–10 h after the administration of topiroxostat. Since the molecular weights of topiroxostat and its metabolites are 248.24 (topiroxostat), 264.24 (*N*-oxide), and 424.37 (N_1-gluculonide and N_2-gluculonide), their plasma concentrations were almost negligible 8–10 h after the single-dose administration of topiroxostat in patients with renal impairments (inulin clearance over 30 mL/min/1.73 m^2) [12]. The plasma concentrations of topiroxostat (active form) and its metabolites, *N*-oxide, N_1-gluculonide, and N_2-gluculonide, were measured at the beginning of hemodialysis and in some cases during hemodialysis. The plasma concentrations of topiroxostat and its metabolites were also measured at the time of dialysis on weeks 4, 12, 26, and 52 in order to assess the possibility of their accumulation during the long-term prescription of the drug.

The clearances of topiroxostat and its metabolites were calculated by sampling of plasma from the arterial and venous side of the dialyzer at 10 min after starting dialysis (arterio-venous method). Ultrafiltration rate was zero during this period for the simplification of chemical kinetics.

Three types of dialyzers were used: type III (clearance of β2-microglobulin 30–50 mL/min), type IV (clearance of β2-microglobulin 50–70 mL/min), and type V (clearance of β2-microglobulin more than 70 mL/min) in 5, 9, and 6 patients, respectively.

The plasma concentrations of topiroxostat and its metabolites, *N*-oxide, N_1-gluculonide, and N_2-gluculonide, were measured using the LC-MS/MS method. Plasma samples were deproteinized by the addition of methanol and an internal standard, mixed, and centrifuged. The resulting supernatant was injected into a LC-MS/MS system with an ESI probe and analyzed by multiple reaction monitoring (MRM) in the negative ion mode. Separation was performed through a Mightysil RP-18 GP column (150 × 2.0 mm, 5 μm) with the mobile phase of 10 mmol/L ammonium acetate and methanol (50/50) for topiroxostat and *N*-oxide and 0.1 % formic acid and methanol (65/35) for N_1-gluculonide and N_2-gluculonide. The standard curves were linear from 0.00403 to 0.403 μmol/L for topiroxostat, from 0.00378 to 0.757 μmol/L for *N*-oxide, and from 0.00403 to 4.03 μmol/L for N_1-gluculonide and N_2-gluculonide. The lower limit of quantification was 0.00403 μmol/L (1.00 ng/mL) for topiroxostat, 0.00378 μmol/L (1.00 ng/mL) for *N*-oxide, and 0.00403 μmol/L (1.00 ng eq/mL) for N_1-glucuronide and N_2-glucuronide.

Samples for the assay of the concentrations of the drug and its metabolites were delivered to the researcher without notification of the name of patients or sampling periods.

Statistical analysis

Statistical analyses were performed using a paired *t* test with Bonferroni corrections, and a *p* value less than 0.05 was considered significant. Data were expressed as the mean ± SD.

Results

Patient profiles

Baseline characteristics and laboratory parameters are listed in Table 1. Twenty participants were enrolled in this study.

Safety and tolerability

One case dropped out at week 12 due to perforation of the colon diverticulum. Nineteen participants were followed up for 52 weeks. Biochemical test results at the baseline and during the follow-up are shown in Table 2. Serum uric acid concentrations decreased from 527 ± 49 to 325 ± 62 μmol/L (week 4; $p < 0.001$), 297 ± 99 μmol/L (week 12; $p < 0.001$), 297 ± 68 μmol/L (week 26; $p < 0.001$), and 296 ± 83 μmol/L (week 52; $p < 0.001$) (Fig. 1). The percentage of patients with serum uric acid concentrations ≤357 μmol/L reached 80.0, 78.9, 84.2, and 78.9 % (weeks 4, 12, 26, and 52, respectively). The dosage of topiroxostat was 20 mg twice per day in all patients. No significant differences were observed in the values obtained in liver function tests or lipid function tests during the entire study period (Table 2).

Plasma concentrations of topiroxostat and its metabolites during hemodialysis at the first and week 4 administration of topiroxostat

The plasma concentrations of topiroxostat were 0.384 ± 0.348 μmol/L (1 h), 0.644 ± 0.374 μmol/L (2 h), 0.435 ± 0.333 μmol/L (3 h), and 0.278 ± 0.265 μmol/L (4 h) with its first administration ($n = 7$) (Fig. 2a). After 4 weeks, the plasma concentrations of topiroxostat were 0.086 ± 0.061 μmol/L (0 h), 0.164 ± 0.093 μmol/L (1 h), 0.460 ± 0.316 μmol/L (2 h), 0.604 ± 0.530 μmol/L (3 h), and 0.367 ± 0.340 μmol/L (4 h) (Fig. 2b). The plasma concentration at week 4 on the 0-h time point

Table 1 Baseline characteristics

Variable	Mean ± SD
Age (years)	62.0 ± 12.3
Sex (male/female)	12/8
Primary disease	
Chronic glomerulonephritis, *n* (%)	7 (35.0)
Diabetic nephropathy, *n* (%)	5 (25.0)
Nephrosclerosis, *n* (%)	3 (15.0)
Unknown, *n* (%)	5 (25.0)
Duration of hemodialysis (years)	7.8 ± 9.6

Table 2 Biochemical test results at the baseline and during the follow-up

Parameter	Baseline	Week 4	Week 12	Week 26	Week 52
Number of participants	20	20	19	19	19
BUN (mmol/L)	25.1 ± 5.2	24.3 ± 5.4	20.8 ± 6.9*	20.8 ± 4.9*	23.5 ± 5.2
Creatinine (μmol/L)	1105.4 ± 244.4	1079.2 ± 210.6	1003.8 ± 286.9	1030.2 ± 281.2*	1018.7 ± 251.8*
Total protein (g/L)	63.2 ± 5.0	64.7 ± 5.4	61.3 ± 4.9	62.4 ± 7.0	63.2 ± 5.4
Albumin (g/L)	37.6 ± 3.1	37.3 ± 4.6	35.8 ± 4.6	36.7 ± 5.3	36.1 ± 3.9
AST (IU/L)	12.6 ± 7.3	11.4 ± 5.2	10.5 ± 4.4	12.1 ± 5.9	11.5 ± 5.3
ALT (IU/L)	10.8 ± 6.3	9.8 ± 4.0	9.2 ± 3.5	10.5 ± 3.0	9.7 ± 5.6
ALP (IU/L)	243.8 ± 94.8	218.9 ± 69.7	213.6 ± 92.4	243.1 ± 133.3	224.9 ± 78.7
Total bilirubin (μmol/L)	4.4 ± 1.5	4.5 ± 1.7	4.4 ± 1.8	4.8 ± 2.3	4.5 ± 1.3
LDH (IU/L)	186.6 ± 25.5	185.0 ± 29.1	184.1 ± 31.9	191.8 ± 40.0	181.7 ± 27.1
Total cholesterol (mmol/L)	4.273 ± 0.710	4.439 ± 0.900	4.266 ± 0.797	4.539 ± 0.918	4.241 ± 1.159
Triglycerides (mmol/L)	1.214 ± 0.414	1.096 ± 0.281	1.036 ± 0.333	1.149 ± 0.386	1.213 ± 0.635
HDL cholesterol (mmol/L)	1.24 ± 0.39	1.38 ± 0.49	1.41 ± 0.52	1.52 ± 0.72	1.30 ± 0.44
LDL cholesterol (mmol/L)	2.41 ± 0.41	2.56 ± 0.66	2.45 ± 0.63	2.53 ± 0.74	2.44 ± 0.89

BUN blood urea nitrogen, *AST* aspartate aminotransferase, *ALT* alanine aminotransferase, *ALP* alkaline phosphatase, *LDH* lactate dehydrogenase
*$p < 0.05$ (paired t test vs. baseline, after Bonferroni corrections). Mean ± SD

was not significantly different from that of the 4-h time point with the first administration ($p > 0.10$). This suggests that the active form of topiroxostat did not accumulate during the 4-week administration in patients receiving hemodialysis.

The concentration of the two metabolites increased after repetitive administration of the drug for 4 weeks when compared with the concentration of 4 h after the first administration of topiroxostat (N_1-glucuronide from 0.57 ± 0.08 to 4.18 ± 1.96 μmol/L, $p < 0.005$; N_2-glucuronide from 0.27 ± 0.07 to 1.12 ± 0.41 μmol/L, $p < 0.001$). These results suggest the accumulation of the two metabolites after the administration of the drug for 4 weeks in patients receiving hemodialysis.

Clearances of topiroxostat and its metabolites by a dialyzer by use of an arterio-venous method

The molecular weight of topiroxostat is 248.24, and *N*-oxide is 264.24. However, the clearance was small in topiroxostat compared with *N*-oxide, possibly because plasma protein binding rates of topiroxostat are higher than those of *N*-oxide. The clearances of *N*-oxide, N_1-glucuronide, and N_2-glucuronide were similar with those of BUN, creatinine, and serum uric acid ($n = 6$) (Table 3).

Long-term effects

The plasma concentration of topiroxostat was 0.094 ± 0.086 μmol/L at week 4 before hemodialysis ($n = 20$). The concentration did not increase further during the study (0.152 ± 0.207 μmol/L at week 52, $n = 19$; $p = 0.733$) (Fig. 3). Similarly, the plasma concentrations of the three metabolites of topiroxostat did not increase further during the study.

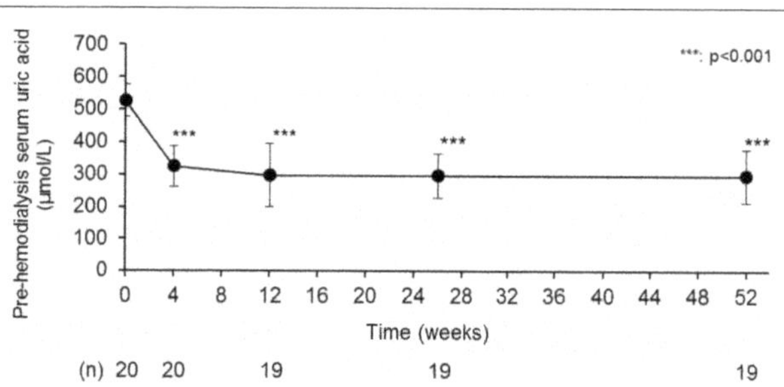

Fig. 1 Pre-hemodialysis uric acid concentrations after repeated administration of 20 mg of topiroxostat twice per day. *p* value; paired *t* test with Bonferroni corrections vs. baseline. Mean ± SD

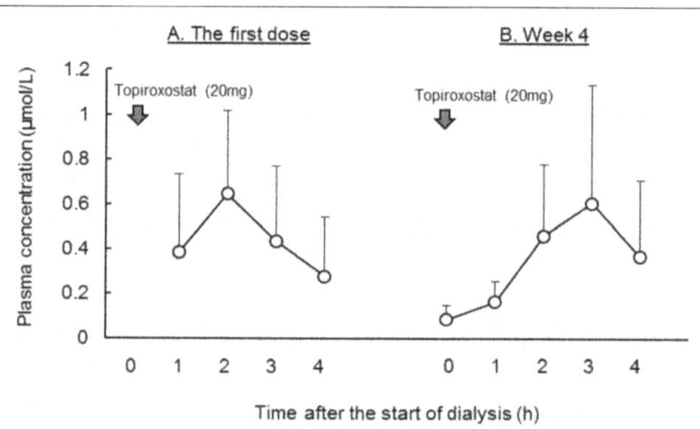

Fig. 2 Plasma concentrations of topiroxostat during hemodialysis ($n = 7$). Plasma concentration of topiroxostat at week 4 on the 0-h time point was not different from that of the 4-h time point with the first dose ($p > 0.1$, paired t test). Topiroxostat was administered at the starting time of dialysis

Table 3 Clearances of topiroxostat and its metabolites by a dialyzer by use of an arterio-venous method

	Pre-dialyzer concentration	Post-dialyzer concentration	Clearance (mL/min)
Topiroxostat(μmol/L)	0.269 ± 0.164	0.216 ± 0.166	55.9 ± 31.1
N-Oxide (μmol/L)	0.0812 ± 0.0277	0.0317 ± 0.0190	143.9 ± 37.0
N_1-Glucuronide (μmol/L)	3.21 ± 1.00	0.81 ± 0.64	179.0 ± 41.1
N_2-Glucuronide (μmol/L)	0.853 ± 0.412	0.144 ± 0.121	192.9 ± 37.0
Albumin (g/L)	32.8 ± 5.2	32.5 ± 5.1	2.3 ± 6.7
BUN (mmol/L)	18.8 ± 7.6	1.3 ± 1.0	217.2 ± 27.8
Creatinine (μmol/L)	769.8 ± 164.4	169.4 ± 40.7	179.4 ± 20.4
Serum uric acid (μmol/L)	224.0 ± 66.4	46.6 ± 17.4	184.0 ± 26.2

Mean ± SD. $n = 6$

Xanthine oxidoreductase-inhibitory activities of topiroxostat and its metabolites in patients on week 52

The xanthine oxidoreductase-inhibitory activities of the metabolites of topiroxostat were 1/1449 and 1/188 that of topiroxostat. The estimated plasma concentrations of topiroxostat based on the relative activity of the plasma concentrations of its metabolites on week 52 were 0.0005 μmol/L (*N*-oxide), 0.002 μmol/L (N_1-glucuronide), and 0.0005 μmol/L (N_2-glucuronide) (Table 4). These biological activities in plasma were considered as negligibly low.

Discussion

Drug safety is typically monitored by chemical parameters, clinical signs, and symptoms. The pharmacokinetics of the metabolites of most drugs have not been investigated in patients receiving hemodialysis. However, drug accumulation may be inevitable in patients with end-stage renal failure. Even if the activities of the metabolites are low, their concentrations may be markedly increased after long periods of anuria. Precise investigations are needed in order to determine the possibility of the accumulation of the metabolites and to rule out adverse effects in patients receiving hemodialysis. We herein demonstrated that topiroxostat at a dose of 20 mg twice per day effectively and safely reduced serum uric acid concentrations in patients receiving hemodialysis. The dose of topiroxostat administered was 40 mg per day in all patients. Uric acid concentrations decreased from week 4 and remained low until week 52. Topiroxostat and its metabolites did not accumulate at concentrations high enough to cease its administration during the 52-week study period.

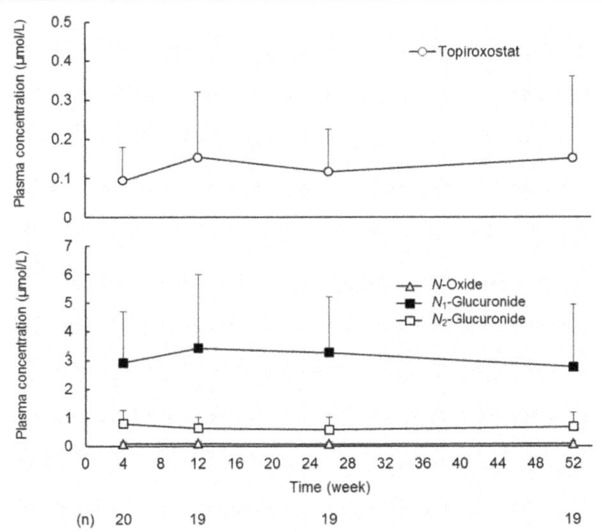

Fig. 3 Plasma concentrations of topiroxostat and its metabolites after repeated administration of 20 mg twice per day of topiroxostat. There were no significant differences between the concentrations of topiroxostat and its three metabolites at weeks 4, 12, 26, and 52 (paired *t* test vs. 4 weeks, after Bonferroni corrections). ($n = 20$, week 4; $n = 19$, weeks 19, 26, and 52). Mean ± SD

The clearance of topiroxostat was slightly small compared with that of the other three metabolites probably because topiroxostat binds albumin in plasma. Even with clearing from a dialyzer, the plasma peak levels of topiroxostat are about 30 % lower when compared with the peak concentration of normal volunteers who were studied in fasting condition (0.926 ± 0.329 μmol/L: data from interview form). The difference between our results and the results of normal volunteers may be due to the removal of the drug by the dialyzer and the delay of drug absorption from the digestive tract in the condition of patients who have taken the drug after meals. This result suggests topiroxostat remains in substantial amounts during the 4-h hemodialysis and also does not accumulate after repeated administration in patients receiving hemodialysis. The clearances of *N*-oxide, N_1-glucuronide, and N_2-glucuronide were similar with those of BUN, creatinine, and serum uric acid. This could have protected against the accumulation of the metabolites to an unexpectedly high concentration in patients receiving hemodialysis.

Forty milligrams per day of topiroxostat may be sufficient to treat hyperuricemia in patients receiving dialysis, possibly because uric acid is removed from the body by hemodialysis in addition to the pharmacological effects of topiroxostat.

Table 4 Xanthine oxidoreductase-inhibitory activities of topiroxostat and its metabolites in patients at week 52

	IC^{a}_{50} (μmol/L)	Relative ratio of IC^{b}_{50}	Plasma concentration[c] (μmol/L)	Concentration[d] (μmol/L)
Topiroxostat	0.069	1	0.152	0.152
N-Oxide	13	1/188	0.0952	0.0005
N_1-Glucuronide	>100	1/1449	2.77	0.002
N_2-Glucuronide	>100	1/1449	0.686	0.0005

[a]Half maximal (50 %) xanthine oxidoreductase (XOR)-inhibitory concentration
[b]The relative ratio of IC_{50} between topiroxostat and its metabolites
[c]Pre-hemodialysis plasma concentrations of topiroxostat and its metabolites at week 52
[d]Estimated plasma concentrations based on the relative ratio of IC_{50} between topiroxostat and its metabolites

Uric acid has been identified as a strong risk factor for myocardial infarction, stroke, and chronic kidney disease progression [3]; however, other studies have not reported a significant relationship between uric acid levels and mortality [4]. Uric acid has been shown to have a function of both an antioxidant and pro-oxidant. Uric acid is a powerful scavenger of carbon-centered and peroxyl radicals in a hydrophilic environment but loses its ability to scavenge lipophilic radicals and cannot break radical chain propagation within lipid membranes. At the same time, peroxynitrous radicals are extremely diffusible through the membrane and the hydrophobic environment is also more favorable for tyrosine nitration. Thus, these physicochemical findings may explain why the antioxidant effects of uric acid only manifested in the hydrophilic environment of biological fluids, such as plasma. This may be a major limitation for the antioxidant function of uric acid. On the other hand, uric acid has a function as pro-oxidant [14, 15]. Reactions between uric acid and oxidants may also produce other radicals that have the ability to propagate radical chain reactions and oxidative damage to cells. A xanthine oxidase inhibitor may be beneficial for reducing uric acid and reactive oxygen species levels. Uric acid may be a marker of oxidants as the result of xanthine oxidases.

Allopurinol, febuxostat, and topiroxostat are the most frequently used drugs to treat hyperuricemic patients with renal dysfunction. Allopurinol is an analog of xanthine used in the treatment of hyperuricemia. This drug is absorbed well orally and is converted to oxipurinol, an analog of xanthine. Oxipurinol binds tightly to xanthine oxidase and inhibits this enzyme, thereby preventing the conversion of hypoxanthine and xanthine to uric acid. Oxipurinol is slowly cleared via the kidney, with a serum half-life of 14 to 26 h in patients with normal renal function. In patients with renal insufficiency, the renal clearance of the major metabolite of allopurinol, oxipurinol, was shown to be directly proportional to the renal clearance of creatinine [16]. The avoidance of treatments with allopurinol in patients with renal insufficiency has been recommended in order to prevent the life-threatening toxicity syndrome (Stevens-Johnson syndrome) of an erythematous, desquamative skin rash, fever, hepatitis, eosinophilia, and deteriorated renal function.

Febuxostat, a xanthine oxidase inhibitor, strongly binds to albumin in blood. It is mainly metabolized to its acyl-glucuronide metabolite and to its active oxidative metabolites 67M-1, 67M-2, and 67M-4 [17]. A once-daily 80-mg dose of febuxostat appears to be safe and tolerated well in different renal function groups and does not appear to require any dose adjustments based on differences in renal function. However, regression analyses for 67M-2 and 67M-4 C_{max} and for the AUC_{24h} of all three metabolites indicated a significant linear relationship with creatinine clearance. Plasma exposure to febuxostat and its metabolites was generally found to be higher in subjects with increasing degrees of renal impairment; therefore, dose adjustments are recommended in patients with severe renal dysfunction. Approximately 2.1–3.8 % of febuxostat and 46.7–49.7 % (glucuronide) and 9.7–12.7 % (oxidative metabolite; active form) of its metabolites are excreted into the urine within 24 h. Mean cumulative excretion was 94 % (49 % urine and 45 % feces) of the dose over 9 days [18]. These findings suggest that active metabolites may accumulate to a critical range, particularly in anuric patients with hemodialysis.

In patients receiving hemodialysis, allopurinol and febuxostat have both been reported to be safe and effectively reduce serum uric acid concentrations [7, 8]. However, the risk of adverse effects due to the accumulation of their active forms and metabolites in patients receiving hemodialysis cannot be excluded yet.

One case (81-year-old male) dropped out of our study due to perforation of the colon diverticulum. He had multiple diverticula in the colon and had been taking prednisolone at 7.5 mg per day for 3 years to treat interstitial pneumonia. Perforated colonic diverticular disease results in high mortality and morbidity. Colonic diverticular disease is rare in developing countries but is common in Western and industrialized societies. Its prevalence has been reported to increase with age, ranging from ~5 % in adults <40 years of age to 65 % among those 80 years of age. In Japan, diverticulum of the colon was detected by plain CT in 57 (41.6 %) out of 137 consecutive chronic kidney disease patients (stage 4 or 5) who were candidates for peritoneal dialysis [19]. In a prospective study comprising 3103 patient months, a total of 44 (15 % of all) episodes of peritonitis with microorganisms of enteral origin occurred in 30 out of 129 patients. Several drug and dietary exposures have potential biological mechanisms of action that cause perforation. Of these, only non-steroidal anti-inflammatory drugs (NSAIDs) have been consistently identified as risk factors in etiological studies. Our case was an 81-year-old male who was receiving hemodialysis for 5 years without peritoneal dialysis. He had taken glucocorticoids, but not NSAIDs. Glucocorticoids may have had some adverse effects leading to perforation of the diverticulum in our patient. Topiroxostat is presumed to be easily dissolved in an acidic milieu such as the stomach based on its physicochemical properties. It is very unlikely to remain in its pill form in the colon. We considered it very unlikely that topiroxostat was the cause of colon perforation in our patient. The causes of perforated colonic diverticular disease remain largely unknown. Further etiological studies are required in order to determine whether cause-effect relationships exist for drug and dietary exposures.

There were several limitations to the present study. It was not designed in a double-blinded fashion, and the participant number was small. Furthermore, our results did not show any benefits concerning mortality because it was only conducted for 52 weeks. However, the safety and effectiveness of topiroxostat have enabled us to investigate the effects of lowering serum uric acid concentrations on mortality in patients receiving hemodialysis for a long period of time in the future. Because this is the first report that measured the concentrations of topiroxostat and its metabolites in patients receiving hemodialysis with collaboration of a pharmaceutical company, these findings need to be further investigated in other studies.

Conclusions

We herein demonstrated that topiroxostat effectively and safely reduced serum uric acid concentrations in patients receiving hemodialysis. Topiroxostat and its metabolites were partly cleared during hemodialysis and were sufficiently low to allow for the continued administration of the drug for 52 weeks.

Abbreviations

ALP: Alkaline phosphatase; ALT: Alanine aminotransferase; AST: Aspartate aminotransferase; BUN: Blood urea nitrogen; LDH: Lactate dehydrogenase

Acknowledgements

The authors thank Sanwa Kagaku Kenkyusho Co., Ltd., for the measurements of topiroxostat and its metabolite concentrations.

Funding

We have no funding to declare.

Authors' contributions

OS and TK were responsible for the research idea and study. HC, HK, SK, and ZJ were responsible for the data acquisition. TM was responsible for the measurements of topiroxostat and its metabolite concentrations. All authors read and approve the final manuscript.

Competing interests

Pharmaceutical Research Laboratories, Sanwa Kagaku Kenkyusho Co., Ltd., measured the concentration of topiroxostat and its metabolites.

Author details

[1]The Chronic Kidney Disease Research Center, Tomei Atsugi Hospital, 232, Funako, Atsugi City, Kanagawa 243-8571, Japan. [2]Pharmaceutical Research Laboratories, Sanwa Kagaku Kenkyusho Co., Ltd., Nagoya 461-8631, Japan.

References

1. Reunanen A, Takkunen H, Knekt P, Aromaa A. Hyperuricemia as a risk factor for cardiovascular mortality. Acta Med Scand Suppl. 1982;668:49–59.
2. Tomita M, Mizuno S, Yamanaka H, Hosoda Y, Sakuma K, Matuoka Y, et al. Does hyperuricemia affect mortality? A prospective cohort study of Japanese male workers. J Epidemiol. 2000;10(6):403–9.
3. Iseki K, Iseki C, Kinjo K. Changes in serum uric acid have a reciprocal effect on eGFR change: a 10-year follow-up study of community-based screening in Okinawa, Japan. Hypertens Res. 2013;36(7):650–4.
4. Sakata K, Hashimoto T, Ueshima H, Okayama A, NIPPON DATA 80 Research Group. Absence of an association between serum uric acid and mortality from cardiovascular disease: NIPPON DATA 80, 1980-1994. National Integrated Projects for Prospective Observation of Non-communicable Diseases and its Trend in the Aged. Eur J Epidemiol. 2001;17(5):461–8.
5. Hsu SP, Pai MF, Peng YS, Chiang CK, Ho TI, Hung KY. Serum uric acid levels show a 'J-shaped' association with all-cause mortality in haemodialysis patients. Nephrol Dial Transplant. 2004;19(2):457–62.
6. Latif W, Karaboyas A, Tong L, Winchester JF, Arrington CJ, Pisoni RL, et al. Uric acid levels and all-cause and cardiovascular mortality in the hemodialysis population. Clin J Am Soc Nephrol. 2011;6(10):2470–7.
7. Tsuruta Y, Nitta K, Akizawa T, Fukuhara S, Saito A, Karaboyas A, et al. Association between allopurinol and mortality among Japanese hemodialysis patients: results from the DOPPS. Int Urol Nephrol. 2014;46:1833–41.
8. Tsuruta Y, Kikuchi K, Tsuruta Y, Sasaki Y, Moriyama T, Itabashi M, et al. Febuxostat improves endothelial function in hemodialysis patients with hyperuricemia: a randomized controlled study. Hemodial Int. 2015;19(4):514–20.
9. Hosoya T, Ohno I, Nomura S, Hisatome I, Uchida S, Fujimori S, et al. Effects of topiroxostat on the serum urate levels and urinary albumin excretion in hyperuricemic stage 3 chronic kidney disease patients with or without gout. Clin Exp Nephrol. 2014;18:876–84.
10. Ichida K, Matsuo H, Takada T, Nakayama A, Murakami K, Shimizu T, et al. Decreased extra-renal urate excretion is a common cause of hyperuricemia. Nat Commun. 2012;3:764.
11. Yano H, Tamura Y, Kobayashi K, Tanemoto M, Uchida S. Uric acid transporter ABCG2 is increased in the intestine of the 5/6 nephrectomy rat model of chronic kidney disease. Clin Exp Nephrol. 2014;18(1):50–5.
12. Nakazawa T, Iwanaga T, Ohashi T, Saito K. Pharmacokinetics and pharmacodynamics study of topiroxostat by oral administration in subjects with renal impairment. Jpn Pharmacol Ther. 2015;43:639–45.
13. Nakazawa T, Miyata K, Omura K, Iwanaga T, Nagata O. Metabolic profile of FYX-051 (4-(5-pyridin-4-yl-1h-[1,2,4]triazol-3-yl)pyridine-2-carbonitrile) in the rat, dog, monkey, and human: identification of N-glucuronides and N-glucosides. Drug Metab Dispos. 2006;34(11):1880–6.
14. Yu MA, Sánchez-Lozada LG, Johnson RJ, Kang DH. Oxidative stress with an activation of the renin-angiotensin system in human vascular endothelial cells as a novel mechanism of uric acid-induced endothelial dysfunction. J Hypertens. 2010;28(6):1234–42.

15. Martinon F, Pétrilli V, Mayor A, Tardivel A, Tschopp J. Gout-associated uric acid crystals activate the NALP3 inflammasome. Nature. 2006;440(7081):237–41.
16. Hande KR, Noone RM, Stone WJ. Severe allopurinol toxicity. Description and guidelines for prevention in patients with renal insufficiency. Am J Med. 1984;76(1):47–56.
17. Mayer MD, Khosravan R, Vernillet L, Wu JT, Joseph-Ridge N, Mulford DJ. Pharmacokinetics and pharmacodynamics of febuxostat, a new non-purine selective inhibitor of xanthine oxidase in subjects with renal impairment. Am J Ther. 2005;12(1):22–34.
18. Grabowski BA, Khosravan R, Vernillet L, Mulford DJ. Metabolism and excretion of [14C] febuxostat, a novel nonpurine selective inhibitor of xanthine oxidase, in healthy male subjects. Clin Pharmacol. 2011;51(2):189–201.
19. Toda S, Ito Y, Mizuno M, Suzuki Y, Ito I, Hiramatsu H, et al. Asymptomatic diverticulosis identified by computed tomography is not a risk factor for enteric peritonitis. Nephrol Dial Transplant. 2012;27(6):2511–6.

Low serum sodium concentration is a prognostic factor related to current blood glucose level in stable hemodialysis patients

Kojiro Nagai[1,4*†], Sayo Ueda[1†], Kenji Tsuchida[2,5], Toshio Doi[1] and Jun Minakuchi[3]

Abstract

Background: A lot of risk factors for mortality have been proposed in hemodialysis patients. However, most of the findings were derived from the analyses using all of the hemodialysis patients. What we really want to know is the prognostic factor in stable hemodialysis patients who have good activities of daily living, because it is difficult to estimate their prognosis by physical appearance.

Methods: This is a 7-year observational study. The study involved registering 631 patients who had undergone hemodialysis for more than 1 year at enrollment and were still alive more than 1 year after it. Demographic and clinical data were collected to analyze the relationship with mortality. Moreover, the patients were age-stratified to investigate age-dependent prognostic factors.

Results: Low serum sodium concentration is an independent risk factor for all-cause and cardiovascular mortality common to a wide range of ages in stable hemodialysis patients. Causes of hyponatremia included the predialysis blood glucose level as well as the variables related to nutrition, inflammation, and fluid overload.

Conclusions: Low serum sodium concentration is a significant prognostic factor in stable hemodialysis patients. Low serum sodium concentration can be a clue to finding current poor glucose control in stable hemodialysis patients. Predialysis blood glucose level is one of the representative factors correlated with serum sodium concentration.

Keywords: Serum sodium concentration, Hemodialysis, Mortality, Diabetes, Blood glucose level

Background

To date, a lot of demographic characteristics and clinical data have been proposed as prognostic factors in hemodialysis (HD) patients. Diabetic patients have an increased mortality compared to non-diabetic patients. The variables related to nutrition and inflammation are also representative risk factors [1]. The dialysis prescription is important to control small- and middle-weight-protein uremic toxins, anemia, and mineral-bone disorder that are associated with the prognosis of HD patients [2]. However, most of these findings were derived from the analyses including all of the HD patients. There are few reports that focus on stable maintenance HD patients who have good activities of daily living (ADLs). In reality, clinicians and medical staff can easily predict the prognosis of patients in poor condition from their age, appearance, and behavior. Conversely, it is difficult to estimate the prognosis of stable HD patients with good ADLs. Consequently, what we really want to know is a common risk factor in such stable HD patients.

Low serum sodium concentration is related to mortality in not only HD patients [3], but also chronic kidney disease (CKD) [4, 5] and peritoneal dialysis patients [6, 7]. However, the reason why hyponatremia induces an increased mortality has yet to be fully examined [8]. Intervention to hyponatremia is challenged by individualized

* Correspondence: knagai@tokushima-u.ac.jp
†Equal contributors
1Department of Nephrology, Institute of Biomedical Sciences, Tokushima University Graduate School, Tokushima, Japan
4Tokushima University Graduate School, 3-18-15, Kuramoto-cho, Tokushima 770-8503, Japan
Full list of author information is available at the end of the article

dialysate sodium prescription [9]. To date, dialysate sodium prescription has an effect on blood pressure and recovery time, while the relationship between dialysate sodium prescription and mortality remains uncertain [10, 11]. There is no solution to preventing a hyponatremia-related mortality risk without unveiling the hidden contributors to hyponatremia.

In this study, we investigated the risk factor for all-cause and cardiovascular mortality in stable HD patients who had undergone HD for more than 1 year at enrollment and were still alive more than 1 year after it, because HD patients have a higher mortality within a year after dialysis initiation [12] and our purpose is to seek for the prognostic marker in stable HD patients with good ADLs. Moreover, we stratified the patients according to their age to clarify the risk factor for mortality common to a wide range of ages. In addition, causes of low serum sodium concentration were evaluated, because low serum sodium was a common risk factor in our analysis.

Methods

Design and subjects

Seven hundred and forty patients received HD at Kawashima Hospital in April 2005. Of these, patients (i) who were visitors and (ii) who had acute illness, significant infection, or malignancy were initially excluded. Because our purpose of this study is to seek for the risk factor in stable maintenance HD patients who have good ADLs, the patients who had less than 1 year dialysis duration in April 2005 or who died before the end of March 2006 were also excluded, because the death rate is high in the first year after the initiation of dialysis treatment [12] and we wanted to avoid including the patients who had an unrevealed serious disease related to short life span.

Finally, 631 patients were included in the first crude analysis. Every patient received HD three times a week. In most patients, high-flux membranes with surface area of 1.4–2.2 m^2 were used according to clinical conditions. The ultrapure dialysate flow was fixed at 500 mL/min. The blood flow rate was between 220 and 280 mL/min, and the length of each HD session was between 3.5 and 5 h. Definition of cardiovascular mortality is deaths by ischemic heart disease, congestive heart failure, cerebrovascular disease, and sudden death used in the previous reports [13, 14]. This observational study was conducted for 7 years ending March 2012.

Next, we stratified the patients according to their age. We excluded 34 patients younger than 40 years old, because no one died within the 7-year observation period. We also excluded 12 patients older than or equal to 85 years old, because life expectancy is short. In fact, among the above mentioned 12 participants, 11 died within 7 years, and one moved 3 years later. The other patients were dichotomized between 40 and 64 years and 65 and 84 years old and defined as "middle-aged" and "older" patients, because the median age for prevalent HD patients was around 65 years old [12]. As a result, 341 patients were included in the middle-aged patient group, and 244 were involved in the older patient group in the second, age-stratified analysis.

Demographic and clinical characteristics were collected in April 2005. Blood samples for biochemical data were obtained from arteriovenous shunt just before starting the first HD session of the week. Cumulative mean predialysis β_2-microglobulin was the average value of serum β_2-microglobulin concentration taken every 6 months. Sodium concentration and interdialytic weight gain (the percentage of body weight gain/dry weight) were the average of the values in the first HD session of the first week in April, May, and June 2005. Kt/V, normalized protein catabolic rate (n-PCR) and creatinine generation rate (CGR) were calculated according to the formula of Shinzato [15, 16]. Serum calcium concentration was adjusted for serum albumin according to the equation: corrected Ca = measured Ca + (4.0 - serum albumin in g/dL) [17].

Statistical analysis

All values are expressed as mean ± SD. Spearman's coefficients are denoted by r_s. Statistical analysis was performed using SPSS for Windows version 13.0 (SPSS, Inc., Chicago, IL, USA). The variables related to patients' survival were initially examined by univariate Cox proportional hazards method. Urea nitrogen, creatinine, and hematocrit were deleted from the analysis because of a strong association ($r_s > 0.7$) with n-PCR, CGR, and hemoglobin, respectively. Multivariate Cox proportional hazards analysis were performed to identify the independent risk factor associated with mortality. In multivariate analysis, age, gender, HD duration, and diabetic nephropathy as the primary disease were unconditionally chosen in both full and final model analysis. The other possible factors associated with mortality that showed P less than 0.15 in univariate analysis were chosen in full model analysis. Variables that showed P less than 0.1 in full model analysis were used in final model analysis. The difference between groups was analyzed using Student's t test or Welch's t test. F test was used for comparing the factors of the total deviation. Categorical data were compared by the chi-square test. Correlation was analyzed by Spearman's rank correlation. Single and multiple regression analyses were also performed to explain serum sodium concentration using the variables above. Predialysis blood glucose level was added instead of diabetic nephropathy as the primary disease. The variables that showed P less than 0.05 in single regression analysis were used as possible factors in multiple regression analysis. Significance was defined by P less than 0.05.

Initially, the analysis was done using sodium concentration in April 2005. To confirm the results, the analysis was re-examined using average sodium concentration. The results were similar so the data obtained using average sodium concentration are shown in this manuscript.

Results

Low serum sodium concentration is a risk factor for 7-year all-cause and cardiovascular mortality of patients enrolled in crude analysis

Six hundred and thirty-one patients undergoing stable maintenance HD in April 2005 were enrolled in the first crude analysis. They were aged 24 to 94 years (mean ± SD, 61.1 ± 12.2 years). There were 395 men and 236 women. The clinical diagnoses of primary renal disease included chronic glomerulonephritis ($n = 286$), diabetic nephropathy ($n = 126$), nephrosclerosis ($n = 22$), polycystic kidney disease ($n = 17$), toxemia of pregnancy ($n = 18$), and others/unknown ($n = 162$). In the following 7-year observation period (actual follow-up period: 68.3 ± 23.3 months), 194 patients (30.7%) died. Among the 194 patients who died, 72 patients (11.4%) died from cardiovascular events. These events consisted of ischemic heart disease ($n = 17$), congestive heart failure ($n = 23$), cerebrovascular disease ($n = 19$), and sudden death ($n = 13$). Non-cardiovascular deaths suffered from infectious disease ($n = 64$), malignancy ($n = 13$), and the others/unknown ($n = 45$) (Table 1). To examine the influential factor for all-cause mortality, univariate analysis with Cox proportional hazard model was performed. The variables analyzed were shown in Table 1. Urea nitrogen, creatinine, and hematocrit were excluded because of a strong correlation with the other variable as described in the "Methods" section. Among them, we found that increased age, male sex, diabetic nephropathy as the primary disease, higher β_2-microglobulin, calcium, lower Kt/V, n-PCR, CGR, hemoglobin, platelet, albumin, uric acid, mean sodium, potassium, phosphate, and smaller interdialytic weight gain were related to mortality which have P less than 0.15 in univariate analysis. Multivariate analysis with Cox proportional hazard model (full model analysis) was performed using the variables above extracted in univariate analysis to identify the independent factor for mortality. As shown in Table 2, increased age, male sex, diabetic nephropathy as the primary disease, longer duration of HD, higher β_2-microglobulin, calcium, and phosphate, lower CGR, hemoglobin, and mean sodium were the possible factors with P less than 0.1 in full-model analysis. Finally, we performed multivariate analysis with Cox proportional hazard model (final model analysis) again with the possible factors. It revealed that all of the factors were the independent predictors of mortality in the final model analysis (P less than 0.05). Concerning cardiovascular mortality, increased age, male sex, diabetic nephropathy as the primary disease, and lower n-PCR, CGR, hemoglobin, albumin, uric acid, mean sodium, and phosphate were related to mortality which have P less than 0.15 in univariate analysis. As shown in Table 3, full and final model analysis revealed that increased age, male sex, diabetic nephropathy as the primary disease, lower hemoglobin, and mean sodium were the independent prognostic factors of mortality. Consequently, hyponatremia was chosen as a risk factor for both all-cause and cardiovascular mortality in the first crude analysis.

Table 1 Demographic and clinical characteristics of stable hemodialysis patients enrolled in crude analysis

Number of patients	631
Deaths during follow-up, *n* (%)	194 (30.7%)
Deaths in cardiovascular disease, *n* (%)	72 (11.4%)
Age, years	61.1 ± 12.2
Female, *n* (%)	236 (37.4%)
Diabetic nephropathy, *n* (%)	126 (20.0%)
Hemodialysis duration, months	110.1 ± 86.2
Body mass index, kg/m^2	22.2 ± 3.2
Kt/V	1.51 ± 0.26
Cumu. mean predia. β_2-M, mg/L	28.7 ± 5.3
Normalized PCR, g/kg/day	1.01 ± 0.18
Creatinine generation rate, %	100.7 ± 22.2
WBC count, 10^3/μL	6.09 ± 1.81
Hemoglobin, g/dL	10.6 ± 1.1
Hematocrit, %	32.4 ± 3.6
Platelet count, 10^3/μL	192.6 ± 56.8
Albumin, g/dL	3.66 ± 0.34
Urea nitrogen, mg/dL	75.3 ± 15.9
Uric acid, mg/dL	7.72 ± 1.18
Creatinine, mg/dL	11.4 ± 2.8
Mean predialysis sodium, mEq/L	139.9 ± 2.8
Potassium, mEq/L	4.86 ± 0.69
Calcium, mg/dL	9.83 ± 0.79
Phosphate, mg/dL	5.16 ± 1.12
Mean interdialytic weight gain, % of DW	4.52 ± 1.31
Actual follow-up period, months	68.3 ± 23.3

Calcium was adjusted for serum albumin according to the equation: corrected Ca = measured Ca + (4.0 - serum albumin in g/dL)
Urea nitrogen, creatinine, and hematocrit were excluded in crude analysis because of a strong association with normalized PCR, creatinine generation rate, and hemoglobin, respectively
Cumu. mean predia. β_2-M cumulative mean predialysis β_2-microglobulin, *PCR* protein catabolic rate. *WBC* white blood cell, *DW* dry weight

Characteristics of stable middle-aged and older patients undergoing HD

Next, we wonder whether hyponatremia is a risk factor common to a wide range of ages or not. Therefore, we

Table 2 Significant independent factors associated with all-cause mortality in stable hemodialysis patients

	Univariate			Multivariate (full model)			Multivariate (final model)		
Variable	HR	95% CI	*P*	HR	95% CI	*P*	HR	95% CI	*P*
Age (per 1 year)	1.089	1.074–1.104	< 0.001	1.100	1.081–1.119	< 0.001	1.098	1.081–1.116	< 0.001
Gender (vs. female)	1.768	1.289–2.425	< 0.001	1.702	1.172–2.471	0.005	1.759	1.264–2.449	0.001
DN (vs. non-DN)	2.149	1.583–2.915	< 0.001	1.687	1.190–2.392	0.003	1.673	1.184–2.363	0.004
HD duration (per 1 month)	0.999	0.997–1.001	0.269	1.003	1.001–1.005	0.002	1.003	1.001–1.005	0.002
β_2M (per 1 mg/L)	1.049	1.023–1.076	< 0.001	1.061	1.033–1.089	< 0.001	1.063	1.037–1.089	< 0.001
CGR (per 1%)	0.979	0.973–0.985	< 0.001	0.980	0.973–0.988	< 0.001	0.980	0.973–0.987	< 0.001
Hemoglobin (per 1 g/dL)	0.803	0.711–0.908	< 0.001	0.866	0.760–0.987	0.032	0.852	0.753–0.964	0.011
Mean sodium (per 1 mEq/L)	0.863	0.822–0.907	< 0.001	0.929	0.885–0.974	0.002	0.919	0.878–0.963	< 0.001
Calcium (per 1 mg/dL)	1.202	0.991–1.457	0.062	1.190	0.983–1.439	0.074	1.236	1.028–1.486	0.024
Phosphate (per 1 mg/dL)	0.771	0.672–0.886	< 0.001	1.213	1.035–1.422	0.017	1.181	1.022–1.365	0.024

In addition to age, gender, hemodialysis duration, and diabetic nephropathy, possible factors that showed *P* less than 0.15 in univariate analysis such as Kt/V, β_2-microglobulin, protein catabolic rate, creatinine generation rate, hemoglobin, platelet, albumin, uric acid, mean sodium, potassium, calcium, phosphate, and mean interdialytic weight gain were chosen in full-model analysis

Final model analysis was done with age, gender, hemodialysis duration, diabetic nephropathy, and the variables with *P* less than 0.1 in full-model analysis such as β_2-microglobulin, creatinine generation rate, hemoglobin, mean sodium, calcium, and phosphate

DN diabetic nephropathy, *HD duration* hemodialysis duration, *β_2M* cumulative mean predialysis β2-microglobulin, *CGR* creatinine generation rate, *HR* hazard ratio, *95% CI* 95% confidence interval

divided the stable HD patients into middle-aged and older patients. As shown in Additional file 1: Table S1, as expected, older patients had a higher mortality. Causes of death were shown in Additional file 2: Table S2. Older patients included a larger percentage of ones diagnosed with diabetic nephropathy and had shorter HD duration, lower n-PCR, CGR, hemoglobin, platelet, albumin, potassium, phosphate, and smaller interdialytic weight gain, suggesting older patients had lower activity and nutrient intake than middle-aged patients.

Low serum sodium concentration was selected as a prognostic factor for 7-year survival of stable middle-aged patients in age-stratified analysis

In stable middle-aged patients, using the same series of analysis, increased age, male sex, longer duration of HD, higher β_2-microglobulin, white blood cell (WBC) count, lower CGR, and mean sodium were the risk factors for mortality as shown in Additional file 3: Table S3. Moreover, higher WBC count and lower mean sodium were chosen as the prognostic factors for cardiovascular mortality as well as increased age and male sex (Additional file 4: Table S4). Therefore, hyponatremia was associated with poor prognosis in stable middle-aged patients.

Low serum sodium concentration was also selected as a prognostic factor for 7-year survival of stable older-aged patients in age-stratified analysis

In stable older patients, increased age, male sex, diabetic nephropathy as the primary disease, higher β_2-microglobulin, WBC count, lower CGR, hemoglobin, and mean sodium were the risk factors for mortality as shown in Additional file 5: Table S5. Moreover, lower hemoglobin and mean sodium as well as increased age and diabetic nephropathy as the primary disease were chosen as the prognostic factors for cardiovascular

Table 3 Significant independent factors associated with cardiovascular mortality in stable hemodialysis patients

	Univariate			Multivariate (Full model)			Multivariate (Final model)		
Variable	HR	95%CI	*P*	HR	95%CI	*P*	HR	95%CI	*P*
Age (per 1 year)	1.086	1.061–1.111	< 0.001	1.089	1.060–1.117	< 0.001	1.087	1.061–1.114	< 0.001
Gender (vs. female)	2.148	1.246–3.700	0.006	2.028	1.151–3.572	0.014	1.984	1.131–3.479	0.017
DN (vs. non-DN)	2.546	1.565–4.142	< 0.001	2.050	1.169–3.595	0.012	2.008	1.178–3.423	0.010
HD duration (per 1 month)	0.999	0.996–1.001	0.349	1.001	0.998–1.004	0.425	1.001	0.998–1.004	0.409
Hemoglobin (per 1 g/dL)	0.737	0.608–0.893	0.002	0.752	0.618–0.915	0.004	0.750	0.620–0.906	0.003
Mean sodium (per 1 mEq/L)	0.789	0.731–0.851	< 0.001	0.830	0.768–0.896	< 0.001	0.826	0.767–0.890	< 0.001

In addition to age, gender, hemodialysis duration, and diabetic nephropathy, possible factors that showed *P* less than 0.15 in univariate analysis such as protein catabolic rate, creatinine generation rate, hemoglobin, albumin, uric acid, mean sodium, and phosphate were chosen in full model analysis

Final model analysis was done with age, gender, hemodialysis duration, diabetic nephropathy and the variables with *P* less than 0.1 in full model analysis such as hemoglobin, and mean sodium

DN diabetic nephropathy, *HD duration* hemodialysis duration, *HR* hazard ratio, *95% CI* 95% confidence interval

mortality (Additional file 6: Table S6). Therefore, hyponatremia was also associated with poor prognosis in stable older patients.

Causes of hyponatremia

Causes of hyponatremia were unclear, so we divided patients by average mean sodium concentration. Then, as shown in Table 4, the low sodium group consisted of larger percentages of male sex, patients diagnosed with diabetic nephropathy, and had higher WBC count, platelet count, potassium, larger interdialytic weight gain, lower CGR, albumin, and uric acid. Concerning age-stratified analysis, in stable middle-aged patients, the low sodium group consisted of a larger percentage of patients diagnosed with diabetic nephropathy and had higher platelet, calcium, larger interdialytic weight gain, and lower albumin (Additional file 7: Table S7). In stable older patients, the low sodium group consisted of larger percentages of male sex, patients diagnosed with diabetic nephropathy, and had higher potassium, larger interdialytic weight gain, lower body mass index, and uric acid (Additional file 8: Table S8). Thus, low sodium concentration was especially detected in patients diagnosed with diabetic nephropathy and/or with larger interdialytic weight gain common to a wide range of ages.

Table 4 Demographic and clinical characteristics of low sodium or high sodium patients

	Low < 139.9	High ≥ 139.9	*P*
Number of patients	274	357	N/A
Deaths during follow-up, *n* (%)	108 (39.4%)	86 (24.1%)	< 0.001
Deaths in cardiovascular disease, *n* (%)	49 (17.9%)	23 (6.4%)	< 0.001
Age, years	60.6 ± 12.7	61.5 ± 11.7	0.387
Female, *n* (%)	89 (32.5%)	147 (41.2%)	0.025
Diabetic nephropathy, *n* (%)	80 (29.2%)	46 (12.9%)	< 0.001
Hemodialysis duration, months	107.4 ± 83.8	112.3 ± 88.0	0.480
Body mass index, kg/m^2	21.9 ± 3.3	22.4 ± 3.2	0.114
Kt/V	1.50 ± 0.24	1.51 ± 0.27	0.887
Cumu. mean predia. β_2-M, mg/L	29.1 ± 5.4	28.4 ± 5.2	0.113
Normalized PCR, g/kg/day	1.01 ± 0.19	1.01 ± 0.17	0.688
Creatinine generation rate, %	97.7 ± 21.8	103.0 ± 22.2	0.003
WBC count, 10^3/μL	6.32 ± 1.86	5.92 ± 1.75	0.006
Hemoglobin, g/dL	10.5 ± 1.2	10.6 ± 1.1	0.239
Hematocrit, %	32.2 ± 3.8	32.6 ± 3.4	0.111
Platelet count, 10^3/μL	199.8 ± 61.7	187.2 ± 52.1	0.006
Albumin, g/dL	3.62 ± 0.36	3.70 ± 0.32	0.003
Urea nitrogen, mg/dL	75.1 ± 17.1	75.4 ± 15.0	0.834
Uric acid, mg/dL	7.59 ± 1.25	7.83 ± 1.11	0.011
Creatinine, mg/dL	11.2 ± 2.7	11.6 ± 2.9	0.064
Mean predialysis sodium, mEq/L	137.3 ± 1.9	141.9 ± 1.3	< 0.001
Potassium, mEq/L	4.93 ± 0.74	4.80 ± 0.66	0.020
Calcium, mg/dL	9.89 ± 0.86	9.78 ± 0.73	0.073
Phosphate, mg/dL	5.11 ± 1.21	5.20 ± 1.05	0.298
Interdialytic weight gain, % of DW	4.81 ± 1.32	4.29 ± 1.26	< 0.001

Calcium was adjusted for serum albumin according to the equation: corrected Ca = measured Ca + (4.0 - serum albumin in g/dL)
Cumu. mean predia. β_2-M cumulative mean predialysis β_2-microglobulin, *PCR* protein catabolic rate, *WBC* white blood cell, *DW* dry weight, *N/A* not applicable

Non-fasting predialysis blood glucose level was inversely correlated with serum sodium concentration

The low sodium group consisted of a larger percentage of patients diagnosed with diabetic nephropathy. Therefore, we investigated the relationship between non-fasting predialysis blood glucose level and serum sodium concentration. Then, we found a weak inverse correlation between non-fasting predialysis blood glucose level and serum sodium concentration (r_s = – 0.209, 0.204, and 0.237 in crude analysis, middle-aged patients, and older patients, respectively) (Fig. 1a–c). Next, we divided the patients with blood glucose level greater than or equal to 140 mg/dL from those with blood glucose level less than 140 mg/dL. We decided the cutoff value according to the diagnostic criteria of diabetes mellitus [18]. Then, as shown in Fig. 1d–f, we found a better correlation between blood glucose level and serum sodium concentration in the patients with blood glucose level greater than or equal to 140 mg/dL (r_s = – 0.296, 0.392, and 0.157 in crude analysis, middle-aged patients, and older patients, respectively) than that in the patients with blood glucose level less than 140 mg/dL (r_s = – 0.036, 0.054, and 0.048 in crude analysis, middle-aged patients, and older patients, respectively. Data not shown.).

The correlation of interdialytic weight gain and the other variables with serum sodium concentration

The low sodium group had a larger interdialytic weight gain common to a wide range of ages. Therefore, we also investigated the correlation of interdialytic weight gain with serum sodium concentration. As shown in Fig. 2, interdialytic weight gain had a weak inverse correlation with serum sodium concentration especially in older patients. The other variables shown in Table 1 were not correlated with serum sodium concentration in all of the crude analysis, middle-aged patients, and older patients (r_s < 0.2).

Single and multiple regression analysis to explain serum sodium concentration

Single and multiple regression analyses were performed to explain serum sodium concentration. However, we could only find low coefficient of determination (at most

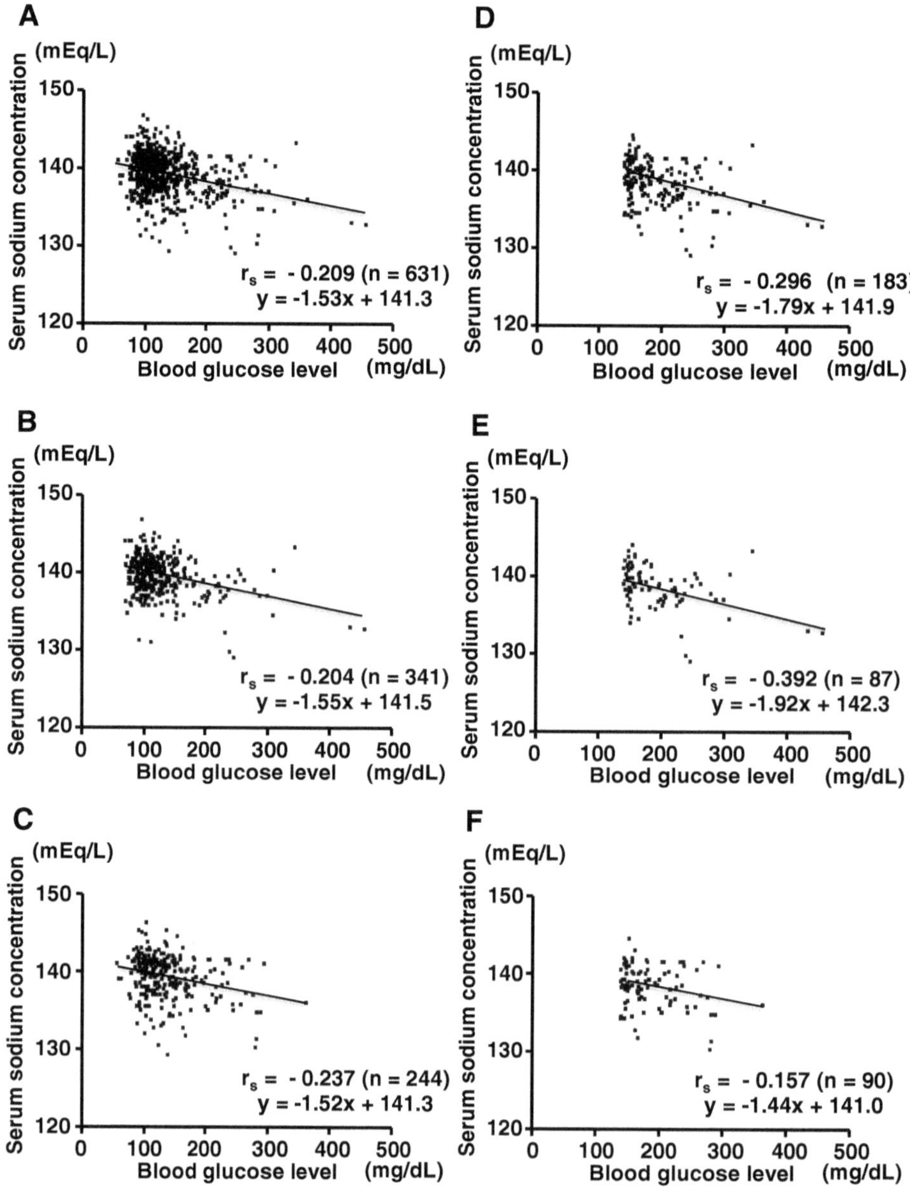

Fig. 1 Non-fasting predialysis blood glucose level was inversely related to serum sodium concentration. **a**–**c** Non-fasting predialysis blood glucose level was inversely related to serum sodium concentration in crude analysis (**a**), middle-aged patients (**b**), and older patients (**c**). **d**–**f** The relationship between serum sodium concentration and non-fasting predialysis blood glucose level in the patients with blood glucose level greater than or equal to 140 mg/dL in crude analysis (**d**), middle-aged patients (**e**), and older patients (**f**). Spearman's coefficients are denoted by r_s. The regression equation was shown in each graph

0.165 in older patients) in all of the crude analysis, middle-aged patients, and older patients (data not shown).

Discussion

In this study, we demonstrated that low serum sodium concentration is related to poor prognosis in stable HD patients. The low sodium group had a larger percentage of patients diagnosed with diabetic nephropathy and with larger interdialytic weight gain common to a wide range of ages. Predialysis blood glucose level affected serum sodium concentration.

The first finding of this study is that hyponatremia is confirmed as an independent prognostic factor for all-cause and cardiovascular mortality in stable HD patients common to a wide range of ages. HD-related guidelines were established based on the data obtained from all of the HD patients. What we really need is to find out the hidden risk factor in stable HD patients with good ADLs and look for the solution to preventing poor prognosis.

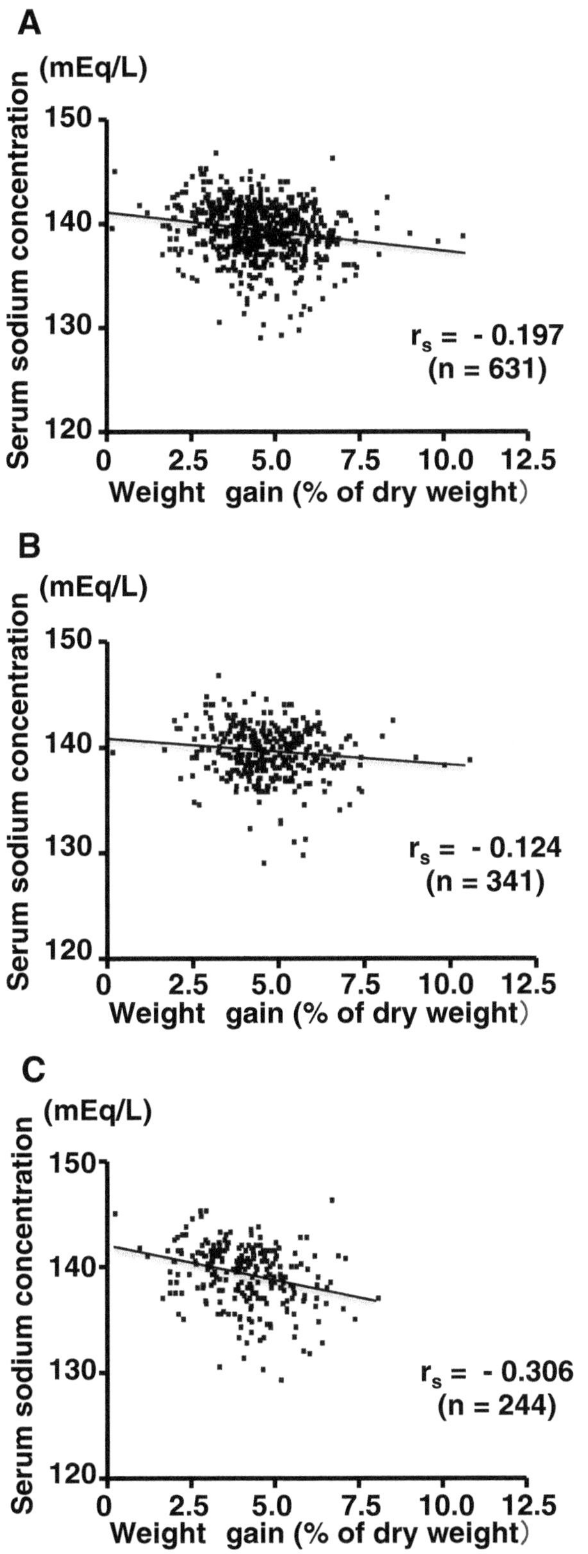

Fig. 2 The relationship between interdialytic weight gain and serum sodium concentration. Interdialytic weight gain was inversely related to serum sodium concentration especially in older patients. **a** crude analysis, **b** middle-aged patients, and **c** older patients

Serum sodium concentration is a widely available blood test item, evaluated on a daily basis. Our study clearly showed that low serum sodium concentration is important to forecast the prognosis in stable HD patients, common to a wide range of ages.

The reason why hyponatremia is associated with poor prognosis was unknown. Hyponatremia is recognized as a risk factor in CKD patients [3–8]. However, is hyponatremia a direct cause of death in HD patients? Chawla et al. discussed the role of hyponatremia in mortality in hospitalized patients [19]. The authors found that more than two thirds of patients who died after a sodium concentration less than 120 mEq/L had acute severe progressive illnesses and only 5.6% of the dead patients could plausibly be related to adverse consequences of hyponatremia. They concluded that the nature of underlying illness, rather than the severity of hyponatremia, best explains mortality associated with hyponatremia. In our study, relatively low sodium concentration within normal range was related to a higher mortality. Therefore, we also assume that hyponatremia is an indirect prognostic factor. We need to find out underlying causes of hyponatremia.

More important findings of this study were the analyses concerning causes of hyponatremia. It is noteworthy that no correlation was found between serum sodium concentration and the variables shown in Table 1 ($r_s < 0.2$) except interdialytic weight gain in older patients (Fig. 2). Next, the low sodium group in our study consisted of more patients diagnosed with diabetic nephropathy than the high sodium group. Actually, serum sodium concentration had a weak inverse correlation with non-fasting predialysis blood glucose level (Fig. 1). Katz et al. described theoretical considerations about hyperglycemia-induced hyponatremia–calculation of expected serum sodium depression, demonstrating the serum sodium concentration decreases by 1.6 mEq/l for every 100 mg/dl increase in glucose concentration due to water shifts from the intracellular to the extracellular compartment [20]. Penne et al. validated the correction factor in HD patients and reported that the mean slope for the relation between serum sodium and glucose concentration -1.47 ± 0.82 mEq/l per 100 mg/dl increase in glucose level [21]. In our study, the regression equations in Fig. 1 were consistent with the previous report, and higher glucose level had better correlation with serum sodium concentration (Fig. 1d–f), suggesting serum sodium concentration was affected by glucose-induced serum osmolarity. Therefore, when we see the HD patients with low serum sodium concentration, it can be a promising clue to diagnosing diabetes newly, because HbA1c and glycated albumin are influenced by alterations in hemoglobin and albumin metabolism, which makes it difficult to interpret these values in HD patients [22]. However, the impact of low serum sodium on survival cannot be explained only by diabetic status, because hyponatremia is an independent risk factor after adjustment of the existence of diabetic nephropathy as the primary disease. Coefficient of determination to explain serum sodium concentration was low in multiple regression analysis even if we added non-fasting predialysis blood glucose level as a possible factor. Therefore, hyponatremia reflects on a mixture of underlying causes. Pérez-García et al. reported that HD patients with hyponatremia have a poor prognosis and present malnutrition or fluid overload [23]. Poulikakos et al. reported that low serum sodium is associated with protein energy wasting and increased interdialytic weight gain in HD patients [24]. Dekker et al. found that hyponatremia is associated with malnutrition, inflammation, and fluid overload [25]. Our study supports their findings because the low sodium group had significantly lower CGR, higher WBC count, and larger interdialytic weight gain (Table 4). Interdialytic weight gain was inversely correlated with serum sodium concentration especially in older patients (Fig. 2). It might be due to the body water compartments with human aging. Intracellular water was reported lower in elderly HD patients than in young HD patients [26]. Thus, fluid overload may be also related to poor prognosis in our low serum sodium group.

Consequently, low sodium concentration is a prognostic marker related to current blood glucose level, as well as interdialytic weight gain, malnutrition, and inflammation. It means that the intervention to resolve the causes described above should be done to correct hyponatremia. Control of serum sodium concentration by dialysate sodium prescription will not have a direct effect on mortality.

The strength of this study is a long observation period. The limitation is a lack of a representative inflammation marker such as C-reactive protein. High WBC count was chosen as a risk factor for all-cause mortality in age-stratified analysis (Additional file 3: Table S3 and Additional file 5: Table S5). It suggested that inflammation is also related to mortality in our cohort. Another limitation of this study is that the finding of this study might not be applied to all patients with HD because the characteristics of enrolled patients were different from national data concerning age and the rate of the patients with diabetic nephropathy [3, 12].

Conclusions

In summary, low serum sodium concentration is an easily detectable and routinely examined prognostic factor in stable HD patients common to a wide range of ages. Causes of hyponatremia are complicated. Causes consist of not only malnutrition, inflammation, and fluid overload but also the predialysis blood glucose level. Our study suggested that current diabetic status should be checked when we see the stable HD patients with low serum sodium concentration.

Additional files

Additional file 1: Table S1. Demographic and clinical characteristics of stable hemodialysis patients analyzed in age-stratified analysis

Additional file 2: Table S2. Causes of death in stable middle-aged and older patients.

Additional file 3: Table S3. Significant independent factors associated with all-cause mortality in stable middle-aged patients.

Additional file 4: Table S4. Significant independent factors associated with cardiovascular mortality in stable middle-aged patients.

Additional file 5: Table S5. Significant independent factors associated with all-cause mortality in stable older patients.

Additional file 6: Table S6. Significant independent factors associated with cardiovascular mortality in stable older patients.

Additional file 7: Table S7. Demographic and clinical characteristics of low sodium or high sodium stable middle-aged patients.

Additional file 8: Table S8. Demographic and clinical characteristics of low sodium or high sodium stable older patients.

Acknowledgments
Not applicable.

Funding
None.

Authors' contributions
KT designed and promoted the study. SU acquired and summarized data. KN statistically analyzed the results and wrote the manuscript. TD gave critical revision of article. JM conceived and reviewed the study. All authors read and approved the final manuscript.

Competing interests
The authors declare that they have no competing interests.

Author details
[1]Department of Nephrology, Institute of Biomedical Sciences, Tokushima University Graduate School, Tokushima, Japan. [2]Department of Dialysis Vascular Surgery, Tsuchida Dialysis Access Clinic, Osaka, Japan. [3]Department of Kidney Disease (Dialysis & Transplantation), Kawashima Hospital, Tokushima, Japan. [4]Tokushima University Graduate School, 3-18-15, Kuramoto-cho, Tokushima 770-8503, Japan. [5]Tsuchida Dialysis Access Clinic, 2-10-18, Fujiidera DH building 4F, Oka, Fujiidera City, Osaka 583-0027, Japan.

References

1. Nakagawa N, Matsuki M, Yao N, Hirayama T, Ishida H, Kikuchi K, Hasebe N. Impact of metabolic disturbances and malnutrition-inflammation on 6-year mortality in Japanese patients undergoing hemodialysis. Ther Aper Dial. 2015;19:30–9.
2. Watanabe Y, Kawanishi H, Suzuki K, Nakai S, Tsuchida K, Tabei K, et al. Japanese society for dialysis therapy clinical guideline for "maintenance hemodialysis: hemodialysis prescriptions". Ther Aper Dial. 2015;19(Suppl 1):67–92.
3. Rhee CM, Ravel VA, Ayus JC, Sim JJ, Streja E, Mehrotra R, et al. Pre-dialysis serum sodium and mortality in a national incident hemodialysis cohort. Nephrol Dial Transplant. 2016;31:992–1001.

4. Huang H, Jolly SE, Airy M, Arrigain S, Schold JD, Nally JV, Navaneethan SD. Associations of dysnatremias with mortality in chronic kidney disease. Nephrol Dial Transplant. 2017;32:1204–10.
5. Chiu DY, Kalra PA, Sinha S, Green D. Association of serum sodium levels with all-cause and cardiovascular mortality in chronic kidney disease: results from a prospective observational study. Nephrology (Carlton). 2016;21:476–82.
6. Chang TI, Kim YL, Kim H, Ryu GW, Kang EW, Park JT, et al. Hyponatremia as a predictor of mortality in peritoneal dialysis patients. PLoS One. 2014;9: e111373.
7. Ravel VA, Streja E, Mehrotra R, Sim JJ, Harley K, Ayus JC, et al. Serum sodium and mortality in a national peritoneal dialysis cohort. Nephrol Dial Transplant. 2017;32:1224–33.
8. Nigwekar SU, Wenger J, Thadhani R, Bhan I. Hyponatremia, mineral metabolism, and mortality in incident maintenance hemodialysis patients: a cohort study. Am J Kidney Dis. 2013;62:755–62.
9. Basile C, Lomonte C. It is time to individualize the dialysate sodium prescription. Semin Dial. 2016;29:24–7.
10. Hecking M, Karaboyas A, Rayner H, Saran R, Sen A, Inaba M, et al. Dialysate sodium prescription and blood pressure in hemodialysis patients. Am J Hypertens. 2014;27:1160–9.
11. Rayner HC, Zepel L, Fuller DS, Morgenstern H, Karaboyas A, Culleton BF, et al. Recovery time, quality of life, and mortality in hemodialysis patients: the Dialysis Outcomes and Practice Patterns Study (DOPPS). Am J Kidney Dis. 2014;64:86–94.
12. Masakane I, Nakai S, Ogata S, Kimata N, Hanafusa N, Hamano T, et al. An overview of regular dialysis treatment in Japan (as of 31 December 2013). Ther Apher Dial. 2015;19:540–74.
13. Kakiya R, Shoji T, Tsujimoto Y, Tatsumi N, Hatsuda S, Shinohara K, et al. Body fat mass and lean mass as predictors of survival in hemodialysis patients. Kidney Int. 2006;70:549–56.
14. Shoji T, Shinohara K, Kimoto E, Emoto M, Tahara H, Koyama H, et al. Lower risk for cardiovascular mortality in oral 1alpha-hydroxy vitamin D3 users in a haemodialysis population. Nephrol Dial Transplant. 2004;19:179–84.
15. Shinzato T, Nakai S, Fujita Y, Takai I, Morita H, Nakane K, Maeda K. Determination of Kt/V and protein catabolic rate using pre- and postdialysis blood urea nitrogen concentrations. Nephron. 1994;67:280–90.
16. Shinzato T, Nakai S, Miwa M, Iwayama N, Takai I, Matsumoto Y, et al. New method to calculate creatinine generation rate using pre- and postdialysis creatinine concentrations. Artif Organs. 1997;21:864–72.
17. Shigematsu T, Akizawa T, Uchida E, Tsukamoto Y, Iwasaki M, Koshikawa S, KRN1493 Study Group. Long-term cinacalcet HCl treatment improved bone metabolism in Japanese hemodialysis patients with secondary hyperparathyroidism. Am J Nephrol. 2009;29:230–6.
18. Committee of the Japan Diabtes Society on the Diagnostic Criteria of Diabetes Mellitus. Report of the committee on the classification and diagnostic criteria of diabetes mellitus. J Diabetes Investig. 2010;1:212–28.
19. Chawla A, Sterns RH, Nigwekar SU, Cappuccio JD. Mortality and serum sodium: do patients die from or with hyponatremia? Clin J Am Soc Nephrol. 2011;6:960–5.
20. Katz MA. Hyperglycemia-induced hyponatremia—calculation of expected serum sodium depression. N Engl J Med. 1973;289:843–4.
21. Penne EL, Thijssen S, Raimann JG, Levin NW, Kotanko P. Correction of serum sodium for glucose concentration in hemodialysis patients with poor glucose control. Diabetes Care. 2010;33:e91.
22. Inoue K, Goto A, Kishimoto M, Tsujimoto T, Yamamoto-Honda R, Noto H, et al. Possible discrepancy of HbA1c values and its assessment among patients with chronic renal failure, hemodialysis and other diseases. Clin Exp Nephrol. 2015;19:1179–83.
23. Pérez-García R, Palomares I, Merello JI, Ramos R, Maduell F, Molina M, et al. Hyponatraemia, mortality and haemodialysis: an unexplained association. Nefrologia. 2016;36:42–50.
24. Poulikakos D, Marks V, Lelos N, Banerjee D. Low serum sodium is associated with protein energy wasting and increased interdialytic weight gain in haemodialysis patients. Clin Kidney J. 2014;7:156–60.
25. Dekker MJ, Marcelli D, Canaud B, Konings CJ, Leunissen KM, Levin NW, et al. Unraveling the relationship between mortality, hyponatremia, inflammation and malnutrition in hemodialysis patients: results from the international MONDO initiative. Eur J Clin Nutr. 2016;70:779–84.
26. Lee JE, Jo IY, Lee SM, Kim WJ, Choi HY, Ha SK, et al. Comparison of hydration and nutritional status between young and elderly hemodialysis patients through bioimpedance analysis. Clin Interv Aging. 2015;10:1327–34.

15

Triglyceride to high-density lipoprotein cholesterol ratio predicts cardiovascular events in maintenance hemodialysis patients

Ayako Hasegawa[1], Fumiko Kojima[1], Mio Ueda[1], Yoshiko Tanaka[1] and Kosaku Nitta[2*]

Abstract

Background: The triglyceride to high-density lipoprotein cholesterol (TG/HDL-C) ratio has been shown to be a predictor of cardiovascular (CV) outcomes in the general population. The aim of this study was to determine whether the TG/HDL-C ratio is a predictor of CV events and all-cause mortality in maintenance hemodialysis (MHD) patients.

Methods: We performed a retrospective, observational cohort study in which we enrolled 193 MHD patients from a single center in Japan who had been followed up for a median of 3.9 years. The outcomes were the occurrence of a CV event and all-cause mortality during the follow-up period. Baseline TG/HDL-C ratios were investigated for associations with outcomes by using Cox regression models adjusted for demographic parameters.

Results: Overall, 88 of the subjects experienced a CV event, and 32 patients had died, of whom 4 died due to CV events. Patients with higher TG/HDL-C levels (tertile 3) had a higher incidence of CV events (adjusted hazard ratio [HR] 1.82, 95 % confidence interval [CI] 1.01–3.35) and higher all-cause mortality (adjusted HR 6.13, 95 % CI 2.13–20.22) than the patients in tertile 1. Kaplan–Meier analyses by the log-rank test showed that the TG/HDL-C ratio had significant predictive power for detecting a CV event.

Conclusions: The TG/HDL-C ratio is a reliable and easily accessible marker for predicting CV events and mortality in MHD patients.

Keywords: Triglyceride to HDL cholesterol ratio, Cardiovascular events, Hemodialysis, Survival

Background

Chronic kidney disease (CKD) is one of the major causes of dyslipidemia [1], and an elevated serum triglyceride (TG) level is a common feature of CKD [2]. The serum concentrations of TG-rich lipoproteins, including very-low-density lipoprotein, start to increase in the early stages of CKD. The predominant mechanism responsible for the increased concentration of TG-rich lipoproteins in CKD is a low catabolic rate [3]. By contrast, several epidemiological studies have demonstrated that high-density lipoprotein cholesterol (HDL-C) is a negative risk factor for atherosclerosis [4].

* Correspondence: knitta@kc.twmu.ac.jp
[2]Department of Medicine, Kidney Center, Tokyo Women's Medical University, 8-1 Kawada-cho, Shinjuku-ku, Tokyo 162-8666, Japan
Full list of author information is available at the end of the article

Dyslipidemia in which there is a combination of a high TG level and low HDL-C level has been reported to strongly predict cardiovascular (CV) morbidity, and coronary artery disease, in particular, in the general population [5, 6]. Several studies have demonstrated a correlation between the TG to HDL-C (TG/HDL-C) ratios and both the severity of insulin resistance and presence of coronary atherosclerotic lesions in the general population [7, 8]. The TG/HDL-C ratio has been shown to predict the occurrence of myocardial infarction, ischemic heart disease [9, 10], and CV mortality, both in women with coronary artery disease and in the general population [11, 12].

Low-density lipoprotein cholesterol (LDL-C) has been found to be a non-sensitive marker for risk of CV events because of its weak association with coronary events in CKD patients who have a low estimated glomerular filtration rate [13, 14], and no CV benefit in HD patients has been clearly demonstrated in response to aggressive LDL-C reduction strategies [15, 16]. Hypertriglyceridemia has been reported to have a U-shaped relationship with mortality in HD patients [17, 18], whereas HDL-C has been reported to have a discordant association with all-cause or CV mortality in HD patients [19, 20].

The aim of this study was to determine if the TG/HDL-C ratio is a predictor of CV events and all-cause mortality in maintenance HD (MHD) patients.

Methods

Subjects

This was a retrospective cohort study conducted at a single center in Japan. The subjects were recruited from among patients who had been routinely dialyzed via an arteriovenous fistula in the dialysis unit of the Shinjuku Ishikawa Clinic for at least 6 months by the procedure [21].

MHD patients with malignancy, active inflammation, liver cirrhosis, gastrointestinal bleeding, or severe illness were excluded from participation as subjects. The patients who were enrolled as subjects ($n = 193$) had been undergoing stable regular HD with a bicarbonate dialysate. The underlying disease was chronic glomerulonephritis in 85 cases, diabetic nephropathy in 68 cases, hypertensive nephrosclerosis in 30 cases, polycystic kidney disease in 8 cases, and chronic pyelonephritis in 2 cases.

Evaluation of demographic and laboratory parameters

All patients were on thrice-weekly HD therapy. Blood pressure (BP) was measured with a mercury sphygmomanometer with the patient in the supine position after resting for 10 to 15 min, and mean values for the 1-month period preceding enrollment were used in the statistical analysis. Dry weight was targeted to achieve a normotensive edema-free state. Information regarding previous CV disease was collected from the patient's medical records. Diabetes mellitus (DM) was recorded as present if the patient had been diagnosed with DM and/or had a fasting plasma glucose concentration >126 mg/dl or HbA1c value >6.5 % or prescription of glucose-lowering agent.

A past history of CV disease was recorded as positive if the patient had a history of stroke, coronary artery disease (including myocardial infarction and unstable angina), or history of decompensated heart failure. Body mass index (BMI) was calculated by dividing body weight in kilograms by body height in meters squared and is expressed in kg/m^2.

Blood samples were collected before dialysis sessions after an overnight fast. Whole blood samples were used to measure hemoglobin, and serum samples were used to measure creatinine, albumin, calcium, phosphorus, TG, total cholesterol (T-Chol), LDL-C, HDL-C levels, and C-reactive protein (CRP) levels with an autoanalyzer (Hitachi Co., Tokyo, Japan) that uses standard laboratory methods. Whole parathyroid hormone (PTH) levels were determined by immunoassay [22].

Outcomes

Primary outcomes were a CV event, which was recorded as having occurred when a new CV event, including a coronary event (nonfatal myocardial infarction, unstable angina, and coronary revascularization) was diagnosed, a patient was hospitalized for heart failure, a patient was hospitalized for incident stroke (either ischemic or hemorrhagic stroke), or an incident peripheral arterial disease requiring surgical intervention was diagnosed. The secondary outcome was all-cause mortality. The outcome information was centrally adjudicated by trained nephrologists based on the above prespecified criteria.

Statistical analysis

Continuous data are reported as the mean value ± SD, and categorical data are reported as percentages. Differences in baseline characteristics and biochemical parameters were assessed using Student's t test and the Mann–Whitney U test. Groups of patients in different TG/HDL-C ratio tertiles were compared in regard to continuous variables by analysis of variance, and in regard to nonnormally distributed continuous variables by the nonparametric Kruskal–Wallis test, and the χ^2 test was used for categorical variables. To evaluate and compare the predictive performance of the TG/HDL-C ratio and non-HDL-C levels, we used receiver operating characteristic (ROC) curves for censored data and the area under the ROC curve (AUC) as the criterion.

We stratified the patients into three groups according to their TG/HDL-C ratio. The primary predictor variable was the TG/HDL-C ratio in each tertile. The outcome analysis was performed by using Cox proportional hazard models. We considered some variables whose P value was <0.10 according to the results of the univariate logistic regression analyses in the multivariate analysis. The adjusted covariates included age, gender, dialysis vintage, presence of DM, previous CV disease, CRP, creatinine, statin use and hemoglobin levels in the analysis of a CV event, and all-cause mortality. The results are expressed as hazard ratios (HRs) and 95 % confidence intervals (CIs). The age- and gender-related odds ratios (ORs) for CV events and all-cause mortality were calculated using logistic regression models. We also selected the non-HDL-C value (calculated by subtracting the HDL-C value from the T-Chol value) [23] and stratified the patients into tertiles accordingly for analysis. We tested for heterogeneity in the relationship between

Table 1 Baseline characteristics of the study subjects according to the TG/HDL-C ratio

	All patients	TG/HDL-C tertile 1 (0.35–1.60) $n = 64$	TG/HDL-C tertile 2 (1.61–3.00) $n = 65$	TG/HDL-C tertile 3 (3.01–64.05) $n = 64$	*P* value
Age, years	60 (50–69)	59 (51–68)	61 (51–70)	57 (49–65)	0.3249
Female sex, %	26.8	28.2	28.2	24.1	0.7819
DM, %	32.3	28.2	31.8	36.8	0.4837
Dialysis vintage, years	9.4 (4.7–15.8)	11.1 (5.7–16.3)	10.8 (4.4–16.9)	8.0 (4.6–13.8)	0.2608
History of hypertension, %	79.7	80.0	76.5	82.6	0.6107
History of previous CVD, %	29.2	23.5	35.3	28.7	0.2394
Systolic BP, mmHg	153 (139–165)	154 (142–165)	152 (138–166)	153 (136–163)	0.7112
Diastolic BP, mmHg	82 (73–91)	83 (76–91)	81 (72–90)	82 (70–93)	0.4152
BMI, kg/m^2	21.8 (19.7–24.4)	20.5 (19.0–22.6)	21.8 (19.7–24.0)	23.2 (21.1–25.7)	<0.0001
Laboratory data					
Hemoglobin, g/dL	10.7 (10.2–11.2)	10.7 (10.2–11.1)	10.6 (10.1–11.2)	10.8 (10.1–11.4)	0.2499
Creatinine, mg/dL	11.8 (10.3–13.5)	11.4 (10.15–12.75)	12.0 (10.15–13.65)	12.3 (10.4–13.9)	0.1032
Calcium (Ca), mg/dL; corrected	9.0 (8.6–9.4)	9.0 (8.6–9.4)	9.1 (8.45–9.4)	9.0 (8.6–9.4)	0.9831
Phosphorus (P), mg/dL	5.4 (4.6–6.1)	5.5 (4.8–6.2)	5.1 (4.4–5.9)	5.5 (4.5–6.1)	0.0967
Ca x P, (mg/dL)^2	48.1 (40.9–55.2)	51.4 (42.1–55.7)	45.6 (40–54.1)	47.8 (41.2–57)	0.0554
Whole PTH, pg/mL	63 (31–103)	68 (28–95)	53 (27–110)	64 (34–114)	0.5728
CRP, mg/L	0.1 (0.1–0.3)	0.1 (0.1–0.2)	0.1 (0.1–0.3)	0.1 (0.1–0.4)	0.1403
Albumin, g/L	3.9 (3.7–4.1)	3.9 (3.7–4.1)	3.9 (3.7–4.1)	3.9 (3.7–4.1)	0.9530
T-CHO, mg/dL	157 (137–178)	156 (136–177)	150 (133–170)	162 (142–188)	0.0341
TG, mg/dL	98 (70–144)	60 (47–73)	98 (83–112)	172 (138–229)	<0.0001
HDL-C, md/dL	44 (37–55)	59 (51–72)	43 (40–49)	37 (31–41)	<0.0001
LDL-C, mg/dL	77 (62–94)	69 (54–86)	79 (65–103)	86 (64–105)	0.0001
TG/HDL-C ratio	2.28 (1.29–3.66)	1.03 (0.76–1.29)	2.27 (1.84–2.61)	4.63 (3.62–6.57)	<0.0001
Medications, %					
ESA	92.5	91.5	90.5	95.4	0.4447
HMG-CoA reductase inhibitors	29.4	22.9	24.7	40.5	0.0228
Antihypertensive agents	79.0	77.7	78.8	80.5	0.9017

DM diabetes mellitus, *CVD* cardiovascular disease, *BP* blood pressure, *BMI* body mass index, *PTH* parathyroid hormone, *CRP* C-reactive protein, *T-Chol* total cholesterol, *TG* triglyceride, *HDL-C* high-density lipoprotein cholesterol, *LDL-C* low-density cholesterol, *ESAs* erythropoiesis-stimulating agents

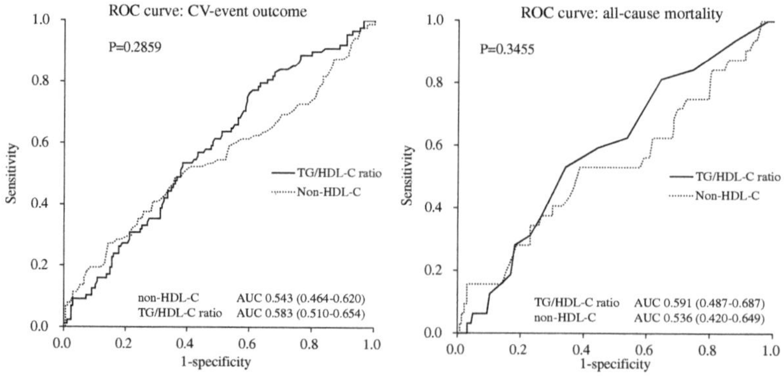

Fig. 1 ROC curve of the TG/HDL-C ratios and non-HDL-C levels as predictors of the outcomes. The TG/HDL-C ratio exhibited a similar predictive performance for cardiovascular events and all-cause mortality

Table 2 Hazard ratios (HRs) of dyslipidemia in predicting the outcomes using Cox proportional hazards regression models with multivariate adjustments

	CV event Adjusted HR (95 % CI)	All-cause mortality Adjusted HR (95 % CI)
TG/HDL-C ratio		
TG/HDL-C ratio tertile		
(Third vs first tertile)	1.82 (1.01–3.35)	6.13 (2.13–20.22)
TG/HDL-C ratio tertile		
(Second vs first tertile)	1.84 (1.05–3.31)	2.64 (0.92–8.38)
TG/HDL-C ratio >1.64 (yes vs no)	1.81 (1.11–3.06)	3.12 (1.30–8.54)
Non-HDL-C		
Non-HDL-C tertile		
(Third vs first tertile)	1.19 (0.71–2.01)	1.32 (0.55–3.20)
Non-HDL-C quartile		
(Second vs first tertile)	0.90 (0.32–2.37)	1.47 (0.49–4.29)
Non-HDL-C >140 mg/dL (yes vs no)	1.51 (0.88–2.51)	1.56 (0.53–4.09)

Adjusted for age, sex, dialysis vintage, presence of DM, concurrent CV disease, CRP, creatinine, statin use, and hemoglobin levels

subgroups by adding a multiplicative interaction term in our statistical model as previously described [24]. The survival analysis was based on the Kaplan–Meier curve with subjects censored for death. A log-rank test was used to compare the survival rates of two groups. *P* values <0.05 were considered evidence of statistical significance. All statistical analyses were performed by using the SAS version 9.2 software program (SAS Institute Inc., Cary, NC, USA) for Windows.

Results

The baseline characteristics of the subjects according to TG/HDL-C tertiles are summarized in Table 1. The study cohort consisted of 193 subjects, 52 females, and 141 males, and their mean age was 59.3 ± 12.7 years. Their mean dialysis vintage was 11.0 ± 7.7 years, and their mean BMI was 22.3 ± 3.7 kg/m^2. All of the subjects had an arteriovenous fistula. None of the subjects had residual renal function (urine volume >100 mL/day). DM was present in 32.3 %. A history of CVD was present in 29.2 %.

The patients in the TG/HDL-C tertiles had different levels of BMI and lipid profiles. There was no significant difference between the median values of TG/HDL-C ratio were 2.28 at the time of entry and 2.31 after 1 month and 2.22 after 2 months. The TG/HDL-

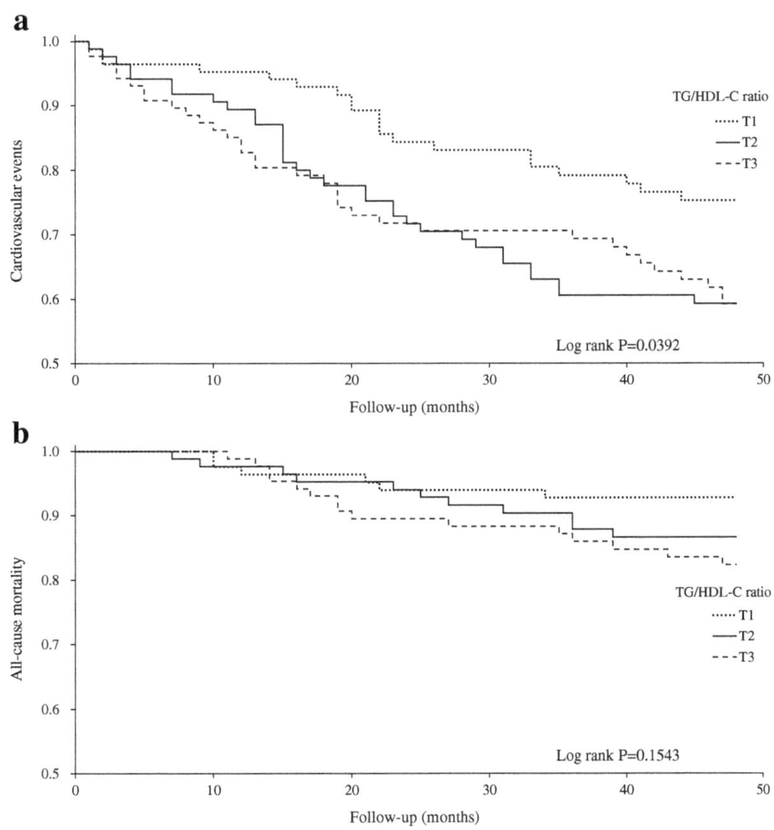

Fig. 2 Kaplan–Meier curves for patients with different TG/HDL-C ratio levels. **a** Cardiovascular events. **b** All-cause mortality

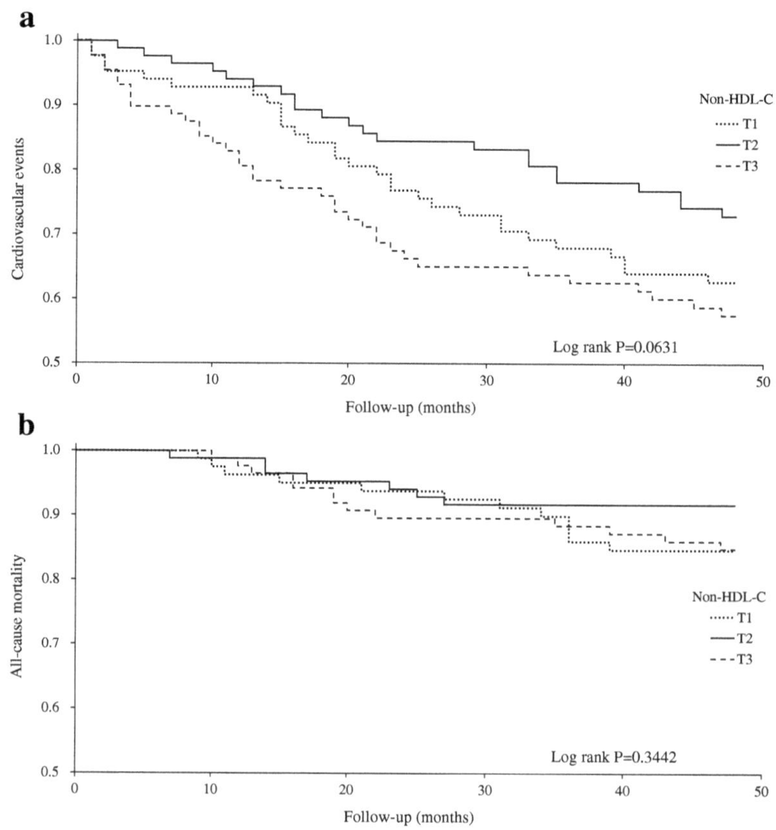

Fig. 3 Kaplan–Meier curves of patients with different non-HDL-C levels. **a** Cardiovascular events. **b** All-cause mortality

C ratio (5.02 ± 8.57) in subjects with statin treatment (29.4 %) was significantly higher than those (2.83 ± 3.09) in subjects without statin treatment (70.6 %) ($P = 0.0028$).

During the mean follow-up period of 43.3 ± 11.0 months, 88 of the subjects experienced a CV event, and 32 patients died, 4 of a CV event. Among the 88 patients who experienced a CV event, 17 had an intracranial hemorrhage or ischemic stroke, 33 had coronary artery disease (either nonfatal acute myocardial infarction or coronary revascularization or coronary bypass surgery), 11 had peripheral arterial disease, 16 were hospitalized for heart failure, and the CV events in the other subjects were unknown. Of the 32 patients who died of any cause, 11 died of an infectious disease, 6 of a sudden cardiac death, 5 of malignancy, and 4 of a cerebrovascular event, and the causes of other death were unknown.

The AUCs for the TG/HDL-C ratio and non-HDL-C level vs. outcomes are shown in Fig. 1. The TG/HDL-C ratio and non-HDL-C levels exhibited similar predictive performance for CV event outcome (AUC 0.583 vs. AUC 0.543, $P = 0.2859$) and all-cause mortality outcome (AUC 0.591 vs. AUC 0.536, $P = 0.3455$).

In the multivariate Cox regression model, the MHD patients with a higher TG/HDL-C level (tertile 3; T3) had a higher incidence of CV events (adjusted HR 1.82, 95 % CI 1.01–3.35) and higher all-cause mortality (adjusted HR 6.13, 95 % CI 2.13–20.22) than the patients in tertile 1 (T1, Table 2). When the TG/HDL-C ratio was used as a dichotomous variable, the group with a TG/HDL-C ratio >1.64 was found to have a higher incidence of CV events (adjusted HR 1.81, 95 % CI 1.11–3.06). Similarly, the group in non-HDL-C tertile 3 also had a higher incidence of CV events and all-cause mortality than the group in non-HDL-C tertile 1. In addition, the group with a TG/HDL-C ratio >1.64 was found to have a higher incidence of cerebrovascular events, although not significant (adjusted HR 2.66, 95 % CI 0.85–3.14).

The Kaplan–Meier survival estimates of CV events and all-cause mortality at different TG/HDL-C ratios are shown in Figs. 2 and 3. The results of the log-rank test showed that the TG/HDL-C ratio had significant predictive power for detecting the CV events (Fig. 2a, $P = 0.0392$). However, the TG/HDL-C ratio did not significantly significant contribute to predicting all-cause mortality (Fig. 2b, $P = 0.1543$). As shown in Fig. 3a, b, there was no significant difference in non-HDL-C level tertiles for predicting CV events ($P = 0.0631$) and all-cause mortality ($P = 0.3442$).

Stratified analyses to detect associations between TG/HDL-C ratios and CV events and all-cause mortality according to gender and presence of DM revealed that the risk of a CV event gradually increased with greater TG-HDL-C ratios ($P = 0.0076$ for interaction, Fig. 4a). However, the risk of all-cause mortality was not associated with greater TG-HDL-C ratios (Fig. 4b).

Discussion

The results of this study showed that the baseline TG/HDL-C ratio was predictive of CV events and all-cause mortality in MHD patients. Dyslipidemia in MHD patients with the TG/HDL-C ratio for stratification of its severity should be recognized as a reliable and readily available tool for predicting long-term CV outcomes and survival.

HD patients have unique lipid profiles, and the associations between their lipid profiles and CV outcomes and mortality are different from the associations in the general population [17]. Several clinical studies of dialysis patients have reported finding unique correlations between the levels of T-CHO and LDL-C levels and CV outcomes, the so-called "cholesterol paradox" [25, 26]. In addition, recent data have shown the absence of a significant association between the HDL-C levels and their risk of CV events of diabetic HD patients [20], and HDL-C and TG did not to predict CV or all-cause mortality in a large HD cohort who were followed up for 3 years [17]. The non-HDL-C level is also easily calculated by subtracting the HDL-C from TC, and non-HDL levels have been found to be a predictor of CV outcomes in MHD patients [27, 28]. The TG/HDL ratio was superior to the non-HDL-C as a predictor of CV event in the present study (Table 2).

We used the TG/HDL-C ratio to predict CV events and all-cause mortality in MHD patients in the present

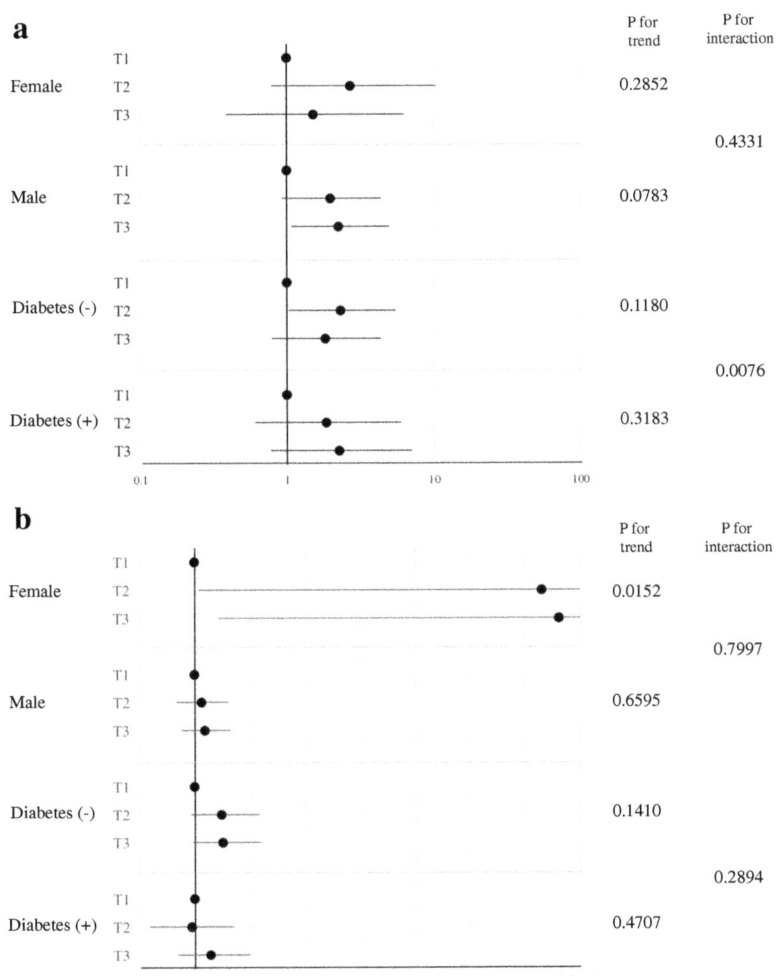

Fig. 4 Odds ratio for CV events (**a**) and all-cause mortality (**b**) according to tertile (T) of TG/HDL-C ratio stratified by gender and presence of diabetes mellitus

study, and the results clearly demonstrated the predictive power of the TG/HDL-C ratio. Chen et al. have recently shown the predictive ability of the TG/HDL-C ratio for CV outcomes and survival in patients undergoing prevalent dialysis [29]. The TG/HDL-C ratio may therefore be the optimal marker for predicting CV outcomes in MHD patients. Moreover, a higher TG/HDL-C ratio including atherogenic lipoprotein particles results in consequent CV events in MHD patients [30].

The cut-off value of TG/HDL-C ratio in prediction of CV event in our study was much lower than that in the previous studies [29, 31]. One of the reasons for lower TG/HDL-C ratio of our patients seems to be based on the good management of food intake by dietitian. In addition, most of the patients came to our dialysis clinic without assistance on foot. Moreover, we could not rule out the effects of statin treatment. The TG/HDL-C ratio (5.02 ± 8.57) in subjects with statin was significantly higher than those (2.83 ± 3.09) in subjects without statin ($P = 0.0028$), suggesting that statin had been administered to patients with increased serum TG.

The mechanisms underlying the association between TG/HDL-C ratios and CV event and all-cause mortality in MHD patients are still unknown. A previous study showed significant associations between increases in TG/HDL ratio and both decreases in LDL particle size and increases in fractional esterification rates of cholesterol in plasma depleted of apoB lipoproteins [32]. Moreover, the TG/HDL-C ratio is already been used as a predictor of insulin resistance [33] and DM [34]. Insulin resistance has been found to increase the serum concentrations of TGs and HDL-C, and the TG/HDL-C ratio was involved in decreased insulin secretion and poor glycemic control among subjects with type 2 DM [35].

We found an interaction between the TG/HDL-C ratio and DM in the prediction of CV events (Fig. 4a). This finding is consistent with the interaction between them in predicting events in the general population, and patients with a high TG/HDL-C ratio have been reported to be predisposed to DM [36]. The diabetic status of patients with both DM and dyslipidemia is crucial when assessing CV outcomes compared with non-diabetic patients with dyslipidemia. As shown in a clinical study [37], manipulation of high TG and low HDL-C levels in DM patients by medical interventions does not reduce their risk of CV outcomes. Consequently, the utility of the TG/HDL-C ratio for predicting long-term CV outcomes in diabetic MHD patients should be carefully assessed in further large-scale investigations.

The present study had several limitations. First, the observational nature of the study precludes drawing conclusions about causal relationships. Second, we did not measure the specific lipoproteins related to atherogenic dyslipidemia, such as apolipoprotein B, which may be more specific to LDL particles, and the relationship between TG/HDL-C ratios and apolipoproteins in MHD patients needs to be validated further. Third, the AUC for TG/HDL-C ratio was 0.583, implying a low accuracy (<0.7). Fourth, this was a single-center study; all of the participants were Japanese and treated by the same physicians, and the same uniform laboratory tests were performed during the observation period, which guaranteed the accuracy of our results, but our conclusions cannot be generalized to other ethnicities.

Conclusions

The results of this study suggest that the TG/HDL-C ratio can independently predict CV events and mortality in MHD patients, especially in diabetic MHD patients.

Abbreviations

BP: Blood pressure; CKD: Chronic kidney disease; DM: Diabetes mellitus; HDL-C: High-density lipoprotein cholesterol; MHD: Maintenance hemodialysis; TG: Triglyceride

Acknowledgements

The authors thank all the participants and medical staff at Shinjuku Ishikawa Clinic.

Funding

This study was supported in part by a Grant-in-Aid from the Japan Promotion Society for Cardiovascular Diseases.

Authors' contributions

AH planned the study, searched the literature, assessed the study protocols, extracted the data, analyzed the data, and prepared the article. YT, FK, and UM searched the literature, assessed the study results, and assisted in the preparation of article. KN planned the study, analyzed the data, and assisted in the preparation of article. All authors read and approved the final manuscript.

Competing interests

The authors declare that they have no competing interests.

Author details

[1]Department of Nephrology, Shinjuku Ishikawa Clinic, Tokyo, Japan.
[2]Department of Medicine, Kidney Center, Tokyo Women's Medical University, 8-1 Kawada-cho, Shinjuku-ku, Tokyo 162-8666, Japan.

References

1. Nitta K. Clinical assessment and management of dyslipidemia in patients with chronic kidney disease. Clin Exp Nephrol. 2012;16:522–9.
2. Attman PO, Samuelsson O. Dyslipidemia of kidney disease. Curr Opin Lipidol. 2009;20:293–9.

3. Prinsen BH, de Sain-van der Velden MG, de Koning EJ, Koomans HA, Berger R, Rabelink TJ. Hypertriglycemia in patients with chronic renal failure: possible mechanisms. Kidney Int Suppl. 2003;84:S121–4.
4. Despres JP, Lemieux I, Dagenais GR, Cantin B, Lamarche B. HDL-cholesterol as a marker of coronary heart disease risk: the Quebec cardiovascular study. Atherosclerosis. 2000;153:263–72.
5. Ballantyne CM, Olsson AG, Cook TJ, Mercuri MF, Pedersen TR, Kjekshus J. Influence of low high-density lipoprotein cholesterol and elevated triglyceride on coronary heart disease events and response to simvastatin therapy in 4S. Circulation. 2001;104:3046–51.
6. Manninen V, Tenkanen L, Koskinen P, Huttunen JK, Manttari M, Heinonen OP, et al. Joint effects of serum triglyceride and LDL cholesterol and HDL cholesterol concentrations on coronary heart disease risk in the Helsinki Heart Study. Implications for treatment. Circulation. 1992;85:37–45.
7. Frohlich J, Dobiasova M. Fractional esterification rate of cholesterol and ratio of triglycerides to HDL-cholesterol are powerful predictors of positive findings on coronary angiography. Clin Chem. 2003;49:1873–80.
8. McLaughlin T, Reaven G, Abbasi F, Lamendola C, Saad M, Waters D, et al. Is there a simple way to identify insulin-resistant individuals at increased risk of cardiovascular disease? Am J Cardiol. 2005;96:399–404.
9. Gaziano JM, Hennekens CH, O'Donnell CJ, Breslow JL, Buring JE. Fasting triglycerides, high-density lipoprotein, and risk of myocardial infarction. Circulation. 1997;96:2520–5.
10. Jeppesen J, Hein HO, Suadicani P, Gymtelberg F. Low triglycerides-high high-density lipoprotein cholesterol and risk of ischemic heart disease. Arch Intern Med. 2001;161:361–6.
11. Barzi F, Patel A, Woodward M, Lawes CM, Ohkubo T, Gu D, et al. A comparison of lipid variables as predictors of cardiovascular disease in the Asia Pacific region. Ann Epidemiol. 2005;15:405–13.
12. Bittner V, Johnson BD, Zineh I, Rogers WJ, Vido D, Marroquin OC, et al. The triglyceride/high-density lipoprotein cholesterol ratio predicts all-cause mortality in women with suspected myocardial ischemia: a report from the Women's Ischemia Syndrome Evaluation (WISE). Am Heart J. 2009;157:548–55.
13. Tonelli M, Muntner P, Lloyd A, Manns B, Klarenbach S, Pannu N, et al. Association between LDL-C and risk of myocardial infarction in CKD. J Am Soc Nephrol. 2013;24:979–86.
14. Wanner C, Tonelli M. Kidney Disease: Improving Global Outcomes Lipid Guideline Development Work Group Members. KDIGO Clinical Practice Guideline for Lipid Management in CKD: summary of recommendation statements and clinical approach to the patient. Kidney Int. 2014;85:1303–9.
15. Wanner C, Krane V, Marz W, Olschewski M, Mann JF, Ruf G, et al. Atorvastatin in patients with type 2 diabetes mellitus undergoing hemodialysis. N Engl J Med. 2005;353:238–48.
16. Fellstrom BC, Jardine AG, Schmieder RE, Holdaas H, Bannister K, Beutler J, et al. Rosuvastatin and cardiovascular events in patients undergoing hemodialysis. N Engl J Med. 2009;360:1395–407.
17. Kilpatrick RD, McAllister CJ, Kovesdy CP, Derose SF, Kopple JD, Kalantar-Zadeh K. Association between serum lipids and survival in hemodialysis patients and impact of race. J Am Soc Nephrol. 2007;18:293–303.
18. Postorino M, Marino C, Tripepi G, Zoccali C, CREDIT Working Group. Abdominal obesity modifies the risk of hypertriglyceridemia for all-cause and cardiovascular mortality in hemodialysis patients. Kidney Int. 2011;79:765–72.
19. Moradi H, Streja E, Kashyap ML, Vaziri ND, Fonarow GC, Kalantar-Zadeh K. Elevated high-density lipoprotein cholesterol and cardiovascular mortality in maintenance hemodialysis patients. Nephrol Dial Transplant. 2014;29:1554–62.
20. Silbernagel G, Genser B, Drechsler C, Scharnagl H, Grammer TB, Stojakovic T, et al. HDL cholesterol, apolipoproteins, and cardiovascular risk in hemodialysis patients. J Am Soc Nephrol. 2014;26:484–92.
21. Kobayashi S, Suzuki K, Ueda M, Tanaka Y, Nitta K. A simple protein-energy wasting score for survival prediction of maintenance hemodialysis patients. Ren Replace Ther. 2015;1:1.
22. Miwa N, Nitta K, Kimata N, Watanabe Y, Suzuki K, Kawashima A, et al. An evaluation of 1-84 PTH measurement in relation to bone alkaline phosphatase and bone Gla protein in hemodialysis patients. Nephron Clin Pract. 2003;94:c29–32.
23. Echida Y, Mochizuki T, Uchida K, Tsuchiya K, Nitta K. Serum non-high-density lipoprotein cholesterol (non-HDL-C) levels and cardiovascular mortality in chronic hemodialysis patients. Clin Exp Nephrol. 2012;16:767–72.
24. Tsuruya K, Yoshida H, Nagata M, Kitazono T, Hirakata H, Iseki K, et al. Association of the triglycerides to high-density lipoprotein cholesterol ratio with the risk of chronic kidney disease: analysis in a large Japanese population. Atherosclerosis. 2014;233:260–7.
25. Suliman ME, Stenvinkel P, Barany P, Heimburger O, Anderstam B, Lindholm B. Hyperhomocysteinemia and its relationship to cardiovascular disease in ESRD: influence of hypoalbuminemia, malnutrition, inflammation, and diabetes mellitus. Am J Kidney Dis. 2003;41(3 Suppl 1):S89–95.
26. Liu Y, Coresh J, Eustace JA, Longenecker JC, Jaar B, Fink NE, et al. Association between cholesterol level and mortality in dialysis patients: role of inflammation and malnutrition. JAMA. 2004;291:451–9.
27. Shoji T, Masakane I, Watanabe Y, Iseki K, Tsubakihara Y, et al. Elevated non-high-density lipoprotein cholesterol (non-HDL-C) predicts atherosclerotic cardiovascular events in hemodialysis patients. Clin J Am Soc Nephrol. 2011;6:1112–20.
28. Echida Y, Ogawa T, Otsuka K, Ando Y, Nitta K. Serum non-high-density lipoprotein cholesterol (non-HDL-C) levels and cardiovascular mortality in chronic hemodialysis patients. Clin Exp Nephrol. 2012;16:767–72.
29. Chen HY, Tsai WC, Chiu YL, Hsu SP, Pai ME, Yang JY, Peng YS. Triglyceride to high-density lipoprotein cholesterol ratio predicts cardiovascular outcomes in prevalent dialysis patients. Medicine (Baltimore). 2015;94:e619.
30. Shoji T, Abe T, Matsuo H, Egusa G, Yamasaki Y, Kashihara N, et al. Chronic kidney disease, dyslipidemia, and atherosclerosis. J Atheroscler Thromb. 2012;19:299–315.
31. Hanak V, Munoz J, Teague J, Stanley Jr A, Bittner V. Accuracy of the triglyceride to high-density lipoprotein cholesterol ratio for prediction of the low-density lipoprotein phenotype B. Am J Cardiol. 2004;94:219–22.
32. Dobiasova M, Frohlich J. The plasma parameter log (TG/HDL-C) as an atherogenic index: correlation with lipoprotein particle size and esterification rate in apoB-lipoprotein-depleted plasma (FER(HDL)). Clin Biochem. 2001;34:583–8.
33. Salazae MR, Carbajal HA, Espeche WG, Leiva Sisnieguez CE, Balbin E, Dulbecco CA, et al. Relation among the plasma triglyceride/high-density lipoprotein cholesterol concentration ratio, insulin resistance, and associated cardio-metabolic risk factors in men and women. Am J Cardiol. 2012;109:1749–53.
34. Shimizu Y, Nakazato M, Sekita T, Kadota K, Yamasaki H, Takamura N, et al. Association of arterial stiffness and diabetes with triglycerides-to-HDL cholesterol ratio for Japanese me: the Nagasaki Islands Study. Atherosclerosis. 2013;228:491–5.
35. Hermans MP, Ahn SA, Rousseau MF. Log (TG)/HDL-C is related to both residual cardiometabolic risk and β-cell function loss in type 2 diabetes males. Cardiovasc Diabetol. 2010;9:88.
36. AIM-HIGH Investigators. The role of niacin in raising high-density lipoprotein cholesterol to reduce cardiovascular events in patients with atherosclerotic cardiovascular disease and optimally treated low-density lipoprotein cholesterol: baseline characteristics of study participants. The atherothrombosis intervention in metabolic syndrome with low HDL/high triglycerides: impact on global health outcomes (AIM-HIGH) trial. Am Heart J. 2011;161:538–43.
37. Keech A, Simes RJ, Barter P, Best J, Scott R, Taskinen MR, et al. Effects of long-term fenofibrate therapy on cardiovascular events in 9795 people with type 2 diabetes mellitus (the FIELD study): randomized controlled trial. Lancet. 2005;366:1849–61.

Is hemodialysis itself a risk factor for dementia? An analysis of nationwide registry data of patients on maintenance hemodialysis in Japan

Shigeru Nakai[1*], Kenji Wakai[2], Eiichiro Kanda[3], Kazunori Kawaguchi[1], Kazuyoshi Sakai[1] and Nobuya Kitaguchi[1]

Abstract

Background: Chronic kidney disease is a major risk factor for dementia, but the influence of hemodialysis itself on the development of dementia remains unclear. We previously reported that non-diabetic patients on maintenance hemodialysis have preserved cognitive function; hemodialysis removes blood amyloid β (Aβ), which is a major cause of Alzheimer's disease in the brain; and the number of Aβ deposits in the postmortem brains of hemodialysis patients was significantly less compared to that in age-matched controls not undergoing hemodialysis. We aimed to evaluate the influence of hemodialysis on the development of dementia.

Methods: We accessed the Japanese Society for Dialysis Therapy Renal Data Registry between December 31, 2009, and December 31, 2010. Dementia was identified in 120,101 patients undergoing maintenance hemodialysis. The association between hemodialysis duration and dementia risk was analyzed using logistic regression analysis.

Results: There was a significant decrease in the dementia risk with an increase in the hemodialysis duration, with odds ratios (95% confidence intervals) of 0.78 (0.74–0.82) and 0.88 (0.78–0.99) for every 10 years in non-diabetic and diabetic patients, respectively. However, in diabetic patients, the correlation between hemodialysis duration and dementia risk was not consistent.

Conclusion: A longer hemodialysis duration was correlated with a lower dementia risk, but the correlation between hemodialysis duration and dementia risk in diabetic patients was much weaker and vaguer than that in non-diabetic patients. This finding does not appear to contradict greatly the assumption that the reduction in dementia risk with a prolonged hemodialysis duration in non-diabetic patients was caused not only by the survivor effect but also by hemodialysis itself.

Keywords: Dementia, Dialysis, Epidemiology, Hemodialysis duration, Amyloid β

Background

Chronic kidney disease (CKD) is a major risk factor for dementia [1, 2]. Fukunishi et al. [3] reported that the annual incidence rate of dementia among elderly patients was 7.4 times higher in those on hemodialysis than in those from the general population. Lin et al. [4] showed that there is no significant difference in dementia risk between patients undergoing hemodialysis and those undergoing peritoneal dialysis. However, the influence of long-term hemodialysis itself on the development of dementia remains unclear.

Alzheimer's disease (AD) is a major cause of dementia [5], and the accumulation of amyloid β (Aβ) protein in the brain in this condition was thought to cause cognitive impairment [6]. Moreover, the metabolic degradation of Aβ and its clearance from the brain are impaired in patients with AD [7]. If Aβ clearance from the brain can be increased, it is considered that AD could be prevented or even treated. To this end, treatment with antibodies

* Correspondence: s-nakai@fujita-hu.ac.jp
[1]Faculty of Clinical Engineering Technology, Fujita Health University School of Health Sciences, Dengakugakubo 1-98, Kutsukake-cho, Toyoake, Aichi 470-1192, Japan
Full list of author information is available at the end of the article

against Aβ has been shown to result in cognitive improvement and reduced Aβ burden in the brain among patients with AD [8]. Furthermore, in a current human clinical trial, patients with AD are being treated with peripheral administration of albumin, which is an Aβ-binding substance, and this phase 2 trial already has reported improved cognitive function in patients with AD [9]. Kato et al. [10] showed that hemodialysis removes Aβ, and Kitaguchi et al. [11] showed that cognitive function was maintained or improved in most patients undergoing maintenance non-diabetic hemodialysis over a period of 18 to 36 months. Sakai et al. [12] reported that the deposition of Aβ in postmortem brain tissue was decreased significantly in patients who had undergone hemodialysis compared to that in age-matched patients who had not undergone hemodialysis. Reusche et al. [13] reported similar results. These reports suggest that hemodialysis itself may prevent development of AD through removal of Aβ from the blood.

The Japanese Society for Dialysis Therapy (JSDT) has been conducting epidemiologic studies in dialysis facilities throughout Japan since 1968. Since 1983, more than 700,000 patients have been registered in an electronic database, including those who have died (JSDT Renal Data Registry [JRDR]) [14]. The influence of hemodialysis therapy itself on the development of dementia is unclear. Therefore, we evaluated the influence of hemodialysis therapy itself on the development of dementia using data from the JRDR.

Methods

Database search

The JSDT has been conducting annual surveys at dialysis facilities in Japan since 1968, and since 1983, all patients undergoing dialysis at the target facilities have been registered in the JRDR for monitoring [14]. The present study used the JRDR.

Subjects

Data from 282,010 patients undergoing chronic hemodialysis therapy at the end of 2009 were extracted from the JRDR (JRDR09002 dataset). At first, we selected the target patients based on their status at the end of 2009. To ensure uniformity of treatment conditions of the target patients, we excluded patients who underwent treatments other than hemodialysis. Cerebrovascular disease (CVD) is known to be a major risk factor for the development of dementia [5], but the type of dementia expected to be responsive to the preventive effects of hemodialysis is AD [10, 11]. Therefore, we excluded patients with preexisting brain infarction or brain hemorrhage. Furthermore, to analyze the dementia incidence, we excluded patients with preexisting dementia and those with missing data at the end of 2009. A total of 149,534 patients were included in the baseline dataset. Next, based on the data obtained at the end of 2010, we excluded patients who had died, were lost to follow-up, and had an unclear history of dementia. To avoid the influence of dementia caused by CVD, we excluded those with newly developed brain infarction or hemorrhage and those without information regarding these conditions. Finally, 120,101 patients were included in the analysis.

Diabetic patients are regarded as a high-risk group for AD and vascular dementia (VaD) [15]. Therefore, we speculated that the effect of blood Aβ removal by hemodialysis might be weakened by diabetes with strong risk of dementia, particularly AD. Further, some parts of dementia among diabetic patients are reported as independent diseases because dementia developed in these patients has unique pathologic conditions [16]. Thus, we analyzed not only the whole target patient group but also patients without (non-diabetic group, $n = 80{,}207$) and with (diabetic group, $n = 39{,}894$) diabetes separately.

The baseline characteristics of these patients are summarized in Tables 1 and 2. The selection process for the target patients is summarized in Fig. 1.

Dementia survey

The presence or absence of concomitant dementia, brain infarction, and brain hemorrhage was investigated through surveys conducted in 2009 and 2010 [14, 17]. The questions and possible answers are shown in Table 3.

A note stating, "A patient's primary doctor should answer this question" was added. When assessing the dementia risk, patients designated as "with dementia (requiring no care)" and "with dementia (requiring care)" at the end of 2010, but not in 2009, were recorded as patients with newly developed dementia.

Covariates

Among the items included in the 2009 and 2010 surveys, the following were used as covariates in a logistic regression analysis: Kt/V for urea calculated with a single pool model (Kt/V) [18]; body mass index (BMI), predialysis serum albumin level (albumin level), predialysis serum C-reactive protein level (CRP level), and predialysis whole blood hemoglobin level (hemoglobin level); history of myocardial infarction, limb amputation, or hip fracture; activities of daily living (ADLs); and place of residence. The response options for the questions regarding history of brain infarction, brain hemorrhage, myocardial infarction, limb amputation, and hip fracture were "Yes" and "No." The response options for the items on ADLs and place of residence are presented in the footnotes of Tables 1 and 2.

Table 1 Baseline characteristics of non-diabetic patients

		Hemodialysis duration (year)															
		0~ 1	(%)	2~4	(%)	5~9	(%)	10~14	(%)	15~19	(%)	20~24	(%)	25~	(%)	Total	(%)
Total		14,787	(100.0)	17,293	(100.0)	19,984	(100.0)	12,479	(100.0)	7452	(100.0)	4138	(100.0)	4074	(100.0)	80,207	(100.0)
Sex	Male	9106	(61.6)	10,515	(60.8)	11,814	(59.1)	7144	(57.2)	4169	(55.9)	2275	(55.0)	2251	(55.3)	47,274	(58.9)
	Female	5681	(38.4)	6778	(39.2)	8170	(40.9)	5335	(42.8)	3283	(44.1)	1863	(45.0)	1823	(44.7)	32,933	(41.1)
Age (years old)	15–64	5980	(40.4)	7584	(43.9)	10,258	(51.3)	7245	(58.1)	4654	(62.5)	2635	(63.7)	2732	(67.1)	41,088	(51.2)
	65–74	4066	(27.5)	4900	(28.3)	5612	(28.1)	3499	(28.0)	2092	(28.1)	1196	(28.9)	1133	(27.8)	22,498	(28.0)
	< 75	4741	(32.1)	4809	(27.8)	4114	(20.6)	1735	(13.9)	706	(9.5)	307	(7.4)	209	(5.1)	16,621	(20.7)
With history of myocardial infarction		630	(4.3)	780	(4.5)	767	(3.8)	467	(3.7)	314	(4.2)	187	(4.5)	190	(4.7)	3335	(4.2)
With history of limb amputation		101	(0.7)	101	(0.6)	137	(0.7)	100	(0.8)	44	(0.6)	33	(0.8)	48	(1.2)	564	(0.7)
With history of hip fracture		181	(1.2)	279	(1.6)	310	(1.6)	175	(1.4)	104	(1.4)	89	(2.2)	190	(4.7)	1328	(1.7)
ADL	No symptoms[†]	8122	(54.9)	10,072	(58.2)	12,140	(60.7)	7742	(62.0)	4553	(61.1)	2282	(55.1)	1733	(42.5)	46,644	(58.2)
	Moderate symptoms[‡]	4512	(30.5)	5153	(29.8)	5896	(29.5)	3641	(29.2)	2269	(30.4)	1414	(34.2)	1518	(37.3)	24,403	(30.4)
	≥ 50% sitting up[§]	1333	(9.0)	1307	(7.6)	1174	(5.9)	704	(5.6)	370	(5.0)	257	(6.2)	466	(11.4)	5611	(7.0)
	≥ 50% in bed[#]	496	(3.4)	429	(2.5)	416	(2.1)	176	(1.4)	125	(1.7)	96	(2.3)	206	(5.1)	1944	(2.4)
	Whole day in bed[¶]	154	(1.0)	100	(0.6)	115	(0.6)	58	(0.5)	42	(0.6)	32	(0.8)	87	(2.1)	588	(0.7)
Place of residence	Homes[§§]	13,836	(93.6)	16,614	(96.1)	19,359	(96.9)	12,138	(97.3)	7250	(97.3)	4022	(97.2)	3838	(94.2)	77,057	(96.1)
	Care facilities[^]	164	(1.1)	203	(1.2)	162	(0.8)	76	(0.6)	38	(0.5)	16	(0.4)	27	(0.7)	686	(0.9)
	Hospitals[¶¶]	694	(4.7)	335	(1.9)	316	(1.6)	170	(1.4)	106	(1.4)	62	(1.5)	163	(4.0)	1846	(2.3)
With dementia at the end of 2010		669	(4.5)	681	(3.9)	599	(3.0)	285	(2.3)	108	(1.4)	58	(1.4)	39	(1.0)	2439	(3.0)
Age (years old)*		66.2	± 14.0	65.1	± 13.8	63.0	± 13.4	61.2	± 12.5	60.2	± 11.4	60.4	± 10.1	60.8	± 8.5	63.3	± 13.1
Kt/V*		1.25	± 0.3	1.39	± 0.3	1.46	± 0.3	1.52	± 0.3	1.54	± 0.3	1.56	± 0.3	1.57	± 0.3	1.43	± 0.3
Body mass index (kg/m^2)*		21.4	± 3.3	21.5	± 3.4	21.3	± 3.3	20.8	± 3.0	20.4	± 2.9	20.2	± 2.7	19.8	± 2.7	21.0	± 3.2
Serum albumin level (g/dl)*		3.70	± 0.4	3.77	± 0.4	3.79	± 0.4	3.80	± 0.3	3.80	± 0.4	3.77	± 0.3	3.71	± 0.4	3.77	± 0.4
Serum CRP level (mg/dl)*		0.46	± 1.6	0.38	± 1.2	0.36	± 1.2	0.36	± 1.3	0.39	± 1.4	0.38	± 1.4	0.47	± 1.4	0.39	± 1.3
Hemoglobin level (g/dl)*		10.5	± 1.3	10.6	± 1.2	10.6	± 1.2	10.7	± 1.2	10.7	± 1.2	10.7	± 1.2	10.6	± 1.3	10.6	± 1.2

ADLs activities of daily living, *CRP* C-reactive protein

*Data are presented as mean ± standard deviation

[†]No symptoms (the patient can perform social activities without symptoms and behave without restrictions)

[‡]Moderate symptoms (the patient has mild symptoms and has trouble with physical work, but can walk and do light and sedentary work, such as light domestic and clerical work)

[§]≥ 50% sitting up (the patient can walk and take care of him/herself, but sometimes requires care. The patient can sit up at least half of the day, but cannot do light work)

[#]≥ 50% in bed (the patient can take care of him/herself to some extent, but often requires care and is in bed at least half of the day)

[¶]Whole day in bed (the patient cannot take care of him/herself and requires constant care. The patient must be in bed all day)

[§§]Patients' own home

[^]Care facilities (e.g., homes with care services; nursing homes, such as private nursing homes without national aid and nursing homes for families with financial difficulties; group homes; vocational centers; or relief facilities)

[¶¶]Hospitals (e.g., health service facilities for the elderly; beds for general patients, patients at chronic stage, patients requiring rehabilitation, and patients with mental illness and infectious diseases, such as tuberculosis)

Table 2 Baseline characteristics of diabetic patients

		Hemodialysis duration (year)															
		0~1	(%)	2~4	(%)	5~9	(%)	10~14	(%)	15~19	(%)	20~24	(%)	25~	(%)	Total	(%)
Total		12,756	(100.0)	13,342	(100.0)	10,273	(100.0)	2785	(100.0)	605	(100.0)	98	(100.0)	35	(100.0)	39,894	(100.0)
Sex	Male	8949	(70.2)	9215	(69.1)	6819	(66.4)	1767	(63.4)	369	(61.0)	61	(62.2)	18	(51.4)	27,198	(68.2)
	Female	3807	(29.8)	4127	(30.9)	3454	(33.6)	1018	(36.6)	236	(39.0)	37	(37.8)	17	(48.6)	12,696	(31.8)
Age (years old)	15–64	6378	(50.0)	6495	(48.7)	5040	(49.1)	1415	(50.8)	276	(45.6)	57	(58.2)	23	(65.7)	19,684	(49.3)
	65–74	3940	(30.9)	4434	(33.2)	3518	(34.2)	970	(34.8)	234	(38.7)	28	(28.6)	8	(22.9)	13,132	(32.9)
	< 75	2438	(19.1)	2413	(18.1)	1715	(16.7)	400	(14.4)	95	(15.7)	13	(13.3)	4	(11.4)	7078	(17.7)
With history of myocardial infarction		913	(7.2)	1154	(8.6)	896	(8.7)	241	(8.7)	57	(9.4)	12	(12.2)	2	(5.7)	3275	(8.2)
With history of limb amputation		383	(3.0)	571	(4.3)	638	(6.2)	220	(7.9)	66	(10.9)	8	(8.2)	5	(14.3)	1891	(4.7)
With history of hip fracture		201	(1.6)	250	(1.9)	251	(2.4)	65	(2.3)	21	(3.5)	4	(4.1)	1	(2.9)	793	(2.0)
ADL	No symptoms[†]	6419	(50.3)	6685	(50.1)	4942	(48.1)	1277	(45.9)	234	(38.7)	43	(43.9)	9	(25.7)	19,609	(49.2)
	Moderate symptoms[‡]	4121	(32.3)	4323	(32.4)	3323	(32.3)	906	(32.5)	193	(31.9)	28	(28.6)	12	(34.3)	12,906	(32.4)
	≥ 50% sitting up[§]	1425	(11.2)	1401	(10.5)	1244	(12.1)	375	(13.5)	100	(16.5)	20	(20.4)	8	(22.9)	4573	(11.5)
	≥ 50% in bed[#]	471	(3.7)	562	(4.2)	496	(4.8)	151	(5.4)	51	(8.4)	3	(3.1)	2	(5.7)	1736	(4.4)
	Whole day in bed[¶]	155	(1.2)	184	(1.4)	133	(1.3)	51	(1.8)	16	(2.6)	3	(3.1)	2	(5.7)	544	(1.4)
Place of residence	Homes[₰]	11,912	(93.4)	12,656	(94.9)	9769	(95.1)	2617	(94.0)	557	(92.1)	93	(94.9)	29	(82.9)	37,633	(94.3)
	Care facilities[^]	136	(1.1)	141	(1.1)	107	(1.0)	29	(1.0)	9	(1.5)	1	(1.0)	0	(0.0)	423	(1.1)
	Hospitals[₸]	619	(4.9)	438	(3.3)	324	(3.2)	125	(4.5)	33	(5.5)	3	(3.1)	5	(14.3)	1547	(3.9)
With dementia at the end of 2010		512	(4.0)	578	(4.3)	375	(3.7)	97	(3.5)	24	(4.0)	4	(4.1)	2	(5.7)	1592	(4.0)
Age (years old)*		64.0	± 11.5	64.2	± 11.1	64.4	± 10.5	63.9	± 10.0	64.5	± 9.9	62.9	± 9.8	60.5	± 10.5	64.2	± 11.0
Kt/V*		1.18	± 0.3	1.32	± 0.3	1.38	± 0.2	1.45	± 0.3	1.49	± 0.3	1.49	± 0.3	1.52	± 0.2	1.30	± 0.3
Body mass index (kg/m^2)*		22.5	± 3.5	22.7	± 3.6	22.4	± 3.5	21.7	± 3.3	20.7	± 3.3	20.6	± 3.4	19.8	± 3.1	22.4	± 3.5
Serum albumin level (g/dl)*		3.66	± 0.4	3.77	± 0.4	3.77	± 0.3	3.74	± 0.4	3.69	± 0.4	3.73	± 0.3	3.63	± 0.4	3.73	± 0.4
Serum CRP level (mg/dl)*		0.45	± 1.5	0.39	± 1.3	0.43	± 1.5	0.53	± 2.0	0.47	± 1.4	0.39	± 0.9	1.02	± 2.3	0.43	± 1.5
Hemoglobin level (g/dl)*		10.5	± 1.3	10.6	± 1.2	10.6	± 1.2	10.6	± 1.3	10.6	± 1.3	10.6	± 1.4	10.6	± 1.4	10.6	± 1.3

ADLs activities of daily living, *CRP* C-reactive protein

*Data are presented as mean ± standard deviation

[†]No symptoms (the patient can perform social activities without symptoms and behave without restrictions)

[‡]Moderate symptoms (the patient has mild symptoms and has trouble with physical work, but can walk and do light and sedentary work, such as light domestic and clerical work)

[§]≥ 50% sitting up (the patient can walk and take care of him/herself, but sometimes requires care. The patient can sit up at least half of the day, but cannot do light work)

[#]≥ 50% in bed (The patient can take care of him/herself to some extent, but often requires care and is in bed at least half of the day)

[¶]Whole day in bed (The patient cannot take care of him/herself and requires constant care. The patient must be in bed all day)

[₰]Patients' own home

[^]Care facilities (e.g., homes with care services; nursing homes, such as private nursing homes without national aid and nursing homes for families with financial difficulties; group homes; vocational centers; relief facilities)

[₸]Hospitals (e.g., health service facilities for the elderly; beds for general patients, patients at chronic stage, patients requiring rehabilitation, and patients with mental illness and infectious diseases, such as tuberculosis)

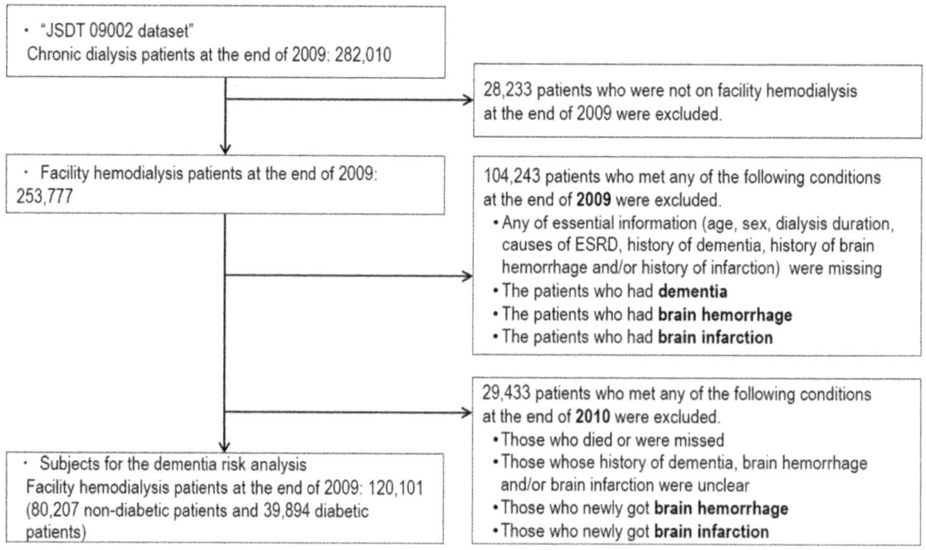

Fig. 1 Selection process for patients. Data from the Japanese Society for Dialysis Therapy (JSDT) Registry were used

Statistical analysis

All analyses were performed using the Statistical Analysis System, version 9.4 (SAS Institute, Inc., Cary, NC, USA). The incidence rate of dementia from the end of 2009 to the end of 2010 was calculated using the following formula: incidence rate of dementia (cases/1000 person-years) = the number of patients with newly developed dementia during the observation period (cases)/the total person-years of the target patients during the observation period (person-years) × 1000.

The time of dementia onset was not recorded in this survey. Therefore, the length of follow-up for patients who suffered dementia during 2010 was assumed to be 0.5 years when the incidence rate of dementia was calculated.

Because of the lack of data on the time of dementia onset, for the analyses of dementia risk, logistic regression models were constructed. All *P* values were two sided. In all models, the hemodialysis duration at the end of 2009 was used as the independent variable and the prevalence of dementia at the end of 2010 was used as the dependent variable. In these analyses, age-adjusted and multifactor models were used.

Table 3 The questions and answer options in the dementia survey

• Questions
Please indicate the presence or absence of dementia in the patient.
Please provide as much information as you can about the conditions of the patient during dialysis treatment or consultation.
(Note that the primary doctor should provide the answer.)
• Answer options
Without dementia
Without dementia (requiring no care)
Without dementia (requiring care)
Unspecified

The age and hemodialysis duration values used in this report were calculated as of the end of 2009. As age is the most independent risk factor of dementia, the age-adjusted model included only age and hemodialysis duration as independent variables. The multifactor model included baseline factors from the age-adjusted model plus additional clinical covariates (i.e., sex; comorbidity of diabetes; Kt/V; BMI; albumin level; CRP level; hemoglobin level; history of myocardial infarction, limb amputation, or hip fracture; ADLs; and place of residence). Age, hemodialysis duration, Kt/V, BMI, albumin level, CRP level, and hemoglobin level were incorporated as continuous variables, whereas the other factors were incorporated as stratified categorical variables (Tables 1 and 2). A missing value of each covariate was treated as "a missing value group" and was analyzed.

In the multifactor model analysis, we analyzed not only the whole target patients but also non-diabetic and diabetic patients separately, to compare the tendency of dementia risk of these two patient groups. In these separated analyses, we incorporated hemodialysis duration as a stratified variable into the analytic model to confirm the dementia risk trend associated with elongation of hemodialysis duration. The hemodialysis duration was stratified into the following intervals: 0 to 1, 2 to 4, 5 to 9, 10 to 14, 15 to 19, 20 to 24, and ≥ 25 years. Because patients initiated on hemodialysis within 2 years frequently have significant residual renal function, we considered hemodialysis duration of < 2 years as a separate category. The mean value of age, which is the most independent risk factor, was quite similar between the hemodialysis duration groups (Tables 1 and 2).

Finally, to evaluate how the exclusion of patients by the end of 2010 affected the results (Fig. 1, $n = 29{,}433$), we conducted the following sensitivity analyses. We analyzed the dementia risk under the assumptions that none of the excluded patients suffered dementia (negative analysis) and that all excluded patients suffered dementia (positive analysis). These analyses were conducted on the non-diabetic and diabetic patients separately, using the multifactor model.

Results

Diabetes and dementia risk

The overall dementia incidence was higher in diabetic than in non-diabetic patients (35.5 cases/1000 person-years; 95% confidence interval [CI], 33.8–37.3 vs. 30.9 cases/1000 person-years, 95% CI, 29.7–32.1; Table 4). In the multifactor model analysis, the diabetic patients did not have significant risk of dementia compared with non-diabetic patients. (Table 5).

Covariates and dementia risk

The associations between the covariates and dementia risk, which were obtained from the whole patient analysis using the multifactor model, are shown in Table 5. Female sex, elder age, and higher CRP level were associated with higher dementia risk. The dementia risk was higher in those with than in those without a history of hip fracture, whereas the risk was lower in those with than in those without a history of amputation. Predictably, reduced ADLs and residence at a hospital or care facility were associated with dementia.

Hemodialysis duration and dementia risk

As shown in Table 4, there was a decrease in the dementia incidence with an increase in hemodialysis duration in non-diabetic patients, but there was no such association in diabetic patients.

When we analyzed the whole target patient group, which included those without and with diabetes simultaneously, longer hemodialysis duration was associated significantly with lower dementia risk in the age-adjusted and multifactor model analyses (Fig. 2a).

On the other hand, when we analyzed patients without and with diabetes separately, the analytic results were different. In non-diabetic patients, longer hemodialysis duration was associated significantly with lower dementia risk in the age-adjusted and multifactor model analyses, similar to the whole patient group analyses (Fig. 2b). However, in diabetic patients, we found no significant association between hemodialysis duration and dementia risk in the age-adjusted model analysis. The multifactor model analysis showed a significant correlation between hemodialysis duration and dementia risk, but the correlation was much weaker than that found in non-diabetic patients (Fig. 2c).

Figure 3 shows the results of the analyses in which hemodialysis duration was treated as a stratified but not as a continuous variable. These analyses were done using a multifactor model. Non-diabetic patients had a consistent decrease in dementia risk with an increase in hemodialysis duration from the shortest to the longest duration strata (Fig. 3a). However, in contrast, diabetic patients had only a vague association between hemodialysis duration and dementia risk. The association between hemodialysis duration and dementia risk was not consistent along with the elongation of hemodialysis duration (Fig. 3b). At less than 5 years of hemodialysis

Table 4 Dementia incidence according to hemodialysis duration

Hemodialysis duration (year)	Non-diabetic patients				Diabetic patients			
	Number of patients	Person-years	Number of patients who developed dementia	Incidence rates of dementia (cases/1000 person-year) (95% CI)	Number of patients	Person-years	Number of patients who developed dementia	Incidence rates of dementia (cases/1000 person-year) (95% CI)
0–1	14,787	14,452.5	669	46.3 (42.9 - 49.9)	12,756	12,500.0	512	35.8 (32.9 - 39.1)
2–4	17,293	16,952.5	681	40.2 (37.3 - 43.3)	13,342	13,053.0	578	39.1 (36.1 - 42.4)
5–9	19,984	19,684.5	599	30.4 (28.1 - 33.0)	10,273	10,085.5	375	32.2 (29.1 - 35.6)
10–14	12,479	12,336.5	285	23.1 (20.6 - 25.9)	2785	2736.5	97	30.1 (24.7 - 36.8)
15–19	7452	7398.0	108	14.6 (12.1 - 17.6)	605	593.0	24	34.5 (23.1 - 51.4)
20–24	4138	4109.0	58	14.1 (10.9 - 18.3)	98	96.0	4	34.9 (13.1 - 93.1)
25–	4074	4054.5	39	9.6 (7.0 - 13.2)	35	34.0	2	50.6 (12.7 - 202.5)
Total	80,207	78,987.5	2439	30.9 (29.7 - 32.1)	39,894	39,098.0	1592	35.5 (33.8 - 37.3)

Incidence rate of dementia (cases/1000 person-years) = the number of patients with newly developed dementia during the observation period (cases)/the total person-years of the target patients during the observation period (person-years) × 1000. The length of follow-up for patients with dementia was assumed to be 0.5 years
CI confidence interval

Table 5 ORs of dementia with covariates

Covariates	Number of patients	Incident number*	OR for development of dementia	(95% CI)	p value	Covariates	Number of patients	Incident number*	OR for development of dementia	(95% CI)	p value
Age						History of myocardial infarction					
For every 10 years old	120,101	4031	1.05	(1.02 - 1.07)	0.0003	No	113,283	3762	1.00	Reference	
Sex						Yes	6610	265	1.02	(0.91 - 1.14)	0.7
Male	74,472	2112	1.00	Reference		No information available	208	4	0.61	(0.30 - 1.25)	0.2
Female	45,629	1919	1.14	(1.08 - 1.21)	0.0001	History of limb amputation					
Comorbidity of diabetes						No	117,449	3911	1.00	Reference	
Without diabetes	80,207	2439	1.00	Reference		Yes	2455	111	0.66	(0.56 - 0.77)	0.0001
With diabetes	39,894	1592	1.00	(0.94 - 1.07)	0.9	No information available	197	9	1.03	(0.53 - 2.00)	0.9
Kt/V						History of hip fracture					
For every 0.1 increase	112,533	3690	1.00	(0.99 - 1.01)	0.5	No	117,467	3789	1.00	Reference	
No information available	7568	341	1.00	(0.83 - 1.19)	1.0	Yes	2121	219	2.38	(2.10 - 2.71)	0.0001
Body mass index						No information available	513	23	1.26	(0.82 - 1.93)	0.3
For every 1 kg/m^2 increase	105,234	3390	0.99	(0.98 - 1.00)	0.2	Activities of daily living					
No information available	14,867	641	1.01	(0.81 - 1.25)	1.0	No symptoms[†]	66,253	1009	1.00	Reference	
Serum albumin level						Moderate symptoms[‡]	37,309	1159	1.13	(1.05 - 1.22)	0.001
For every 1.0 g/dl increase	116,318	3923	0.96	(0.89 - 1.04)	0.3	≥ 50% sitting up[§]	10,184	1050	4.49	(4.14 - 4.88)	0.0001
No information available	3783	108	0.76	(0.55 - 1.06)	0.1	≥ 50% in bed[#]	3680	548	9.60	(8.69 - 10.6)	0.0001
CRP level						Whole day in bed[¶]	1132	224	21.70	(18.7 - 25.2)	0.0001
For every 1.0 mg/dl increase	58,498	2276	1.02	(1.00 - 1.04)	0.03	No information available	1543	41	0.95	(0.66 - 1.37)	0.8
No information available	61,603	1755	0.94	(0.88 - 1.02)	0.1	Place of residence					

Table 5 ORs of dementia with covariates *(Continued)*

Covariates	Number of patients	Incident number*	OR for development of dementia	(95% CI)	p value	Covariates	Number of patients	Incident number*	OR for development of dementia	(95% CI)	p value
Hemoglobin level						Homes[¶¶]	114,690	3286	1.00	Reference	
For every 1.0 g/dl increase	118,829	3967	0.99	(0.97 – 1.01)	0.5	Care facilities[^]	1109	191	10.95	(9.53 – 12.6)	0.0001
No information available	1272	64	1.18	(0.84 – 1.65)	0.3	Hospitals[‡‡]	3393	526	5.32	(4.86 – 5.84)	0.0001
						No information available	909	28	1.15	(0.73 – 1.82)	0.5

The associations between the covariates and dementia risk, which were obtained from the whole patient group analysis using a multifactor model, are shown

ADLs activities of daily living, *CI* confidence interval, *CRP* C-reactive protein, *OR* odds ratio

*Number of patients with dementia

[†]No symptoms (the patient can perform social activities without symptoms and behave without restrictions)

[‡]Moderate symptoms (the patient has mild symptoms and has trouble with physical work, but can walk and do light and sedentary work, such as light domestic and clerical work)

[§]≥ 50% sitting up (the patient can walk and take care of him/herself, but sometimes requires care. The patient can sit up at least half of the day, but cannot do light work)

[#]≥ 50% in bed (the patient can take care of him/herself to some extent, but often requires care and is in bed at least half of the day)

[¶]Whole day in bed (the patient cannot take care of him/herself and requires constant care. The patient must be in bed all day)

[¶¶]Patients' own home

[^]Care facilities (e.g., homes with care services; nursing homes, such as private nursing homes without national aid and nursing homes for families with financial difficulties; group homes; vocational centers; or relief facilities)

[‡‡]Hospitals (e.g., health service facilities for the elderly; beds for general patients, patients at chronic stage, patients requiring rehabilitation, and patients with mental illness and infectious diseases, such as tuberculosis)

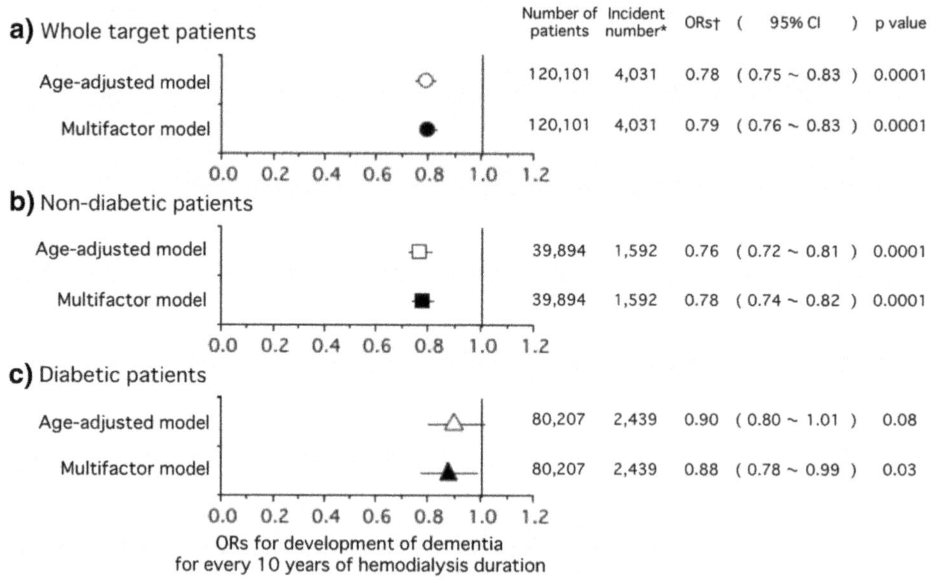

Fig. 2 Dementia risk for hemodialysis duration. The dementia risk for hemodialysis duration was analyzed for each different patient group using the age-adjusted or multifactor model. The age-adjusted model included only age and hemodialysis duration as independent variables. The multifactor model included baseline factors from the age-adjusted model plus additional clinical covariates (i.e., sex, comorbidity of diabetes, Kt/V, BMI, albumin level, CRP level, hemoglobin level, history of myocardial infarction, limb amputation, or hip fracture, ADLs, and place of residence). The duration of hemodialysis was treated as a continuous variable. Please note that the *X* axis is a linear plot. **a** The target patients of the analysis were the whole target patients. **b** The target patients of the analysis were only the non-diabetic patients. **c** The target patients of the analysis were only the diabetic patients. Asterisk indicates the number of patients who suffered dementia. Dagger indicates ORs for development of dementia for every 10 years of hemodialysis duration. ADLs activities of daily living, BMI body mass index, CI confidence interval, CRP C-reactive protein, OR odds ratio

duration, the dementia risk seemed to increase along with the elongation of the hemodialysis duration, but, on the contrary, from five to 19 years, it seemed to decrease. At over 20 years of hemodialysis duration, the dementia risk seemed to increase again along with elongation of the duration.

Figure 4 shows the result of sensitivity analysis. In the negative and positive analyses in the non-diabetic patients, the dementia risk decreased with increasing hemodialysis duration (Fig. 4a). However, in the positive analysis of diabetic patients, the risk of dementia tended to increase with prolongation of hemodialysis duration (Fig. 4b).

Discussion

Our study showed that the dementia risk in non-diabetic patients decreased with prolongation of hemodialysis duration. However, we must consider the survivor effect when analyzing the relationship between hemodialysis duration and dementia incidence.

The survivor effect is a bias caused by a prolonged period of observation for incidence in the target cohort. As the observation period increases, more patients with risk factors will drop out from the target cohort upon reaching the designated endpoints. As a result, the incidence rate tends to decrease with an increase in the observation period. In our study, hemodialysis duration also was the exposure period, with hemodialysis as a risk factor. Therefore, we must consider the survivor effect of hemodialysis duration in this study.

On the other hand, CKD is a reported risk factor of dementia [1, 2]. If we consider hemodialysis duration as the exposure period and consider CKD as a risk factor, a longer hemodialysis duration may be expected to increase dementia risk. However, in our study, the dementia risk in non-diabetic patients decreased as the hemodialysis duration increased. This result may suggest that the risk-reducing power of the survivor effect overcame the risk-enhancing power of CKD in non-diabetic patients throughout the entire hemodialysis period. However, we could not necessarily identify a clear relationship between dialysis duration and dementia risk in diabetic patients.

In general, the survivor effect appears to be stronger when more patients drop out from the target cohort as they reach the designated endpoints. For example, the dementia risk was significantly lower in patients with a history of limb amputation (odds ratio [OR], 0.66 [95% CI, 0.56–0.77]; the OR compares patients "with limb amputation history" to those "without limb amputation history"; Table 5). Moreover, previous research has shown that the survival rate was low in hemodialysis

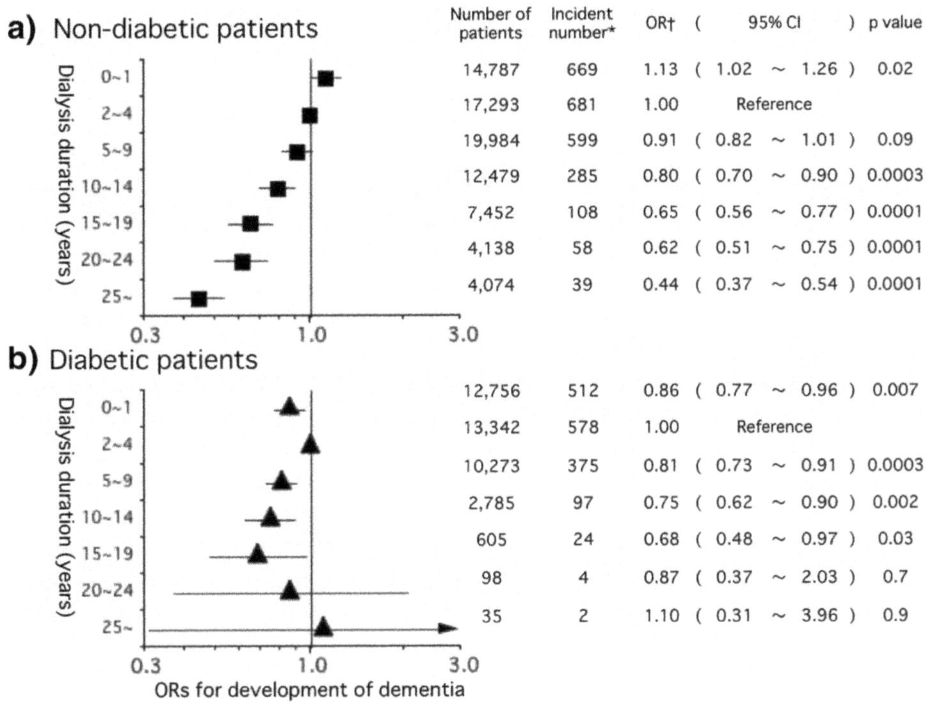

Fig. 3 Dementia risk for hemodialysis duration as a stratified variable. The dementia risk for hemodialysis duration was analyzed as a stratified variable using the multifactor model. The multifactor model included the following factors as independent variables: hemodialysis duration, age, sex, comorbidity of diabetes, Kt/V, BMI, albumin level, CRP level, hemoglobin level, history of myocardial infarction, limb amputation, or hip fracture, ADLs, and place of residence. Please note that the *X* axis is a log-linear plot. **a** The target patients of the analysis were only the non-diabetic patients. **b** The target patients of the analysis were only the diabetic patients. Asterisk indicates the number of patients who suffered dementia. Dagger indicates ORs for development of dementia. ADLs activities of daily living, BMI body mass index, CI confidence interval, CRP C-reactive protein, OR odds ratio

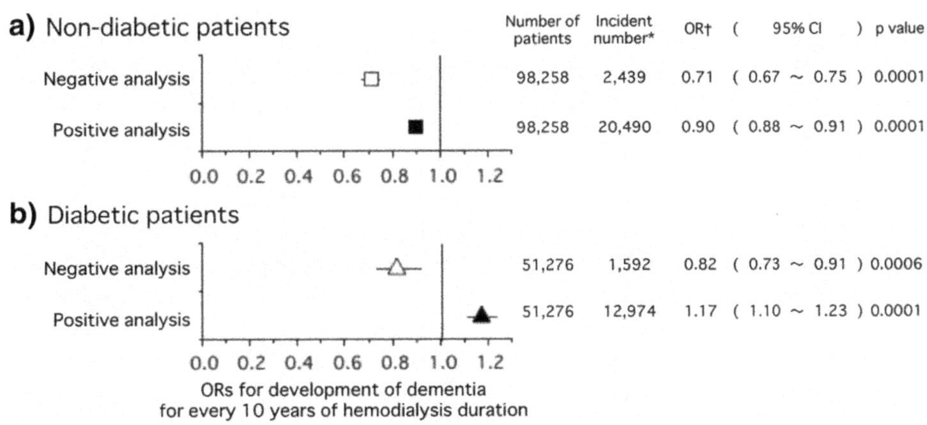

Fig. 4 Sensitivity analyses for the excluded patients' influence evaluation. The sensitivity analyses were conducted to evaluate how the exclusion of patients affected the results. We analyzed the dementia risk under the assumptions that none of the excluded patients had dementia (negative analysis) and that all the excluded patients had dementia (positive analysis). These analyses were conducted using the multifactor model, which included the following factors as independent variables; hemodialysis duration, age, sex, comorbidity of diabetes, Kt/V, BMI, albumin level, CRP level, hemoglobin level, history of myocardial infarction, limb amputation, or hip fracture, ADLs, and place of residence. Please note that the *X* axis is a linear plot. **a** The target patients of the analysis were only the non-diabetic patients. **b** The target patients of the analysis were only the diabetic patients. Asterisk indicates the number of patients with dementia. Dagger indicates ORs for development of dementia for every 10 years of hemodialysis duration. ADLs activities of daily living, BMI body mass index, CI confidence interval, CRP C-reactive protein, OR odds ratio

patients with a history of limb amputation [19]. This also is confirmed in our mortality risk analysis (Additional file 1: Table S1). The mortality risk increased significantly when hemodialysis duration increased in non-diabetic and diabetic (Additional file 1: Table S2). However, the relationship between mortality risk and hemodialysis duration was much stronger in the diabetic patients than in non-diabetic patients. Based on these findings, we may be able to assume that the survivor effect was stronger in diabetic patients than in non-diabetic patients. However, the relationship between dementia risk and hemodialysis duration in diabetic patients was much weaker or vaguer than that in non-diabetic patients (Figs. 2 and 3). Therefore, we might be able to consider that the reduction in dementia risk with prolonged hemodialysis duration in non-diabetic patients was caused not only by the survivor effect but also by some other factors, such as hemodialysis itself.

AD is a major cause of dementia [5], in which accumulation of Aβ in the brain results in cognitive impairment [6]. Moreover, in these patients, the metabolic degradation of Aβ and its clearance from the brain are impaired [7]. If Aβ clearance from the brain can be increased, AD might be prevented or even treated. It has been shown that hemodialysis removes Aβ [10] and that the cognitive function of non-diabetic patients was maintained or improved among those undergoing maintenance hemodialysis over a period of 18 to 36 months [11]. Additionally, Aβ deposition was significantly weaker in the postmortem brains of patients who had undergone hemodialysis than in age-matched controls who had not undergone hemodialysis [12], and this finding is comparable to the finding in the study by Reusche et al. [13]. Although Lin et al. [4] showed that there is no significant difference in dementia risk between patients undergoing hemodialysis and those undergoing peritoneal dialysis, Jin et al. [20] showed that Aβ removal from the blood by peritoneal dialysis also reduces Aβ in the brain interstitial fluid. These reports suggest that hemodialysis might reduce the dementia risk through removal of Aβ from the blood of patients.

It is known that hemodialysis patients have a high morbidity risk of cerebrovascular events [21], and CVD is a major risk factor for VaD. We excluded patients with a clear history of CVD (Fig. 1). Therefore, we may assume that most cases in our analysis had a type of dementia other than VaD. In the study by Sekita et al. [22] on dementia in the general population in Japan, approximately 46% of individuals had AD and 30% had VaD. If we apply this finding to our study in which patients with CVD were excluded, we might be able to assume that approximately two thirds of our patients with dementia had AD. However, we may have to consider the possibility that patients suffered VaD without presenting with clear symptoms of CVD, and it is known that patients with CKD tend to experience VaD rather than AD [23]. Therefore, we may have to consider that the patients with dementia among our target patients still include many with VaD. However, it is reported that the vascular lesion of patients with CKD also is a risk for AD [24]. Furthermore, it has been reported that many patients with cerebrovascular dementia have concomitant AD [5]; thus, we believe that hemodialysis may suppress the development of dementia in this patient group to some extent.

In this survey, despite the notification that the primary physician should determine the presence or absence of dementia, no standard criteria were specified and there was no information on dementia severity. We cannot exclude the possibility that this ambiguity of dementia diagnosis influenced the analytic results. Patients with long hemodialysis duration might be well known by their own physicians in charge. This situation might make it easier for the physicians to be aware of their patients' dementia. On the other hand, the physicians might tend to answer "without dementia" from force of habit. However, even if we suppose the possibility of "negative diagnosis bias" of long-term dialysis patients, we cannot explain the reason why the risk suppression effect of hemodialysis duration in diabetic patients is weaker than that of non-diabetic patients.

On assessing patients in this study, we found no apparent relationship between hemodialysis duration and age (Tables 1 and 2). Moreover, the influence of age was adjusted using the logistic regression analysis. Therefore, it is difficult to consider that a deviation in age with a prolonged hemodialysis duration affected the analytical results.

The discontinuation of dialysis after dementia onset by a substantial number of patients could exacerbate the survivor effect. However, among the 8367 patients excluded from our analytical cohort due to death during 2010, only 33 (0.4%) died due to discontinuation of dialysis. Thus, discontinuation of dialysis does not appear to contribute substantially to the survivor effect.

Considering the aforementioned findings, the assumption that hemodialysis itself may prevent development of AD in non-diabetic patients does not appear to have a major conflict with our results. Our results may not show clearly the dementia-preventing effect of hemodialysis therapy. However, if we can interpret this result as "the first finding," showing the dementia-preventing effect of hemodialysis therapy based on the real clinical data obtained from a large cohort of patients, this result may have important implications in the prevention of dementia. Therefore, we reported this result in this study.

Although hemodialysis is considered to be preventive against the incidence of dementia, it does not imply that the incidence of dementia in the hemodialysis patients is absolutely lower than that in the general population. The incidence of dementia in the > 65-year-old target patients was 50.0 and 59.0 cases/1000 person-years among those without and with diabetes, respectively (Additional file 1: Table S3). On the other hand, it is reported that the incidence of dementia in the > 65-year-old Japanese general population was 30.5–35.6 cases/1000 person-years [25]. This finding suggests that the absolute value of the incidence of dementia in hemodialysis patients is still higher than that in the general population. This may suggest that the dementia risk-reducing effect of hemodialysis did not overcome the risk caused by CKD itself, which every hemodialysis patient faced.

Because it is known that renal failure patients without hemodialysis have a 2.86 times higher risk of cognitive impairment than healthy subjects [2], we consider that the high dementia risk of hemodialysis patients may not have resulted from hemodialysis therapy but from their renal failure. There may be some patients who had dementia or cognitive impairment prior to dialysis initiation. Therefore, in this study, we evaluated the relationship between dementia risk and the patients' hemodialysis duration.

In the present analysis, we found no significant risk of dementia related to Kt/V (Table 5). Kt/V is considered to be the dialysis efficiency indicator of the small substance because the target substance of Kt/V is urea and its molecular weight is only 60 Da. On the other hand, the molecular weight of Aβ, which is considered to be related to the occurrence of AD, is 4 kDa and is much heavier than urea. Recently, Kawaguchi et al. [26] reported that dialyzers remove Aβ from the blood, not by the dialysis phenomenon but by adsorption during hemodialysis therapy [26]. Kato et al. [10] also reported that the reduction rate of blood Aβ concentration of a 4-h hemodialysis session is approximately 34.9 to 53.0%. Based on these reports, we may be able to assume that the reduction rate of Aβ in our target patients was similar to that reported by Kato et al. [10]. These findings suggest that our result of Kt/V having no dementia risk does not necessarily conflict with our hypothesis that the hemodialysis prevents development of AD through removing Aβ.

Regarding removal of large molecular weight substances from the blood, the hemodiafiltration therapy, which uses dialysis and the filtration phenomenon, generally is considered to have a higher efficiency than hemodialysis. However, because the main mechanism of removing Aβ from blood is not dialysis but the adsorption phenomenon of the dialyzer membrane, we may be able to consider that the choice of blood purification method, such as hemodialysis or hemodiafiltration, may not make much difference in the dementia preventive effect.

Diabetes is a known risk factor for dementia [15]. Hanyu et al. [16] recently mentioned that dementia in diabetic patients should be regarded as an independent disease (i.e., diabetes-related dementia) because it results from pathologic conditions related to diabetes. Following their concept, we separated the target patients based on their comorbidity of diabetes in our study. A unique disease entity causing dementia also may explain the weak or absent association between hemodialysis duration and dementia risk in diabetic patients. In our analysis, the multifactor model showed no significant dementia risk in diabetic patients compared with non-diabetic patients (Table 5). When we tentatively analyzed the dementia risk for the comorbidity of diabetes using a simple analytic model that contains only age and hemodialysis duration as covariates other than comorbidity of diabetes, we showed that diabetic patients had a significant OR for dementia of 1.13 (95% CI, 1.07–1.20, $P = 0.0001$; Additional file 1: Table S4). We considered that this finding may show that the influence of the comorbidity of diabetes was confounded by other covariates in the multifactor model analysis.

We conducted a sensitivity analysis to evaluate how the exclusion of patients by the end of 2010 affected the results. In the negative and positive analyses of non-diabetic patients, the dementia risk decreased with increasing hemodialysis duration (Fig. 4a). This result suggested that the exclusion of patients by the end of 2010 did not affect the relationship between dementia risk and hemodialysis duration among the non-diabetic patients. Although the negative analysis of diabetic patients showed that the dementia risk decreased with prolongation of hemodialysis duration, the positive analysis of diabetic patients showed to the contrary that the risk of dementia increased with prolongation of hemodialysis duration (Fig. 4b). This result showed that the dementia risk possibly may increase along with prolongation of hemodialysis duration in diabetic patients. But the diabetic patients may also have a weak negative relationship between the dementia risk and their hemodialysis duration because the multifactor model analysis of the diabetic patients showed a weak but significant negative relationship between the dementia risk and hemodialysis duration (Fig. 2c).

Our analysis showed that advancing age, female sex, a high CRP level, history of hip fracture, low ADLs, and admission to facilities or hospitals were significant risk factors for dementia (Table 5). These risk factors have been reported as significant for dementia in previous studies [27–30]. Anemia has been reported to be a risk factor for cognitive impairment [31]. However, our analysis did not show a significant association between hemoglobin level and dementia risk. We considered that the effects of hemoglobin on dementia probably were confounded by other covariates (Additional file 1: Table S5).

Our study had several limitations. First, the diagnostic criteria for dementia were not specified clearly, and the assessment of dementia was based on a simple query to the respondents at each facility. Despite the notification that the primary physician should determine the presence or absence of dementia, no standard criteria were specified and there was no information on dementia severity. Second, the database used did not include many factors, including hypertension, hyperlipidemia, low socioeconomic status, and low education status, which have been reported to affect dementia risk in patients with CKD [32]. Third, we could not completely exclude survivor bias despite our efforts to mitigate the effect by incorporating many covariates in the regression model. To resolve these problems in the future, extensive cohort studies should be performed among patients undergoing hemodialysis and care should be taken to collect detailed information related to the onset of AD.

Conclusion

A longer hemodialysis duration was correlated with a lower dementia risk in non-diabetic patients, but not in diabetic patients. This finding does not appear to contradict greatly the assumption that the reduction in dementia risk with a prolonged hemodialysis duration in non-diabetic patients was caused not only by the survivor effect but also by hemodialysis itself.

Abbreviations

AD: Alzheimer's disease; ADLs: Activities of daily living; Aβ: Amyloid β; BMI: Body mass index; CI: Confidence interval; CKD: Chronic kidney disease; CRP: C-reactive protein; CVD: Cerebrovascular disease; ESRD: End-stage renal disease; JRDR: Japanese Society for Dialysis Therapy Renal Data Registry; JSDT: Japanese Society for Dialysis Therapy; OR: Odds ratio; VaD: Vascular dementia

Acknowledgements

We are grateful to Dr. Takayuki Hamano, Dr. Takeshi Hasegawa, Dr. Shoichi Maruyama, and Dr. Takahiro Shinzato, for their advice and encouragement. We also appreciate Ms. Shinobu Hattori for her kind English editing.

Funding

The authors did not receive any funding for this study.

Authors' contributions

SN, KW, and NK devised the study design. SN and EK analyzed the data. KS assisted with the pathophysiologic assessment. KK assisted with the etiologic assessment. SN wrote the original draft, prepared the tables and figures, and searched the literature. All authors interpreted the data and reviewed the manuscript. All authors read and approved the final manuscript.

Authors' information

S.N. and E.K. are present members of Committee of Renal Data Registry of JSDT, and K.W. was a previous member of this committee.

Competing interests

The authors declare that they have no competing interests.

Author details

[1]Faculty of Clinical Engineering Technology, Fujita Health University School of Health Sciences, Dengakugakubo 1-98, Kutsukake-cho, Toyoake, Aichi 470-1192, Japan. [2]Department of Preventive Medicine, Nagoya University Graduate School of Medicine, Tsurumai-cho 65, Showa-ku, Nagoya, Aichi 466-8550, Japan. [3]Department of Nephrology, Tokyo Kyosai Hospital, Nakameguro 2-3-8, Meguro-ku, Tokyo 153-8934, Japan.

References

1. Yaffe K, Ackerson L, Kurella Tamura M, Le Blanc P, Kusek JW, Sehgal AR, et al. Chronic kidney disease and cognitive function in older adults: findings from the chronic renal insufficiency cohort cognitive study. J Am Geriatr Soc. 2010;58:338–45.
2. Kurella M, Chertow GM, Fried LF, Cummings SR, Harris T, Simonsick E, et al. Chronic kidney disease and cognitive impairment in the elderly: the health, aging, and body composition study. J Am Soc Nephrol. 2005;16:2127–33.
3. Fukunishi I, Kitaoka T, Shirai T, Kino K, Kanematsu E, Sato Y. Psychiatric disorders among patients undergoing hemodialysis therapy. Nephron. 2002;91:344–7.
4. Lin YT, Wu PH, Kuo MC, Chen CS, Chiu YW, Yang YH, et al. Comparison of dementia risk between end stage renal disease patients with hemodialysis and peritoneal dialysis—a population based study. Sci Rep. 2015;5:8224. https://doi.org/10.1038/srep08224.
5. World Health Organization and Alzheimer's disease international. Dementia: a public health priority. http://www.who.int/mental_health/publications/dementia_report_2012/en/. Accessed 5 Nov 2017.
6. Selkoe DJ. Alzheimer's disease: genes, proteins, and therapy. Physiol Rev. 2001;81:741–66.
7. Mawuenyega KG, Sigurdson W, Ovod V, Munsell L, Kasten T, Morris JC, et al. Decreased clearance of CNS beta-amyloid in Alzheimer's disease. Science. 2010;330:1774.
8. Hock C, Konietzko U, Streffer JR, Tracy J, Signorell A, Müller-Tillmanns B, et al. Antibodies against beta-amyloid slow cognitive decline in Alzheimer's disease. Neuron. 2003;38:547–54.
9. Boada M, Ramos-Fernández E, Guivernau B, Muñoz FJ, Costa M, Ortiz AM, et al. Treatment of Alzheimer disease using combination therapy with plasma exchange and haemapheresis with albumin and intravenous immunoglobulin: rationale and treatment approach of the AMBAR (Alzheimer management by albumin replacement) study. Neurologia. 2016;31:473–81.
10. Kato M, Kawaguchi K, Nakai S, Murakami K, Hori H, Ohashi A, et al. Potential therapeutic system for Alzheimer's disease: removal of blood Aβs by hemodialyzers and its effect on the cognitive functions of renal-failure patients. J Neural Transm. 2012;12:1533–44.
11. Kitaguchi N, Hasegawa M, Ito S, Kawaguchi K, Hiki Y, Nakai S, et al. A prospective study on blood Aβ levels and the cognitive function of patients with hemodialysis: a potential therapeutic strategy for AD. J Neural Transm. 2015;122:1593–607.
12. Sakai K, Senda T, Hata R, Kuroda M, Hasegawa M, Kato M, et al. Patients that have undergone hemodialysis exhibit lower amyloid deposition in the brain: evidence supporting a therapeutic strategy for ad by removal of blood amyloid. J Alzheimers Dis. 2016;51:997–1002.

13. Reusche E, Koch V, Lindner B, Harrison AP, Friedrich HJ. Alzheimer morphology is not increased in dialysis-associated encephalopathy and long-term hemodialysis. Acta Neuropathol. 2001;101:211–6.
14. Nakai S, Iseki K, Itami N, Ogata S, Kazama JJ, Kimata N, et al. An overview of regular dialysis treatment in Japan (as of 31 December 2010). Ther Apher Dial. 2012;16:483–521.
15. Kopf D, Frölich L. Risk of incident Alzheimer's disease in diabetic patients: a systematic review of prospective trials. J Alzheimers Dis. 2009;16:677–85.
16. Hanyu H, Hirose D, Fukasawa R, Hatanaka H, Namioka N, Sakurai H. Guidelines for the clinical diagnosis of diabetes mellitus-related dementia. J Am Geriatr Soc. 2015;63:1721–3.
17. Nakai S, Iseki K, Itami N, Ogata S, Kazama JJ, Kimata N, et al. Overview of regular dialysis treatment in Japan (as of 31 December 2009). Ther Apher Dial. 2012;16:11–53.
18. Shinzato T, Nakai S, Fujita Y, Takai I, Morita H, Nakane K, et al. Determination of Kt/V and protein catabolic rate using pre- and postdialysis blood urea nitrogen concentrations. Nephron. 1994;67:280–90.
19. Constantinescu MI, Constantinescu DP, Chiş B, Andercou A, Mironiuc IA. Influence of risk factors and comorbidities on the successful therapy and survival of patients with critical limb ischemia. Clujul Med. 2013;86:57–64.
20. Jin WS, Shen LL, Bu XL, Zhang WW, Chen SH, Huang ZL, et al. Peritoneal dialysis reduces amyloid-beta plasma levels in humans and attenuates Alzheimer-associated phenotypes in an APP/PS1 mouse model. Acta Neuropathol. 2017;134:207–20.
21. Fu J, Huang J, Lei M, Luo Z, Zhong X, Huang Y, et al. Prevalence and impact on stroke in patients receiving maintenance hemodialysis versus peritoneal dialysis: a prospective observational study. PLoS One. 2015;10:e0140887.
22. Sekita A, Ninomiya T, Tanizaki Y, Hata J, Yonemoto K, Arima H, et al. Trends in prevalence of Alzheimer's disease and vascular dementia in a Japanese community: the Hisayama study. Acta Psychiatr Scand. 2010;122:319–25.
23. Naganuma T, Takemoto Y. New aspects of cerebrovascular diseases in dialysis patients. Contrib Nephrol. 2015;185:138–46.
24. Hardy JA, Mann DM, Wester P, Winblad B. An integrative hypothesis concerning the pathogenesis and progression of Alzheimer's disease. Neurobiol Aging. 1986;7:489–502.
25. Kishimoto H, Ohara T, Hata J, Ninomiya T, Yoshida D, Mukai N, et al. The long-term association between physical activity and risk of dementia in the community: the Hisayama study. Eur J Epidemiol. 2016;31:267–74.
26. Kawaguchi K, Saigusa A, Yamada S, Gotoh T, Nakai S, Hiki Y, et al. Toward the treatment for Alzheimer's disease: adsorption is primary mechanism of removing amyloid β protein with hollow-fiber dialyzers of the suitable materials, polysulfone and polymethyl methacrylate. J Artif Organs. 2016;19:149–58.
27. Moser VA, Pike CJ. Obesity and sex interact in the regulation of Alzheimer's disease. Neurosci Biobehav Rev. 2016;67:102–18.
28. Monastero R, Palmer K, Qiu C, Winblad B, Fratiglioni L. Heterogeneity in risk factors for cognitive impairment, no dementia: population-based longitudinal study from the Kungsholmen project. Am J Geriatr Psychiatry. 2007;15:60–9.
29. Lilamand M, Cesari M, del Campo N, Cantet C, Soto M, Ousset PJ, et al. Brain amyloid deposition is associated with lower instrumental activities of daily living abilities in older adults. Results from the MAPT study. J Gerontol A Biol Sci Med Sci. 2016;71:391–7.
30. Guerra C, Hua M, Wunsch H. Risk of a diagnosis of dementia for elderly medicare beneficiaries after intensive care. Anesthesiology. 2015;123:1105–12.
31. Grimm G, Stockenhuber F, Schneeweiss B, Madl C, Zeitlhofer J, Schneider B. Improvement of brain function in hemodialysis patients treated with erythropoietin. Kidney Int. 1990;38:480–6.
32. Kurella Tamura M, Yaffe K. Dementia and cognitive impairment in ESRD: diagnostic and therapeutic strategies. Kidney Int. 2011;79:14–22.

17

Hemodynamic response to orthostatic stress immediately after dialysis session in chronic hemodialysis patients

Toshiyuki Mochizuki[1*], Yoshimi Matsuo[2], Mayumi Sasaki[3], Kenichi Morihisa[1], Sakuyoshi Tabata[4], Toyofumi Fukuda[5] and Ibuki Yajima[5]

Abstract

Orthostatic hypotension is a risk factor for falls among chronic hemodialysis (HD) patients. This study aimed to investigate the hemodynamic response to orthostatic stress immediately after an HD session. Twenty-one HD patients (mean age, 70.2 ± 8.1 years; HD duration, 7.5 ± 6.4 years) participated in this study. Each 5-min hemodynamic monitoring was performed in the supine, semi-recumbent, and sitting positions immediately after an HD session. Hemodynamic variables were measured using a noninvasive beat-to-beat monitoring device during the test. Patients were divided into an intradialytic hypotension (IDH) group and a non-IDH group according to the presence or absence of IDH on the day of the measurements, and intra- and intergroup comparisons were performed. In the IDH group, the nadir values of systolic blood pressure in the semi-recumbent and sitting positions were significantly lower than those in the supine position and the last systolic blood pressure in the semi-recumbent position. The nadir of stroke volume in the sitting position was significantly lower than that in the supine position. There were no statistically significant intergroup differences in the changes for any positions. These results suggest that patients with IDH require special attention when getting out of bed to prevent post-dialytic falls.

Keywords: Hemodialysis, Hypotension, Noninvasive continuous hemodynamic monitoring, Postural change

Background

Orthostatic hypotension (OH) is caused by an excessive decrease in cardiac output (CO) and/or compensatory vasoconstrictor mechanisms such as autonomic failure and age-related physiologic changes [1]. OH is a risk factor for falls among chronic hemodialysis (HD) patients. The cross-sectional prevalence of OH in HD patients is reportedly higher than that in the general population. Previous studies reported a 42% prevalence of OH in the introductory phase of HD [2] versus 5–30% in unselected individuals aged ≥ 65 years [3].

In the post-dialysis period, there are several HD-related risk factors for OH such as the rapid removal of intravascular volume and several hours of bed rest during HD therapy, in addition to other common risk factors such as advanced age, autonomic failure, and frailty. Previous studies demonstrated that the incidences of OH and falls were higher in the post- than pre-dialysis. Roberts et al. reported that 69.6% of patients had post-dialysis OH versus 34.8% with pre-dialysis OH [4]. The incidences of falls pre- and post-dialysis session are reportedly 9–41% [5] and 27–73% [6], respectively. These findings suggest the risk for post-dialytic falls. Furthermore, post-HD OH and intradialytic hypotension (IDH) are significant and independent factors that affect mortality in HD patients [7]. Therefore, studying hemodynamic responses to orthostatic stress after dialysis is important to manage the fall risk in the care for HD patients. However, to our knowledge, little is known about hemodynamic response during postural change immediately after an HD session.

A manual sphygmomanometer is most frequently used to measure OH; however, this device provides only a single blood pressure value unless repeated measurements are taken to identify clinically relevant OH [8]. Continuous beat-to-beat blood pressure measurements are increasingly available in hospital settings [9]. Beat-to-beat

* Correspondence: ekisaimochizuki@yahoo.co.jp
[1]Physical Therapy Service, Ibuki Clinic, 1-37 Kofuku-cho, Kadoma, Osaka 571-0066, Japan
Full list of author information is available at the end of the article

methods have been validated against intra-arterial recordings, meet acceptable criteria for bias and precision [10], and identified a higher prevalence of OH than sphygmomanometry [11]. Furthermore, beat-to-beat technology is reportedly more effective for detecting OH and discriminating blood pressure responses in fallers and non-fallers compared to intermittent manual sphygmomanometer assessments [12].

This study aimed to investigate hemodynamic responses to orthostatic stress immediately after an HD session using continuous beat-to-beat blood pressure measurements. We hypothesized that the decreases in blood pressure upon orthostatic stress immediately after an HD session would be larger in patients with IDH than in those without IDH.

Methods

Patients

This observational study was conducted in a single dialysis center (Ibuki Clinic, Osaka, Japan). Twenty-five HD patients (mean age, 70.8 ± 8.6 years; male/female ratio, 10/15) who underwent maintenance HD three times a week at Ibuki Clinic, Osaka, Japan, participated in this study. None of the patients had common risk factors for falls such as gait disorder, visual impairment, or neurologic disease [13], and all were able to walk into the clinic unassisted and had a history of hypotensive episodes immediately after HD session within the previous year. We excluded patients with severe heart disease (New York Heart Association III or IV) or peripheral artery disease (Fontaine III or IV) as well as those with neurological diseases that induce OH.

This study was approved by the Ethics Committee of Mukogawa Women's University, and written informed consent was obtained from each participant after a detailed explanation of the study protocol was provided.

Demographic and clinical characteristics

The demographic and clinical characteristics obtained from patients' medical records included age, sex, body mass index, presence of underlying diabetes mellitus (DM), HD vintage, dry weight, cardiothoracic ratio, left ventricular ejection fraction (LVEF) by echocardiography, and hemoglobin (Hb), hematocrit (Ht), blood urea nitrogen, creatinine, albumin (Alb), total cholesterol, triglyceride, high-density lipoprotein cholesterol, and C-reactive protein levels in a blood sample obtained before HD. Serum B-type natriuretic peptide (BNP) level was measured before and after the HD session. Parameters concerning arterial stiffness included ankle-brachial index (ABI), toe-brachial index, brachial-ankle pulse wave velocity, and skin perfusion pressure. The body fluid removal rate (%) during the HD session was assessed according to the following equation: body fluid removal rate (%) = (pre-dialysis body weight – post-dialysis body weight)/post-dialysis body weight × 100 [14].

Study protocol

Hemodynamic monitoring was performed on the day of the HD session after a 1-day interval at the timing of getting out of the dialysis bed for returning home. Arterial blood pressure was recorded every 30 min during the HD session by the cuff method with an automatic blood pressure monitor. IDH was defined as a decrease of ≥ 20 mmHg in systolic blood pressure (SBP) during the HD session [15]. Patients were divided into an IDH group and a non-IDH group according to the aforementioned definition of IDH on the day of the measurement.

Immediately after the HD session and detachment of the dialysis circuit, subjects were maintained in the supine position in the dialysis bed for 5 min and then passively moved into a semi-recumbent position by repositioning the head of the bed to 60° and maintained the position for 5 min (semi-recumbent position phase). Next, the subjects were asked to move unassisted into a chair placed beside the dialysis bed and remain there for 5 min (chair sitting position phase). Each postural change occurred within 10 s.

Hemodynamics measurement

During the aforementioned postural changes, we continuously recorded noninvasive beat-to-beat arterial blood pressure (Portapres, Finapres Medical Systems, Amsterdam, The Netherlands) from the pointer or middle finger of the hand without vascular access. The finger cuff of the Portapres was sized to each participant per the manufacturer's specifications after a calibration procedure. Participant height, weight, and age were entered before starting the device to ensure accurate determination of stroke volume (SV) and CO using the Modelflow algorithm (Modelflow, TNO Biomedical Instrumentation, Amsterdam, The Netherlands) [16]. A hydrostatic height correction sensor was placed at the level of the heart to compensate for any hand movements relative to the heart that could impact the blood pressure recordings.

Assessment of hemodynamics

SBP and diastolic blood pressure (DBP) were derived from the arterial pressure waveform. Heart rate (HR) was computed as the inverse of the inter-beat interval and expressed as beats per minute. Beat-to-beat left ventricular SV was estimated by modeling flow from the arterial pressure waveform (16). CO was the product of estimated SV and HR. Total peripheral resistance (TPR) was computed by mean blood pressure at the heart level divided by the computed CO.

Data processing

The data were exported to Microsoft Excel spreadsheets with BeatScope software using the 5-s average method [9], which was reported to show the best association with fall history using various mean times.

Outcome measures

SBP measurements at the following time points were analyzed:

1. Baseline: SBP of the final 5-s average of the supine position phase before the semi-recumbent position phase
2. Semi-recumbent nadir: the lowest 5-s average SBP obtained within the first 3 min of the semi-recumbent position phase
3. Semi-recumbent recovery: SBP of the final 5-s average of the semi-recumbent position phase before the chair sitting position phase
4. Sitting nadir: lowest 5-s average SBP obtained within the first 3 min of the chair sitting position phase

Values for DBP, HR, SV, CO, and TPR at the same time point of SBP obtained according to the above definition were used in the analysis. Data acquired during postural changes were excluded to avoid any effect from body motion.

Statistical analysis

Values for SBP, DBP, HR, SV, CO, and TPR between each time point were analyzed by two-way analysis of variance with the repeated measures or Kruskal-Wallis and Bonferroni test as the post hoc test in each group. The two groups in each time point were compared using an unpaired t test or the Mann-Whitney test after converting to the difference from the baseline values (i.e., ΔSBP, ΔDBP) and percentage changes relative to the baseline values (i.e., %HR, %SV, %CO, %TPR). Clinical characteristics in each group were compared using an unpaired t test or the Mann-Whitney test or chi-square test. Values are shown as mean ± SD. P values < 0.05 were considered statistically significant. All statistical analyses were performed using IBM SPSS version 19 (IBM Japan Inc., Tokyo, Japan).

Results

Clinical and demographic characteristics

We evaluated 21 patients (mean age, 70.3 ± 8.0; male/female ratio, 9/12); three patients were excluded before the hemodynamic monitoring because of discomfort including nausea just after the HD session. In the three patients, SBP decreased by ≥ 20 mmHg in two patients and by < 20 mmHg in one patient during the HD session. Another patient was excluded because of syncope with SBP decrease of ≥ 20 mmHg during the HD session. The underlying kidney diseases were diabetic nephropathy (n = 15), chronic glomerulonephritis (n = 4), polycystic kidney disease (n = 1), and chronic nephritis (n = 1). The body fluid removal rate during the HD in all participants was < 5%. No patient was administered midodrine to prevent IDH before and during the HD session or complained of hypotensive symptoms including dizziness and faintness during the hemodynamic monitoring. Eleven patients were categorized into the IDH group, and the other 10 were categorized into the non-IDH group.

Clinical and demographic characteristics for each group are shown in Table 1. Hb and Ht levels in the IDH group were significantly higher than those in the non-IDH group (P = 0.009 and P = 0.033, respectively). The mean Alb level in the IDH group was significantly lower than that in the non-IDH group (P = 0.040). There were no significant intergroup differences in cardiac function markers or body fluid removal rates (Table 2).

Hemodynamics during postural changes

The changes of hemodynamic parameters between each time point are shown in Fig. 1. SBP for semi-recumbent nadir in the IDH group were significantly lower than those for baseline and semi-recumbent recovery. The SBP for sitting nadir in the IDH group was significantly lower than that for semi-recumbent recovery. The SV for sitting nadir in the IDH group was significantly lower than that for baseline.

There were no statistically significant intergroup differences between the two groups in changes at any time point.

Discussion

In the present study, hemodynamic monitoring during postural changes was performed immediately after an HD session in both the semi-recumbent and sitting positions using noninvasive beat-to-beat blood pressure monitoring. OH has been traditionally measured on active standing or on a head-up tilt table at an angle of 60°. In patients who are unable to stand or who are at risk for symptomatic standing postural hypotension, evaluating postural hypotension in a sitting position is recommended. Advanced age, significant bed rest, and hypertension are reportedly the most important predisposing factors for seated postural hypotension [1]. The effectiveness of the orthostatic stress test in the sitting position was demonstrated in a study by Shaw et al., in which passive seated orthostatic stress and head-up tilt testing produced blood pressure responses of similar magnitudes and no difference was seen in cerebral blood

Table 1 Characteristics of subjects

	IDH group (*n* = 11)	Non-IDH group (*n* = 10)	*P* value
Characteristics			
Age (years)	71.1 ± 8.7	70.4 ± 7.1	0.852
HD vintage (years)	7.5 ± 5.6	7.4 ± 7.2	0.888
Male/female	5/6	4/6	0.617
DM (+/−)	8/3	7/3	0.705
BMI	23.4 ± 2.4	22.2 ± 3.2	0.354
CTR	51.1 ± 3.4	49.2 ± 3.4	0.246
Medications			
ACEI/ARB (%)	9.1	10.0	0.739
β-blocker (%)	9.1	10.0	0.739
Ca antagonist (%)	36.4	20.0	0.145
Laboratory parameters			
Hb	11.8 ± 0.6	10.6 ± 1.2	0.009
Ht	36.3 ± 2.3	32.7 ± 4.4	0.033
BUN	56.3 ± 17.7	59.2 ± 13.1	0.689
Cr	9.79 ± 4.41	9.23 ± 1.23	0.369
Alb	3.4 ± 0.3	3.6 ± 0.2	0.040
TC	163.1 ± 43.9	171.3 ± 37.9	0.669
TG	109.3 ± 48.8	104.3 ± 35.6	0.815
HDL-c	42.9 ± 11.4	42.8 ± 10.6	0.983
CRP	0.24 ± 0.23	0.09 ± 0.08	0.128
Atherosclerotic parameters			
ABI	0.95 ± 0.21	1.10 ± 0.13	0.087
TBI	0.59 ± 0.15	0.63 ± 0.13	0.596
ba-PWV	2233.3 ± 460.0	2087.1 ± 584.4	0.530
SPP	63.3 ± 16.1	63.1 ± 11.9	0.979

Data are expressed as means ± SD

BMI body mass index, *DM* diabetes mellitus, *CTR* cardiothoracic ratio, *ACEI* angiotensin-converting-enzyme inhibitor, *ARB* angiotensin receptor blocker, *Ca* calcium, *Hb* hemoglobin, *Ht* hematocrit, *BUN* blood urea nitrogen, *Cr* creatinine, *Alb* albumin, *TC* total cholesterol, *TG* triglycerides, *HDL-c* high-density lipoprotein cholesterol, *CRP* C-reactive protein, *ABI* ankle-brachial index, *TBI* toe-brachial index, *ba-PWV* brachial-ankle pulse wave velocity, *SPP* skin perfusion pressure

Table 2 Markers of cardiac function and removed body fluid rate

	IDH group (*n* = 11)	Non-IDH group (*n* = 10)	*P* value
LVEF (%)	67.8 ± 7.8	71.1 ± 12.5	0.495
BNP (pre-HD session)	177.7 ± 120.4	109.4 ± 67.9	0.160
BNP (post-HD session)	83.7 ± 53.6	61.4 ± 30.8	0.297
Removed body fluid rate (%)	3.48 ± 1.07	2.96 ± 0.45	0.187

flow velocity in the middle cerebral artery between the two tests in healthy volunteers [8].

In this study, patients with IDH had orthostatic intolerance upon postural change from a supine to a semi-recumbent position immediately after an HD session. This finding supports our assumption that HD therapy negatively affected orthostatic tolerance in HD patients with IDH. Furthermore, the nadir SBP in the sitting position was significantly lower than that in the semi-recumbent position in the patients with IDH, that is, the change from the semi-recumbent to the sitting position decreased the SBP.

In the IDH group, compensatory responses to orthostatic stress such as increases in HR and TPR for stabilizing arterial pressure did not reach statistical significance in spite of significant SBP and SV decrease. Since the orthostatic HR response may be a useful marker of cardiac baroreflex function [10], this result suggests that autonomic dysfunction including diabetic and/or uremic neuropathy was a possible factor for those poor responses considering the lack of a significant intergroup difference in major risk factors for orthostatic intolerance such as age, cardiac function measured by LVEF and BNP level, and body fluid removal rate. Further studies are needed to investigate the effect of those factors on orthostatic intolerance immediately after an HD session.

The post-dialysis period includes not only a higher risk for postural hypotension but also other factors that may increase the risk for accidental falls. Cook et al. revealed that HD treatment altered motor function in older HD patients, weakening their strength and decreasing their mobility after the HD session [7]. Soangra et al. reported decreased sit-to-walk test performance pre- versus post-HD session [17]. Furthermore, a greater postural sway in the post- versus pre-HD session was observed [18] in addition to poorer postural control in HD patients than in age-matched controls, which was further exacerbated by the simultaneous performance of a cognitive task [19]. These results suggest that the immediate post-HD period is particularly unsafe, so medical staff in dialysis units should be sure to provide the necessary support [18]. Accordingly, dialysis staff should consider such alterations concerning physical function post-dialysis as well as the probability of the aforementioned postural hypotension immediately after the HD session. It is likely that dialysis staff already knows about the increased risk for post-dialysis falls; however, only a few studies have reported hemodynamic data from that period. This study is the first to use beat-to-beat technology immediately after an HD session to capture rapid and transient hemodynamic fluctuations.

There were significant differences in Hb, Ht, and Alb levels between the IDH and non-IDH groups. It is

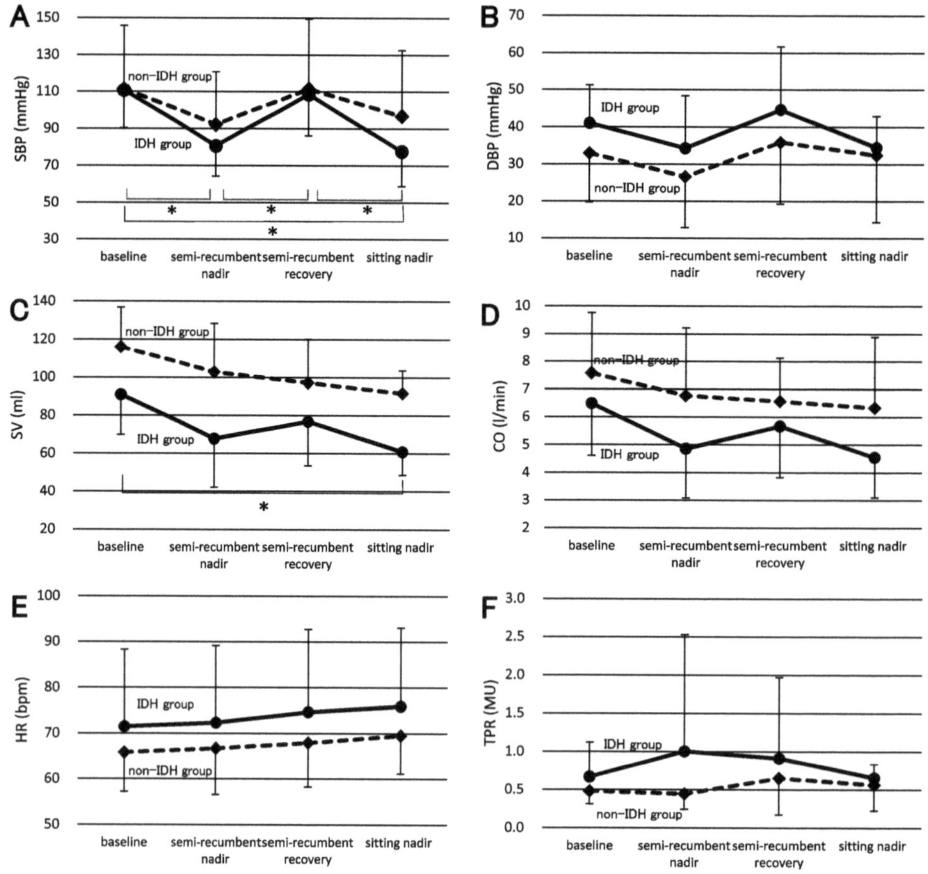

Fig. 1 Hemodynamic responses to postural changes immediately after dialysis session. **a** SBP. **b** DBP. **c** SV. **d** CO. **e** HR. **f** TPR. Data are expressed as means ± SD. *$P < 0.05$

known that anemia is one of the factors that aggravate OH in the general population [20]. However, Hb and Ht level measurements in both groups in this study were within the target range recommended by the Japanese Society of Dialysis Therapy guideline [21], which suggests that even patients with target Hb and Ht levels could develop OH immediately after HD. Meanwhile, the K/DOQI guidelines [15] include hypoalbuminemia as a factor related to IDH; however, whether the intergroup difference in Alb has clinically relevant significance remains unclear because of a lack of evidence.

There are several limitations to this study. First, the small sample size may have affected its ability to show a statistically significant difference in some measures. In addition, we could not evaluate the impact of DM which is the most common disease associated with peripheral damage to the autonomic nerves [22] and could not evaluate patients with hypotensive symptoms before hemodynamic monitoring, who might have had orthostatic intolerance just after HD session. Second, the correlation between IDH and orthostatic intolerance immediately after dialysis was not fully clarified. It is well known that intradialytic and orthostatic hypotension have multifactorial causes. Future studies to identify factors related to post-dialysis OH are needed to enable the earlier detection of fall risk. Third, there is a diverse pattern of orthostatic BP decay [11] such as initial and delayed OH in which a blood pressure decrease occurs within 15 s and after 3 min, respectively [23]; however, we could not investigate the blood pressure patterns and recovery times. Further studies on blood pressure decrease timing are needed to develop more effective strategies to reduce the probability of post-dialytic falls in HD patients upon returning home.

Conclusion

In patients with IDH, postural changes from the supine to the semi-recumbent position immediately after an HD session may significantly decrease SBP. Postural changes from a semi-recumbent to a sitting position may also significantly decrease SBP. These results suggest that beat-to-beat hemodynamic monitoring during HD session provides useful information to identify the patients with a potential risk for post-dialytic falls and that dialysis care team members should provide support to patients with IDH who are transferring out of bed to prevent post-dialytic falls.

Abbreviations

ABI: Ankle-brachial index; Alb: Albumin; BNP: B-type natriuretic peptide; CO: Cardiac output; DBP: Diastolic blood pressure; DM: Diabetes mellitus; Hb: Hemoglobin; HD: Hemodialysis; HR: Heart rate; Ht: Hematocrit; IDH: Intradialytic hypotension; LVEF: Left ventricular ejection fraction; OH: Orthostatic hypotension; SBP: Systolic blood pressure; SV: Stroke volume; TPR: Total peripheral resistance

Acknowledgements

The authors thank the hospital staff and patients who participated in this study.

Funding

The authors declare that there is no funding related to this manuscript.

Authors' contributions

TM and YM were involved in the study design and article writing of the manuscript. TM, MS and KM participated in the study procedure implementation and data collection. ST, TF, and IY kindly reviewed and revised the manuscript. All authors read and approved the final manuscript.

Competing interests

The authors declare that they have no competing interests.

Author details

[1]Physical Therapy Service, Ibuki Clinic, 1-37 Kofuku-cho, Kadoma, Osaka 571-0066, Japan. [2]Graduate School of Health and Sports Sciences, Mukogawa Women's University, 6-46 Ikebiraki, Nishinomiya, Hyogo 663-8558, Japan. [3]Nursing Department, Ibuki Clinic, 1-37 Kofuku-cho, Kadoma, Osaka 571-0066, Japan. [4]Department of Internal Medicine, Ibuki Clinic, 1-37 Kofuku-cho, Kadoma, Osaka 571-0066, Japan. [5]Department of Urology, Ibuki Clinic, 1-37 Kofuku-cho, Kadoma, Osaka 571-0066, Japan.

References

1. Gorelik O, Cohen N. Seated postural hypotension. J Am Soc Hypertens. 2015;12:985–92.
2. Sasaki O, Nakahama H, Nakamura S, et al. Orthostatic hypotension at the introductory phase of haemodialysis predicts all-cause mortality. Nephrol Dial Transplant. 2005;20:377–81.
3. Low PA. Prevalence of orthostatic hypotension. Clin Auton Res. 2008; 18(Suppl 1):8–13.
4. Roberts RG, Kenny RA, Brierley EJ. Are elderly haemodialysis patients at risk of falls and postural hypotension? Int Urol Nephrol. 2003;35:415–21.
5. Polinder-Bos HA, Emmelot-Vonk MH, Gansevoort RT, Diepenbroek A, Gaillard CA. High fall incidence and fracture rate in elderly dialysis patients. Neth J Med. 2014;72:509–15.
6. Cook WL, Tomlinson G, Donaldson M, et al. Falls and fall-related injuries in older dialysis patients. Clin J Am Soc Nephrol. 2006;1:1197–204.
7. Shoji T, Tsubakihara Y, Fujii M, Imai E, et al. Hemodialysis-associated hypotension as an independent risk factor for two-year mortality in hemodialysis patients. Kidney Int. 2004;66:1212–20.
8. Shaw BH, Loughin TM, Mackey DC, Robinovitch SN, Claydon VE. The effect of orthostatic stress type on cardiovascular control. Blood Press Monit. 2014; 19:327–38.
9. van der Velde N, van den Meiracker AH, Stricker BH, van der Cammen TJ. Measuring orthostatic hypotension with the Finometer device: is a blood pressure drop of one heartbeat clinically relevant? Blood Press Monit. 2007;12:167–71.
10. Shaw BH, Claydon VE. The relationship between orthostatic hypotension and falling in older adults. Clin Auton Res. 2014;24:3–13.
11. Cooke J, Carew S, Quinn C, et al. The prevalence and pathological correlates of orthostatic hypotension and its subtypes when measured using beat-to-beat technology in a sample of older adults living in the community. Age Ageing. 2013;42:709–14.
12. Shaw BH, Loughin TM, Robinovitch SN, et al. Cardiovascular responses to orthostasis and their association with falls in older adults. BMC Geriatr. 2015;15:174.
13. Abdel-Rahman EM, Turgut F, Turkmen K, Balogun RA. Falls in elderly hemodialysis patients. QJM. 2011;104:829–38.
14. Yamamoto K, Kobayashi N, Kutsuna T, et al. Excessive fall of blood pressure during maintenance hemodialysis in patients with chronic renal failure is induced by vascular malfunction and imbalance of autonomic nervous activity. Ther Apher Dial. 2012;16:219–25.
15. K/DOQI workgroup. K/DOQI clinical practice guidelines for cardiovascular disease in dialysis patients. Am J Kidney Dis. 2005;45(Suppl 3):S1–153.
16. Wesseling KH, Jansen JR, Settels JJ, Schreuder JJ. Computation of aortic flow from pressure in humans using a nonlinear, three-element model. J Appl Physiol. 1993;74:2566–73.
17. Soangra R, Lockhart TE, Lach J, Abdel-Rahman EM. Effects of hemodialysis therapy on sit-to-walk characteristics in end stage renal disease patients. Ann Biomed Eng. 2013;41:795–805.
18. Magnard J, Lardy J, Testa A, Hristea D, Deschamps T. The effect of hemodialysis session on postural strategies in older end-stage renal disease patients. Hemodial Int. 2015;19:553–61.
19. Shin S, Chung HR, Fitschen PJ, et al. Postural control in hemodialysis patients. Gait Posture. 2014;39:723–7.
20. Figueroa JJ, Basford JR, Low PA. Preventing and treating orthostatic hypotension: as easy as A, B, C. Cleve Clin J Med. 2010;77:298–306.
21. Yamamoto H, Nishi S, Tomo T, et al. 2015 Japanese Society for Dialysis Therapy: guidelines for renal anemia in chronic kidney disease (in Japanese). Touseki Kaishi. 2016;49:89–158.
22. Shibao C, Lipsitz LA, Biaggioni I. American Society of Hypertension Writing Group. Evaluation and treatment of orthostatic hypotension. J Am Soc Hypertens. 2013;7:317–24.
23. Freeman R, Wieling W, Axelrod FB, et al. Consensus statement on the definition of orthostatic hypotension, neurally mediated syncope and the postural tachycardia syndrome. Clin Auton Res. 2011;21:69–72.

18

Usefulness of the Japanese version of the 5-D itch scale for rating pruritus experienced by patients undergoing hemodialysis

Naoko Takahashi[1*], Taku Yoshizawa[1], Aiko Okubo[1], Junko Kumagai[1], Hideki Kawanishi[2], Shinichiro Tsuchiya[2], Misaki Moriishi[3], Takao Masaki[4] and Toshiya Ebata[5]

Abstract

Background: Pruritus in patients undergoing hemodialysis reduces quality of life via insomnia and depression, and negatively affects prognosis. For diagnosing pruritus, selecting therapeutic strategies, and determining therapeutic outcomes, methods are needed for objectively quantifying the degree of itchiness. In 2015, the Japanese version of the 5-D itch scale (5D-J), originally developed in the USA in 2010, was developed as a simple self-administered questionnaire; it evaluated the degree of itchiness based on five components: (1) duration of itchiness, (2) degree of itchiness, (3) direction of itchiness, (4) disability caused by itchiness, and (5) distribution of itchiness. 5D-J is useful for comprehensively assessing multiple elements related to itchiness. We used 5D-J to assess the degree of itchiness experienced by patients undergoing hemodialysis to investigate its clinical usefulness.

Methods: Subjects were 336 patients undergoing maintenance hemodialysis at our facility in October 2016; they were selected from 383 patients, of whom 20 were excluded because their itchiness had a dermatologic origin and 27 were excluded because their localized itchiness was related to vascular access, respectively. The status of itchiness (duration, degree, direction, disability, and distribution) of the patients was surveyed in October 2016 using 5D-J; total scores were calculated and used for assessing the itchiness experienced by patients. We additionally investigated whether 5D-J scores correlated with visual analog scale (VAS) and Shiratori severity scores for pruritus.

Results: Degree was reported as "not present" by 124 patients (36.9%), "mild" by 164 (48.8%), "moderate" by 46 (13.7%), "severe" by 2 (0.6%), and "unbearable" by 0 (0%). Total score was 5 points in 55 patients (16.4%), 6–9 in 176 (52.4%), 10–14 in 95 (28.3%), 15–19 in 9 (2.7%), 20–24 in 1 (0.3%), and 25 in 0 (0%). The 5D-J total and VAS scores were strongly correlated ($r = 0.7159$; $p < 0.001$). The 5D-J total score correlated with "daytime itchiness" ($r = 0.6441$; $p < 0.001$) and "nighttime itchiness" ($r = 0.6352$; $p < 0.001$) on the Shiratori severity score.

Conclusions: 5D-J may be useful for objectively assessing itchiness experienced by patients undergoing hemodialysis.

Keywords: Japanese 5-D itch scale, 5-D itch scale, Visual analog scale, Shiratori severity score, Hemodialysis, Pruritus, Quality of life

* Correspondence: u-23naoko@hi3.enjoy.ne.jp
[1]Akane-Foundation Omachi Tsuchiya Clinic, 2-8-35 Omachi Higashi, Asa Minami-ku, Hiroshima 731-0124, Japan
Full list of author information is available at the end of the article

Background

Approximately 60–80% of patients undergoing hemodialysis have pruritus, and many cases are refractory to treatment [1–8]. Moreover, degree of itchiness and sleep disorders are strongly correlated. Sleep disorders were previously identified in patients with moderate or worse itchiness at a rate of 1.9- to 3.7-fold higher than in patients without itchiness [5]. In addition, patients reporting moderate or severe itchiness that affects daily life also have depression at a rate of 1.3- to 1.7-fold higher than patients reporting no itchiness [2]. The degree of itchiness and survival rate are negatively correlated in patients undergoing hemodialysis [2, 3]. Thus, because pruritus in patients undergoing hemodialysis reduces quality of life (QOL) owing to sleep disorders, depression, and other adverse effects and negatively impacts prognosis, it is a major complication that requires careful treatment.

When diagnosing pruritus, selecting therapeutic strategies, and predicting therapeutic outcomes, both the patient's individual and subjective sense of the degree of itchiness needs to be assessed numerically based on the use of a uniform scale and quantitatively based on an objective measure. The scales used for assessing itchiness include the visual analog scale (VAS) [9–12], numerical rating scale (NRS) [10–12], and verbal rating scale (VRS) [10–12]. VAS and the Shiratori severity score for pruritus (Shiratori score) [13], divided into a type of VRS, and the Kawashima classification [14], a simplified version of the Shiratori score, are commonly used in Japan. However, because VAS rates itchiness in increments along a 100-mm line and NRS uses integers from 0 to 10 to indicate the degree of itchiness, problems such as "the degree of itchiness is difficult to accurately express because the standard is vague," "it is impossible to assess multiple aspects of itchiness with a single number," and "the score is influenced by the symptoms of itchiness and the patient's emotional state immediately before taking the test" have been reported [11, 15]. VRS, in which patients express the degree of itchiness by selecting words, has received the following criticism: "There are too few categories with which the patient is required to express minute changes in itchiness, and the differences between the categories are unclear, which results in quantitative inaccuracy" [12].

By contrast, the Japanese version of the 5-D itch scale (5D-J), developed by Ebata et al. in 2015 [16], is based on the 5-D itch scale that was originally developed in the USA in 2010 [17] and uses a point system to assess the duration, degree, direction, and distribution of itchiness as well as the disability caused by itchiness. Each component is rated on a scale of 1–5, giving a maximum score of 25. The 5D-J is a self-administered questionnaire that the patient can complete quickly and easily, with a scoring system that allows for quantification. While the VAS and the Shiratori score evaluate only the degree of pruritus, the 5D-J evaluates pruritus multidimensionally by assessing duration, direction, effect on QOL, and distribution of itchiness, in addition to degree of itchiness. This detailed assessment of pruritus is an advantage of the 5D-J that may make it useful in routine clinical practice and enables an overall evaluation of multiple factors associated with pruritus [17]. In Japan, a validation study in adult atopic dermatitis patients has already confirmed the reliability, validity, and responsiveness of the 5D-J [18].

In this study, we used 5D-J to assess the degree of itchiness experienced by patients undergoing hemodialysis and assessed its clinical usefulness.

Methods

Subjects were 336 patients undergoing maintenance hemodialysis at our facility in October 2016. The patients were selected from 383 patients, of whom 20 were excluded because their itchiness was identified as being dermatologic in origin and an additional 27 were excluded because their localized itchiness was related to vascular access. Table 1 summarizes the baseline characteristics of the patients. There were 213 men and 123 women; median age was 70 years, median number of months on dialysis was 66 months, and primary illnesses were diabetes ($n = 152$), chronic glomerulonephritis ($n = 87$), nephrosclerosis ($n = 35$), other ($n = 35$), and unknown ($n = 27$).

The itchiness of all patients was assessed in terms of five components (duration, degree, direction, disability, and distribution) using 5D-J in October 2016 (Fig. 1). Responses were used to calculate total scores, which were then used to indicate the status of itchiness among patients undergoing hemodialysis at our facility. We also investigated the possibility of a correlation between 5D-J and itchiness determined using VAS and Shiratori scores, which the patients completed at the same time as 5D-J.

VAS is designed as a horizontal line with markings that range from "no itchiness" (0 mm) on the extreme left to "worst possible (or "unbearable") itchiness" (100 mm) on the extreme right. In cases of "worst possible itchiness," patients further indicated the degree of itchiness on a vertical line. The distance (in mm) from the extreme left side to the marking on the vertical line was determined.

The Shiratori score separately indicates itchiness during daytime and nighttime. Daytime itchiness is rated on the following 5-point scale: 0, no itchiness (no symptoms); 1, bearable without scratching (negligible); 2, subsides with some scratching (slight); 3, subsides with

Table 1 Patient baseline characteristics and comparison between groups with 5D-J score ≥ 9 and ≤ 8

	Total (n = 336)	5D-J total scores		
	Number (%)	≥ 9 (n = 145) number (%)	≤ 8 (n = 191) number (%)	p value
Male/female	213 (63.4)/123 (36.6)	93 (64.1)/52 (35.9)	120 (62.8)/71 (37.2)	0.801*
Median, IQR age (years)	70, 63–77	71, 61–78	69, 62–77	0.226**
Median, IQR duration of hemodialysis (months)	66, 33–131	67, 38–119	64, 27–151	0.889**
Primary illness of chronic kidney disease				
Diabetes mellitus	152 (45.2)	74 (51.0)	78 (40.8)	0.063*
Chronic glomerulonephritis	87 (25.9)	33 (22.8)	54 (28.3)	0.253*
Nephrosclerosis	35 (10.4)	14 (9.7)	21 (11.0)	0.691*
Other	35 (10.4)	12 (8.3)	23 (12.0)	0.263*
Unknown	27 (8.0)	12 (8.3)	15 (7.9)	0.888*
Comorbidities				
Hypertension	312 (92.9)	134 (92.4)	178 (93.2)	0.783*
Ischemic heart disease	79 (23.5)	45 (31.0)	34 (17.8)	< 0.005*
Congestive heart failure	64 (19.1)	26 (17.9)	38 (19.9)	0.650*
Cerebral vascular disease	85 (25.3)	41 (28.3)	44 (23.0)	0.274*
Peripheral arterial disease	39 (11.6)	19 (13.1)	20 (10.5)	0.456*
Chronic lung disease	24 (7.1)	12 (8.3)	12 (6.3)	0.482*
Chronic liver disease	19 (5.7)	11 (7.6)	8 (4.2)	0.182*
Malignant neoplasm	19 (5.7)	9 (6.2)	10 (5.2)	0.703*
Medication for pruritus				
Moisturizers	142 (42.3)	79 (54.5)	63 (33.0)	< 0.001*
Topical steroids	83 (24.7)	54 (15.2)	29 (10.0)	< 0.001*
Other topical drugs	35 (10.4)	22 (15.2)	13 (6.8)	< 0.001*
Oral antihistamines	13 (3.9)	8 (5.5)	5 (2.6)	0.172*
Anti-allergy injections	2 (0.6)	2 (1.4)	0 (0.0)	0.186***
Nalfurafine	39 (11.6)	19 (13.1)	20 (10.5)	0.456*
Laboratory parameters (median, IQR)				
Serum albumin (g/dL)	3.6, 3.4–3.8	3.5, 3.3–3.7	3.6, 3.4–3.8	0.070**
Serum corrected calcium (mg/dL)	8.4, 8.1–8.8	8.9, 8.4–9.2	8.8, 8.4–9.1	0.974**
Phosphorus (mg/dL)	4.9, 4.1–5.4	4.9, 4.1–5.4	4.9, 4.1–5.4	0.823****
Whole PTH (pg/mL)	76.4, 51.7–116.2	79.2, 56.7–124.7	71.9, 47.2–109.7	0.101**
Hemoglobin (g/dL)	11.3, 10.7–11.9	11.2, 10.7–11.8	11.4, 10.7–11.9	0.283**
β2-microglobulin (mg/L)	22.9, 20.0–26.4	23.1, 20.4–27.0	22.8, 19.6–25.9	0.174**
Kt/V	1.5, 1.4–1.6	1.5, 1.4–1.6	1.5, 1.4–1.6	0.801**

Data are presented as n (%), unless stated otherwise. p values were calculated using χ^2 test*, Mann-Whitney U test**, Fisher's exact test***, and Student's t test****, respectively

considerable scratching (moderate); and 4, does not subside with scratching and leads to more scratching (severe). Nighttime itchiness is rated on the following 5-point scale: 0, no itchiness (no symptoms); 1, very little itchiness noticed when in bed, not particularly aware of itchiness, and able to sleep (negligible); 2, some itchiness that subsides when scratched, not waking up because of itchiness (slight); 3, waking up because of itchiness, can sleep after scratching but unconscious scratching while asleep (moderate); and 4, almost completely unable to sleep because of itchiness, frequent scratching but itchiness only worsens (severe).

We investigated the correlation between 5D-J, VAS, and Shiratori (daytime and nighttime) scores using Spearman's rank correlation coefficient. The results were determined as follows: $r = 0$, no correlation; $0 < |r| \le 0.2$, almost no correlation; $0.2 < |r| \le 0.4$, weak correlation; $0.4 < |r| \le 0.7$, moderate correlation; $0.7 < |r| < 1.0$, strong correlation; and $r = 1.0$ or -1.0, perfect correlation. We used the χ^2, Mann-Whitney U, Fisher's exact, and

1. Duration
During the last 2 weeks, how many hours a day did you experience itchiness?
1) < 6 h/day, 2) 6–12 h/day, 3) 12–18 h/day, 4) 18–23 h/day, 5) all day
2. Degree
Please rate the intensity of your itchiness over the past 2 weeks.
1) Not present, 2) Mild, 3) Moderate, 4) Severe, 5) Unbearable
3. Direction
Over the past 2 weeks, has your itchiness improved or worsened compared with that in the previous month?
1) Completely resolved, 2) Much better, but still present, 3) Little bit better, but still present, 4) Unchanged, 5) Getting worse
4. Disability
Please rate the impact of your itchiness on the following activities over the last 2 weeks.
・Sleep
1) Never affects sleep, 2) Occasionally delays falling asleep, 3) Frequently delays falling asleep, 4) Delays falling asleep and occasionally wakes me up at night, 5) Delays falling asleep and frequently wakes me up at night
・Leisure/Social activities
1) Never affects this activity, 2) Rarely affects this activity, 3) Occasionally affects this activity, 4) Frequently affects this activity, 5) Always affects this activity, *) Not applicable
・Housework/Errands
1) Never affects this activity, 2) Rarely affects this activity, 3) Occasionally affects this activity, 4) Frequently affects this activity, 5) Always affects this activity, *) Not applicable
・Work/School
1) Never affects this activity, 2) Rarely affects this activity, 3) Occasionally affects this activity, 4) Frequently affects this activity, 5) Always affects this activity, *) Not applicable
5. Distribution
Please indicate the sites on your body where itchiness has been present over the last 2 weeks. If the relevant body part is not listed, choose the site that is anatomically closest. Head/Scalp ( ), Face ( ), Chest ( ), Abdomen ( ), Back ( ), Buttocks ( ), Thighs ( ), Lower legs ( ), Tops of feet/toes ( ), Soles ( ), Palms ( ), Tops of hands/fingers ( ), Forearms ( ), Upper arms ( ), Points of contact with clothing (e.g. waistband, undergarment) ( ), Groin ( )

(Ebata, Toshiya et al.: Creation of a Japanese version of the 5D itch scale. Japanese Journal of Dermatology 2015;125:1035-1040

Method of calculating each score and the total score

- Responses 1–5 for questions 1–5 are rated from 1 to 5 points.
- In Question 4 (Disability), the highest score of each subsection (sleep, leisure/social activities, housework/errands, and work/school) is used.
- For the distribution of itchiness in Question 5, a total of 0–2 sites of itchiness equates to 1 point, 3–5 to 2 points, 6–10 sites to 3 points, 11–13 sites to 4 points, and 14–16 sites to 5 points.
- The total score ranges from 5 to 25 points.

Fig. 1 Japanese version of the 5-D itch scale

Student's t tests for the other analyses. In all analyses, p values less than 0.05 were considered statistically significant. All statistical analyses were performed with SPSS version 23.0 (IBM Japan, Ltd., Tokyo, Japan).

This study was conducted with the approval of the Tsuchiya General Hospital Institutional Review Board for Human Investigation (approval number: E170619-2) and performed according to the principles of the Declaration of Helsinki. Prior verbal consent was obtained from all patients enrolled in this study. The fact that patients provided consent was recorded in their medical records. The need for written informed consent was waived due to the strict maintenance of patients' anonymity and the observational nature of the study.

Results

Assessment of itchiness using 5D-J

Duration

In total, 307 patients (91.4%) reported "less than 6 h," 17 (5.1%) reported "6–12 h," 8 (2.4%) reported "12–18 h," 1 (0.3%) reported "18–23 h," and 3 (0.9%) reported "all day."

Degree

Overall, 124 patients (36.9%) reported "not present," 164 (48.8%) reported "mild," 46 (13.7%) reported "moderate," 2 (0.6%) reported "severe," and 0 (0%) reported "unbearable."

In addition, we divided the patients into two groups, those who reported pruritus as "not present" (124 patients) and those who reported at least "mild" (212 patients) pruritus. Comparison of baseline characteristics and laboratory parameters between the two groups revealed that patients with "at least mild" pruritus had a significantly higher rate of chronic liver disease ($p < 0.05$) and significantly more use of moisturizers, topical steroids, and other topical drugs for pruritus treatment ($p < 0.001$ for each) (Table 2). As for laboratory parameters, patients with "at least mild" pruritus had significantly higher whole PTH levels ($p < 0.05$) (Table 2).

Direction

Among all patients, 62 (18.5%) reported "completely resolved," 71 (21.1%) reported "much better, but still present," 61 (18.2%) reported "a little bit better, but still

Table 2 Comparison of baseline characteristics between the "not present" and "at least mild" groups

	Not present ($n = 124$) number (%)	Mild or above ($n = 212$) number (%)	p value
Male/female	74 (59.7)/50 (40.3)	139 (65.6)/73 (34.4)	0.280*
Median, IQR age (years)	69, 62–76	71, 63–78	0.275**
Median, IQR duration of hemodialysis (months)	72, 30–152	63, 34–123	0.301**
Primary illness of chronic kidney disease			
Diabetes mellitus	50 (40.3)	102 (48.1)	0.166*
Chronic glomerulonephritis	38 (30.6)	49 (23.1)	0.128*
Nephrosclerosis	12 (9.7)	23 (10.8)	0.734*
Other	15 (12.1)	20 (9.4)	0.441*
Unknown	9 (7.3)	18 (8.5)	0.688*
Comorbidities			
Hypertension	114 (91.9)	198 (93.4)	0.616*
Ischemic heart disease	24 (19.4)	55 (25.9)	0.169*
Congestive heart failure	27 (21.8)	37 (17.5)	0.330*
Cerebral vascular disease	28 (22.6)	57 (26.9)	0.381*
Peripheral arterial disease	15 (12.1)	24 (11.3)	0.830*
Chronic lung disease	8 (6.5)	16 (7.5)	0.707*
Chronic liver disease	3 (2.4)	16 (7.5)	< 0.05*
Malignant neoplasm	6 (4.8)	13 (6.1)	0.620*
Medication for pruritus			
Moisturizers	27 (21.8)	115 (54.2)	< 0.001*
Topical steroids	5 (4.0)	78 (36.8)	< 0.001*
Other topical drugs	3 (2.4)	32 (15.1)	< 0.001*
Oral antihistamines	2 (1.6)	11 (5.2)	0.143***
Anti-allergy injections	0 (0.0)	2 (0.9)	0.533***
Nalfurafine	10 (8.1)	29 (13.7)	0.121*
Laboratory parameters (median, IQR)			
Serum albumin (g/dL)	3.7, 3.5–3.8	3.6, 3.4–3.8	0.164**
Serum corrected calcium (mg/dL)	8.8, 8.5–9.2	8.8, 8.4–9.2	0.949**
Phosphorus (mg/dL)	4.9, 4.2–5.4	4.8, 3.9–5.5	0.937****
Whole PTH (pg/mL)	63.6, 47.4–101.4	81.8, 55.0–124.9	< 0.05**
Hemoglobin (g/dL)	11.4, 10.7–12.0	11.3, 10.8–11.9	0.557**
β2-microglobulin (mg/L)	22.9, 19.9–25.9	23.0, 20.1–26.5	0.571**
Kt/V	1.5, 1.4–1.6	1.5, 1.4–1.6	0.760*****

Data are presented as n (%), unless stated otherwise. p values were calculated using χ^2 test*, Mann-Whitney U test**, Fisher's exact test***, Student's t test****, and Welch's test*****, respectively

present," 139 (41.4%) reported "unchanged," and 3 (0.9%) reported "getting worse."

Disability

Sleep "Never affects sleep" was reported by 239 patients (71.1%), "occasionally delays falling asleep" by 73 (21.7%), "frequently delays falling asleep" by 9 (2.7%), "delays falling asleep and occasionally wakes me up at night" by 10 (3.0%), and "delays falling asleep and frequently wakes me up at night" by 5 (1.5%).

Leisure/social activities "Never affects leisure/social activities" was reported by 268 patients (79.8%), "rarely affects leisure/social activities" by 23 (6.8%), "occasionally affects leisure/social activities" by 23 (6.8%), "frequently affects leisure/social activities" by 3 (0.9%), "always affects leisure/social activities" by 2 (0.6%), and "not applicable" by 17 (5.1%).

Housework/errands “Never affects housework/errands” was reported by 273 patients (81.3%), “rarely affects housework/errands” by 25 (7.4%), “occasionally affects housework/errands” by 17 (5.1%), “frequently affects housework/errands” by 1 (0.3%), “always affects housework/errands” by 2 (0.6%), and “not applicable” by 18 (5.4%).

Work/school Among all patients, “never affects work/school” was reported by 256 patients (76.2%), “rarely affects work/school” by 25 (7.4%), “occasionally affects work/school” by 10 (3.0%), “frequently affects work/school” by 3 (0.9%), “always affects work/school” by 2 (0.6%), and “not applicable” by 40 (11.9%).

Distribution

Almost half of the patients ($n = 150$; 44.6%) reported “back,” followed by “head/scalp” ($n = 82$; 24.4%), “abdomen” ($n = 62$; 18.5%), and “lower legs” ($n = 54$; 16.1%) (Fig. 2).

Total scores

Total score was 5 points in 55 patients (16.4%), 6–9 points in 176 patients (52.4%), 10–14 points in 95 patients (28.3%), 15–19 points in 9 patients (2.7%), 20–24 points in 1 patient (0.3%), and 25 points in 0 (0%).

The median total score of all patients was 8 points. We divided the patients into two groups based on their total score, with 145 patients in the “≥ 9 points” group and 191 patients in the “≤ 8 points” group. Comparison of baseline characteristics and laboratory parameters of the two groups revealed that the “≥ 9 points” group included significantly more patients with ischemic heart disease ($p < 0.005$) and significantly more patients who had been prescribed moisturizers, topical steroids, and other topical drugs for the treatment of pruritus ($p < 0.001$ for each medication; Table 1).

Correlation between 5D-J and VAS

A strong correlation was observed between degree on 5D-J and VAS score ($r = 0.7588$; $p < 0.001$). Correlations were also found between both disability ($r = 0.6005$; $p < 0.001$) and distribution and the VAS score ($r = 0.4945$; $p < 0.001$; Table 3). The 5D-J total scores and VAS scores were also strongly correlated ($r = 0.7159$; $p < 0.001$; Fig. 3).

Correlation between 5D-J and Shiratori score

Daytime

A strong correlation was observed between degree on 5D-J and the Shiratori score ($r = 0.7457$; $p < 0.001$). Correlations were also found between both disability ($r = 0.5201$; $p < 0.001$) and distribution and the Shiratori score ($r = 0.4674$; $p < 0.001$; Table 4). In addition, a correlation was observed between the 5D-J total score and Shiratori score ($r = 0.6441$; $p < 0.001$; Fig. 4).

Nighttime

Correlations were found between degree, disability, and distribution on 5D-J and the Shiratori score ($r = 0.6099$, $r = 0.5811$, and $r = 0.4097$, respectively; $p < 0.001$; Table 5). A correlation was also observed between the 5D-J total score and Shiratori score ($r = 0.6352$; $p < 0.001$; Fig. 5).

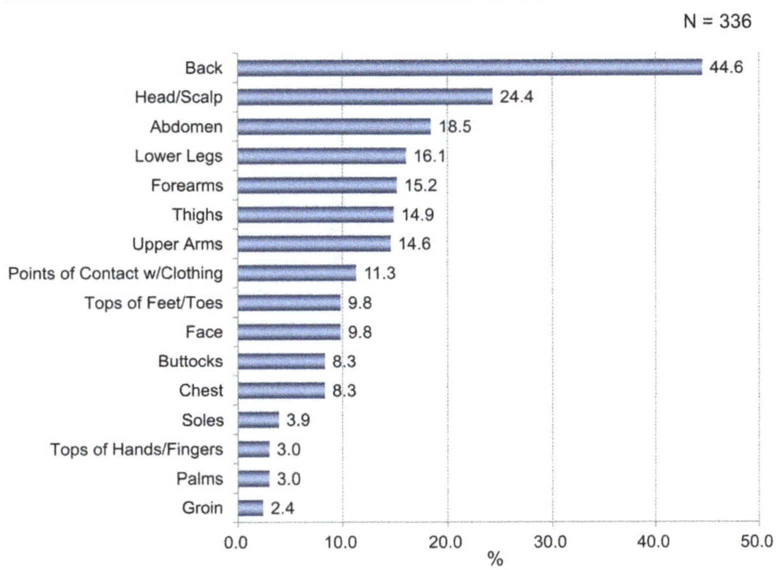

Fig. 2 Distribution of itchiness

Table 3 Correlation between 5D-J and VAS

	Spearman's rank correlation coefficient	
	r	*p* value
Duration	0.3845	< 0.001
Degree	0.7588	< 0.001
Direction	0.2330	< 0.001
Disability	0.6005	< 0.001
Distribution	0.4945	< 0.001
Total	0.7159	< 0.001

Table 4 Correlation between 5D-J and the Shiratori score (daytime)

	Spearman's rank correlation coefficient	
	r	*p* value
Duration	0.2251	< 0.001
Degree	0.7457	< 0.001
Direction	0.2309	< 0.005
Disability	0.5201	< 0.001
Distribution	0.4674	< 0.001
Total	0.6441	< 0.001

Correlation between 5D-J and objective parameters

We examined the relationship between 5D-J score and objective parameters, and no correlation was found (Table 6).

Discussion

In this study, we assessed the status of pruritus among patients undergoing hemodialysis at our facility using 5D-J, which is a new assessment scale for itchiness. We also investigated the usefulness of 5D-J by determining whether correlations existed between 5D-J and VAS and Shiratori scores, which the patients completed at the same time as 5D-J.

In summary, our assessment of the status of itchiness using 5D-J provided the following results. For duration, 91.4% of the patients reported < 6 h/day. For degree, 63.1% reported mild or more severe itchiness, which is comparable to the 60–80% previously reported [1–8]. However, 14.3% of the patients in our study reported moderate or more severe itchiness, which was lower than the 30–50% previously reported [1–8]. In addition, no patients reported unbearable itchiness. For disability, the percentages of patients who reported "never affects (this activity)" were as follows: sleep, 71.1%; leisure/social activities, 79.8%; housework/errands, 81.3%; and work/school, 76.2%. These results indicate that itchiness did not negatively affect the QOL of 70 to 80% of the patients at our facility. An assessment of the total scores indicated that > 95% scored ≤ 14 points (of a possible maximum 25 points). In the high-scoring group, comprising patients with total scores > 8, the number of patients with comorbid ischemic heart disease was significantly higher; the reason for this is unclear. Moreover, in the high-scoring group, significantly more patients were prescribed moisturizers, topical steroids, and other topical drugs. We believe the reason for this difference is that, compared with the low scoring group, factors that worsen pruritus such as dry skin, inflammation due to scratching, and secondary rashes may have been more prevalent in the high-scoring group.

In the group with "at least mild" pruritus, whole PTH level was significantly higher, as was the rate of chronic liver disease. Secondary hyperparathyroidism [3, 5] and viral hepatitis [19] have been reported to cause pruritus

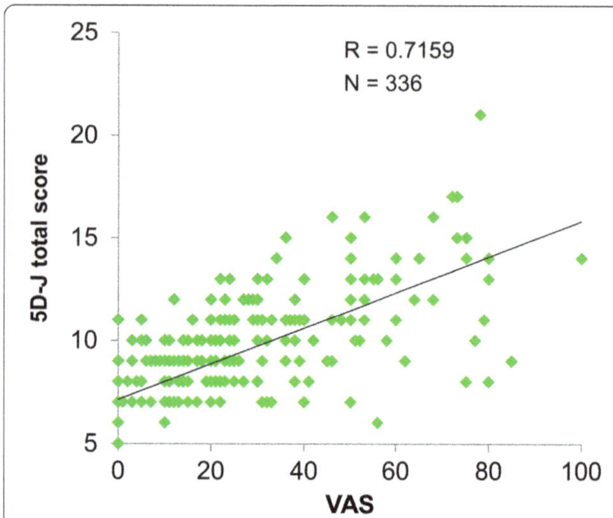

Fig. 3 Correlation between the 5D-J total score and VAS score

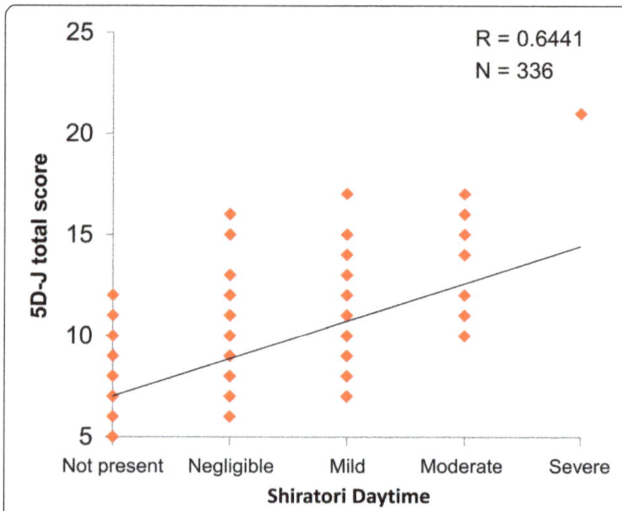

Fig. 4 Correlation between the 5D-J total score and the Shiratori score (daytime)

Table 5 Correlation between the 5D-J total score and Shiratori score (nighttime)

	Spearman's rank correlation coefficient	
	r	*p* value
Duration	0.3000	< 0.001
Degree	0.6099	< 0.001
Direction	0.2265	< 0.001
Disability	0.5811	< 0.001
Distribution	0.4097	< 0.001
Total	0.6352	< 0.001

Table 6 Correlation between 5D-J total score and objective parameters

	Spearman's rank correlation coefficient	
	r	*p* value
Albumin (g/dL)	− 0.140	< 0.05
Corrected calcium (mg/dL)	0.067	0.222
Phosphorus (mg/dL)	0.022	0.690
Whole PTH (pg/mL)	0.096	0.083
Hemoglobin (g/dL)	− 0.042	0.442
β2-microglobulin (mg/L)	0.043	0.448
Kt/V	− 0.026	0.648

in hemodialysis patients. Thus, we believe clinicians should take particular note of pruritus in hemodialysis patients with secondary hyperparathyroidism or viral hepatitis.

The therapeutic strategy for pruritus experienced by patients undergoing hemodialysis was revised at our facility in June 2009 by creating and introducing a new treatment algorithm. In particular, in addition to investigating dialysis techniques (e.g., protein adsorptive dialysis with a polymethylmethacrylate membrane and predilution online hemodiafiltration), as well as pharmacotherapies including the selective κ-opioid receptor agonist nalfurafine hydrochloride, we actively promoted skin care using moisturizers and provided lifestyle guidance. This treatment algorithm has been reported to be useful [20, 21]. In the current study, we found that in general, the duration of itchiness was short, degree was mild or less severe, and few patients experienced a negative effect on QOL owing to moderate or more severe itchiness or disability. We believe that these results

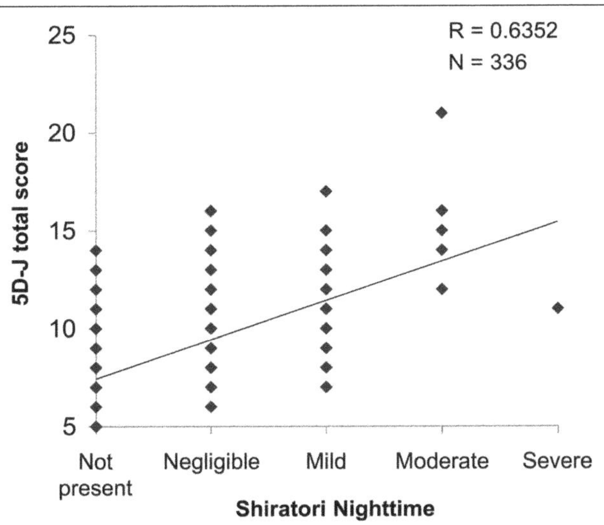

Fig. 5 Correlation between the 5D-J total score and the Shiratori score (nighttime)

reflect the success of the treatment algorithm currently being used at our facility.

Our study of itchiness distribution indicated that almost half of the patients reported "back," which is consistent with previous findings [1, 4]; after this body location, patients reported the head/scalp, abdomen, and lower legs. The distribution section comprises 16 detailed sites on the body where itchiness can be experienced. Because this allows patients to indicate the precise sites of itchiness, such data would be useful in appropriately selecting sites that require treatment.

Our study of the correlation between 5D-J, VAS, and Shiratori scores indicated that degree, disability, and distribution were all correlated, in some cases moderately or strongly. Our analysis of direction showed that 139 patients (41.4%) reported "unchanged." However, we believe that this reflects the fact that no change occurred in the symptoms experienced by patients who originally reported "no itchiness" or "mild itchiness." Furthermore, the correlation coefficients between these sections, VAS scores, and Shiratori scores were $r = 0.2330$, $r = 0.2309$, and $r = 0.2265$, respectively, indicating weak correlation. Thus, these results may not allow for an objective assessment of itchiness.

A strong correlation was observed between 5D-J total scores and VAS scores, as well as a correlation between 5D-J total scores and both daytime and nighttime Shiratori scores. In their study of 409 patients undergoing hemodialysis, Lai et al. reported a strong correlation between the 5-D itch scale and NRS ($r = 0.831$; $p < 0.001$) and also reported that the 5-D itch scale was a reliable multidimensional assessment scale of itchiness for use in patients undergoing hemodialysis [22]. In the present study, a strong or moderate correlation was found between multiple components, as well as 5D-J total scores, VAS scores, and Shiratori scores, possibly indicating that 5D-J is useful for comprehensively assessing itchiness experienced by patients undergoing hemodialysis.

Limitations of this study should be considered. As a result of continued treatment of pruritus based on our treatment algorithm, the number of patients with "severe" pruritus has gradually decreased over the years. At the time of our study in October 2016, of the 336 study patients, only 2 (0.6%) had "severe" itchiness and none had "unbearable" itchiness. The scarcity of patients with "severe" or "unbearable" pruritus may have influenced our study results and may have limited the assessment of this scoring system. In addition, because we did not compare 5D-J with other scales such as NRS or VRS to identify whether correlations exist between these scales, we are unable to comment further on the reliability of 5D-J.

Conclusions

The 5D-J is a simple, yet comprehensive, assessment system for pruritus that evaluates not only the degree but also the overall status of pruritus based on multiple features. Thus, it may be more useful than the VAS and the Shiratori score as an objective assessment scale of pruritus in hemodialysis patients.

Abbreviations

5D-J: Japanese version of the 5-D itch scale; NRS: Numerical rating scale; QOL: Quality of life; VAS: Visual analog scale; VRS: Verbal rating scale

Acknowledgements

The authors are grateful to all the medical staff who participated in this study.

Authors' contributions

NT conceived the study and wrote the first draft of this manuscript. TY contributed to the study design, coordinated the study, and conducted the statistical analysis. AO, JK, HK, ST, MM, and TM contributed to the study design and were involved in the production of the first draft of parts of this manuscript. TE developed the Japanese version of the 5-D itch scale and contributed to the study design and drafting parts of this manuscript. All authors read and approved the final manuscript.

Competing interests

The authors declare that they have no competing interests.

Author details

[1]Akane-Foundation Omachi Tsuchiya Clinic, 2-8-35 Omachi Higashi, Asa Minami-ku, Hiroshima 731-0124, Japan. [2]Department of Artificial Organs, Akane-Foundation, Tsuchiya General Hospital, Hiroshima, Japan. [3]Akane-Foundation Nakajima Tsuchiya Clinic, Hiroshima, Japan. [4]Department of Nephrology, Hiroshima University Hospital, Hiroshima, Japan. [5]Chitofuna Dermatology Clinic, Tokyo, Japan.

References

1. Omori K, Aoike I, Aoyagi H, Aoyagi R, Imai K, Iwafuchi Y, et al. Risk factors for uremic pruritus in long-term hemodialysis patients. J Jpn Soc Dial Ther. 2001;34:1469–77. (in Japanese)
2. Pisoni RL, Wikström B, Elder SJ, Akizawa T, Asano Y, Keen ML, et al. Pruritus in haemodialysis patients: international results from the Dialysis Outcomes and Practice Patterns Study (DOPPS). Nephrol Transplant. 2006;21:3495–505.
3. Narita I, Alchi B, Omori K, Sato F, Ajiro J, Saga D, et al. Etiology and prognostic significance of severe uremic pruritus in chronic hemodialysis patients. Kidney Int. 2006;69:1626–32.
4. Yamada S, Sakurai H, Kasuga H, Kawahara H. Investigation of the status of uremic pruritus in hemodialysis patients and the efficacy of nalfurafine hydrochloride—questionnaire administered to 1,936 patients from 17 clinics in Tokai area of Japan. J Jpn Soc Dial Ther. 2012;45:1133–40. (in Japanese)
5. Kimata N, Fuller DS, Saito A, Akizawa T, Fukuhara S, Pisoni RL, et al. Pruritus in hemodialysis patients: results from the Japanese Dialysis Outcomes and Practice Patterns Study (JDOPPS). Hemodial Int. 2014;18:657–67.
6. Remakrishnan K, Bond TC, Claxton A, Sood VC, Kootsikas M, Agnese W, et al. Clinical characteristics and outcomes of end-stage renal disease patients with self-reported pruritus symptoms. Int J Nephrol Renovasc Dis. 2014; 7:1–12.
7. Mathur VS, Lindberg J, Germain M, Block G, Tumlin J, Smith M, et al. ITCH National Registry Investigators: a longitudinal study of uremic pruritus in hemodialysis patients. Clin J Am Soc Nephrol. 2010;5:1410–9.
8. Shirazian S, Aina O, Park Y, Chowdhury N, Leger K, Hou L, et al. Chronic kidney disease-associated pruritus: impact on quality of life and current management challenges. Int J Nephrol Renovasc Dis. 2017;10:11–26.
9. Furue M, Ebata T, Ikoma A, Takeuchi S, Kataoka Y, Takamori K, et al. Verbalizing extremes of the visual analogue scale for pruritus: a consensus statement. Acta Derm Venereol. 2013;93:214–21.
10. Williamson A, Hoggart B. Pain: a review of three commonly used pain rating scales. J Clin Nurs. 2005;14:798–804.
11. Reich A, Heisig M, Phan NQ, Taneda K, Takamori K, Takeuchi S, et al. Visual analogue scale: evaluation of the instrument for the assessment of pruritus. Acta Derm Venereol. 2012;92:497–501.
12. Phan NQ, Blome C, Fritz F, Gerss J, Reich A, Ebata T, et al. Assessment of pruritus intensity: prospective study on validity and reliability of the visual analogue scale, numerical rating scale and verbal rating scale in 471 patients with chronic pruritus. Acta Derm Venereol. 2012;92:502–7.
13. Shiratori A. Therapeutic outcomes of the use of mequitazine (LM-209) in severe dermatological diseases. Nishinihon J Dermatol. 1983;45:470–3. (in Japanese)
14. Kawashima M, Tango T, Noguchi T, Inagi M, Nakagawa H, Harada S. Addition of fexofenadine to a topical corticosteroid reduces the pruritus associated with atopic dermatitis in a 1-week randomized, multicentre, double-blind, placebo-controlled, parallel-group study. Br J Dermatol. 2003; 148:1212–21.
15. Ständer S, Augustin M, Reich A, Blome C, Ebata T, Phan NQ, et al. Pruritus assessment in clinical trials: consensus recommendations from the International Forum for the Study of Itch (IFSI) Special Interest Group Scoring Itch in Clinical Trials. Acta Derm Venereol. 2013;93:509–14.
16. Ebata T, Ishiuji Y, Saeki H, Nakagawa H. Creation of a Japanese version of the 5D itch scale. Jpn J Dermatol. 2015;125:1035–40. (in Japanese)
17. Elman S, Hynan LS, Gabriel V, Mayo MJ. The 5-D itch scale: a new measure of pruritus. Br J Dermatol. 2010;162:587–93.
18. Ebata T. Recent advances in the evaluation of itch and introduction of the Japanese version of the 5D-itch scale in adult patients with atopic dermatitis; Atopic Dermatitis Treatment Study Group. Skin Res. 2015;14:S1–6. (in Japanese)
19. Chiu YL, Chen HY, Chuang YF, Hsu SP, Lai CF, Pai MF, et al. Association of uraemic pruritus with inflammation and hepatitis infection in haemodialysis patients. Nephrol Dial Transplant. 2008;23:3685–9.
20. Takahashi N, Yoshizawa T, Kumagai J. Efficacy and safety of long-term (104-week) administration of nalfurafine hydrochloride. J Jpn Soc Dial Ther. 2013; 46:371–8. (in Japanese)
21. Takahashi N, Yoshizawa T, Kumagai J, Kawanishi H, Moriishi M, Masaki T, et al. Response of patients with hemodialysis-associated pruritus to new treatment protocol with nalfurafine hydrochloride: a retrospective survey-based study. Ren Replac Ther. 2016;2:27.
22. Lai JW, Chen HC, Chou CY, Yen HR, Li TC, Sun MF, et al. Transformation of 5-D itch scale and numerical rating scale in chronic hemodialysis patients. BMC Nephrol. 2017;18:56.

19

Hypereosinophilic syndrome manifested as eosinophilic gastroenteritis and colitis in a patient undergoing hemodialysis

Eri Amano[1], Taro Horino[1*], Osamu Ichii[2], Satoshi Inotani, Tatsuki Matsumoto[1], Kazu Hamada-Ode[1], Yoshiko Shimamura[1], Kosuke Inoue[1] and Yoshio Terada[1]

Abstract

Background: Hypereosinophilic syndrome (HES) consists of a group of disorders characterized by abnormal accumulation of eosinophils in the blood or peripheral tissues, independent of known secondary causes of eosinophilia. Clinical manifestations of HES are highly variable, ranging from asymptomatic eosinophilia to severe tissue damage and end-organ failure.

Case presentation: We herein present the case of a 65-year-old female with a 38-year history of hemodialysis who presented with lower leg pain, fever, skin eruption with leg edema, and diarrhea. Two months before admission, she underwent placement of a stent made of nickel and titanium for abdominal aortic stenosis. Lower leg pain occurred during hemodialysis, followed by fever, pedal edema with skin eruption, and diarrhea. Gastrointestinal endoscopy, colonoscopy, and biopsy histopathology revealed colitis with massive infiltration of eosinophils, compatible with eosinophilic gastroenteritis and colitis. The patient was treated with prednisolone at an initial dose of 40 mg daily and later reduced to 10 mg daily, after which her symptoms improved and her laboratory parameters normalized. She has not experienced a relapse after 1 year of follow-up.

Conclusions: Our case of HES manifested as eosinophilic gastroenteritis and colitis and was successfully treated with corticosteroids. Clinicians should consider the differential diagnosis of HES when faced with similar cases in order to effect timely and appropriate treatment.

Keywords: Hypereosinophilic syndrome (HES), Metal stent placement, Nickel allergy, Peripheral arterial disease (PAD)

Background

Hypereosinophilic syndrome (HES) is defined as a group of disorders characterized by abnormal accumulation of eosinophils in the blood or peripheral tissues. Clinical manifestations vary considerably, ranging from asymptomatic eosinophilia to severe tissue damage and end-organ failure. The prevalence of eosinophilia has been reported to vary from 13 to 52% in hemodialysis patients and can increase with time spent undergoing dialysis [1]. Eosinophilia from any other cause has also been reported to cause life-threatening reactions in patients undergoing hemodialysis due to the release of interleukins and eosinophil peroxidase due to the degranulation of eosinophils [1]. Severe reactions to dialysis secondary to hypereosinophilia and the therapy provided for such patients have not been reported frequently [1]. We herein report a case of HES that manifested as eosinophilic gastroenteritis and colitis on long-term maintenance hemodialysis and was successfully treated with corticosteroids.

Case presentation

A 65-year-old female with a 38-year history of hemodialysis presented with lower leg pain, fever, skin eruption with leg edema, and diarrhea. Two months before admission, she had undergone placement of a stent made of nickel and titanium for abdominal aortic stenosis with lower leg pain during hemodialysis. "She received chronic maintenance hemodialysis with Vitamin E immobilized

* Correspondence: horinott@yahoo.co.jp
[1]Department of Endocrinology, Metabolism and Nephrology, Kochi Medical School, Kochi University, Kohasu, Oko-cho, Nankoku, Kochi 783-8505, Japan
Full list of author information is available at the end of the article

Table 1 Laboratory data at admission of our patient

			(Reference range)
CBC			
RBC	309	$\times 10^4/\mu L$	(435–555)
Ht	26.1	%	(40.7–50.1)
Hb	8.3	g/dL	(13.7–16.8)
Plt	25.4	$\times 10^4/\mu L$	(15.8–34.8)
WBC	27.4	$\times 10^3/\mu L$	(3.3–8.6)
neu	49	%	(41.2–74.7)
lym	2	%	(21.2–51.0)
mon	1	%	(3.1–8.0)
eos	48	%	(0.2–4.8)
bas	0	%	(0.1–1.0)
Proteinogram			
IgG	2540	mg/dL	(870–1700)
IgA	147	mg/dL	(110–410)
IgM	106	mg/dL	(35–220)
IgE	1913	IU/mL	(< 100.0)
Serological examinations			
CRP	4.73	mg/dL	(< 0.14)
ANA	< 40	×	(< 40)
MPO-ANCA	(–)		(–)
PR3-ANCA	(–)		(–)
GBM Ab	(–)		(–)
sIL2R	4834	U/mL	(127–582)
Blood chemistry			
TP	7.3	g/dL	(6.6–8.1)
FBS	89	mg/dL	(73–109)
Alp	350	U/L	(106–322)
t-Cho	122	mg/dL	(142–322)
γ-GTP	18	U/L	(13–64)
t-Bil	0.3	mg/dL	(0.4–1.5)
d-Bil	0.1	mg/dL	(< 0.4)
ChE	147	U/L	(240–486)
Glb	5.1	g/dL	(2.2–3.4)
Alb	2.2	g/dL	(4.1–5.1)
ALT	13	U/L	(10–42)
AST	17	U/L	(13–30)
LDH	324	U/L	(124–222)
CPK	159	U/L	(59–248)
SCr	5.6	mg/dL	(0.65–1.07)
BUN	43	mg/dL	(8–20)
UA	5.6	mg/dL	(3.7–7.8)
Amy	51	U/L	(44–132)
HbA1c	5.8	%	(4.6–6.2)
Infection			
HCV Ab	(+)		(–)
HBs Ag	(–)		(–)

CBC complete blood cell count, *RBC* red blood cell count, *Hb* hemoglobin, *Ht* hematocrit, *Plt* platelet, *WBC* white blood cell count, *neu* neutrophils, *lym* lymphocytes, *mon* monocytes, *eos* eosinophils, *bas* basophils, *IgG* immunoglobulin G, *IgA* immunoglobulin A, *IgM* immunoglobulin M, *IgE* immunoglobulin E, *CRP* C-reactive protein, *ANA* anti-nuclear antibody, *MPO-ANCA* myeloperoxidase-anti-neutrophil cytoplasmic antibody, *PR3-ANCA* serine proteinase3-anti-neutrophil cytoplasmic antibody, *GBM Ab* anti-glomerular basement membrane antibody, *sIL2R* soluble interleukin 2 receptor, *TP* total protein, *FBS* fasting blood sugar, *Alp* alkaline phosphatase, *t-Cho* total cholesterol, *γ-GTP* g-glutamyltransferase, *t-Bil* total bilirubin, *d-Bil* direct bilirubin, *ChE* cholinesterase, *Glb* globulin, *Alb* albumin, *ALT* alanine transaminase, *AST* aspartate aminotransferase, *LDH* lactate dehydrogenase, *CPK* creatine phosphokinase, *SCr* serum creatinine, *BUN* blood urea nitrogen, *UA* uric acid, *Amy* amylase, *HbA1c* hemoglobin A1c, *HCV Ab* hepatitis C virus antibody, *HBs Ag* hepatitis B surface antigen

polysulfone dialyzer VPS-18HA® (AsahiKASEI, Tokyo, JAPAN) and heparin sodium as anticoagulant. The condition of hemodialysis did not change during her clinical course, and she has not indicated hypereosinophilia while performing the same hemodialysis condition so far."

After stent placement, her lower leg pain continued, and subsequently, fever, pedal edema with skin eruption, and diarrhea occurred. She was treated with meropenem hydrate 0.5 g daily after hemodialysis due to the initial suspicion of cellulitis. However, her symptoms progressed rapidly; therefore, she was transferred to our hospital.

On admission, physical examination revealed muscle weakness and pedal edema with eruption. As shown in Table 1, laboratory examination revealed elevated levels of C-reactive protein (CRP) (4.73 mg/dL) and white blood cell count (WBC) (27,400/μL) with eosinophils (13,152/μL), hemoglobin (Hb) (8.3 g/dL), and IgE (1913.0 IU/mL). Fecal examination revealed that occult blood was positive but parasites were negative. Tumor markers including carcinoembryonic antigen and α-fetoprotein were all negative. Serological testings including anti-nuclear antibody, myeloperoxidase-anti-neutrophil cytoplasmic antibody, and serine proteinase3-anti-neutrophil cytoplasmic antibody were all negative. Bone marrow examination was performed to exclude chronic myeloid disorders and revealed no remarkable abnormalities. Abdominal computed tomography (CT) scan revealed peripheral arterial disease (PAD) as well as the abdominal aortic stenosis with intra-aortic stent (Fig. 1). Echocardiogram and electrocardiography showed no remarkable findings (Fig. 2). Erythrocyte transfusion equivalent to 400 mL blood was performed for progression of anemia (Hb 6.4 g/dL). Fever and skin eruption continued. One month after admission, diarrhea and melena occurred, and subsequently, anemia

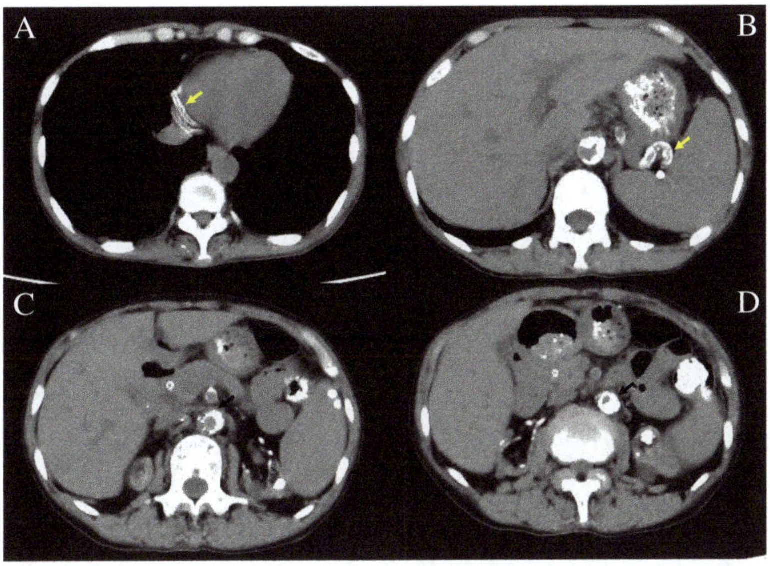

Fig. 1 Abdominal computed tomography revealing **a**, **b** peripheral arterial disease (PAD) (yellow arrows) and **c**, **d** abdominal aortic stenosis with intra-aortic stent (red arrows)

progressed. Her antibiotic treatment was changed to levofloxacin 250 mg every other day; however, her symptoms did not change. Colonoscopy revealed colitis, and biopsy histopathology revealed colitis with massive infiltration of eosinophils, compatible with eosinophilic colitis (Fig. 3a, b). As shown in Fig. 4, prednisolone (PSL) 40 mg daily was started, after which her symptoms, including fever and skin eruption, improved and her laboratory parameters, including CRP, WBC, and eosinophil count, normalized. PSL was then tapered to 5 mg daily; however, the melena recurred. Gastrointestinal endoscopy revealed enteritis in the small intestine, and biopsy histopathology confirmed eosinophilic gastroenteritis (Fig. 3c, d). Therefore, PSL was increased to 10 mg daily, after which her symptoms improved. After discharge, she was followed up in an outpatient clinic for 1 year without relapse.

Discussion

Eosinophilia is defined as an elevation in the absolute eosinophil count (AEC). Definition and classification of the severity of eosinophilia is shown in Table 2 [2–4]. First used in 1968 [5], the term "hypereosinophilic syndrome" was coined to describe this set of symptoms [6]. Subsequently, formal diagnostic criteria for HES were established in 1975, in which HES was defined as having no secondary causes of eosinophilia [7]. To date, with the accumulation of knowledge contributed by multiple researchers, not only have improved diagnostic techniques led to the identification of previously unrecognized causes of HES, but also the availability of effective therapies has led to a marked decrease in morbidity and mortality in patients with HES who are treated early. Therefore, HES has recently been categorized as a syndrome that includes

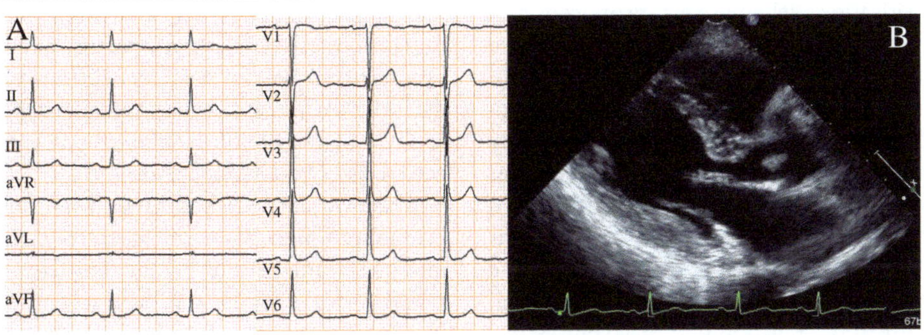

Fig. 2 The findings of echocardiogram and electrocardiography. **a** The echocardiogram revealed no remarkable findings. **b** Electrocardiography showed no remarkable abnormalities

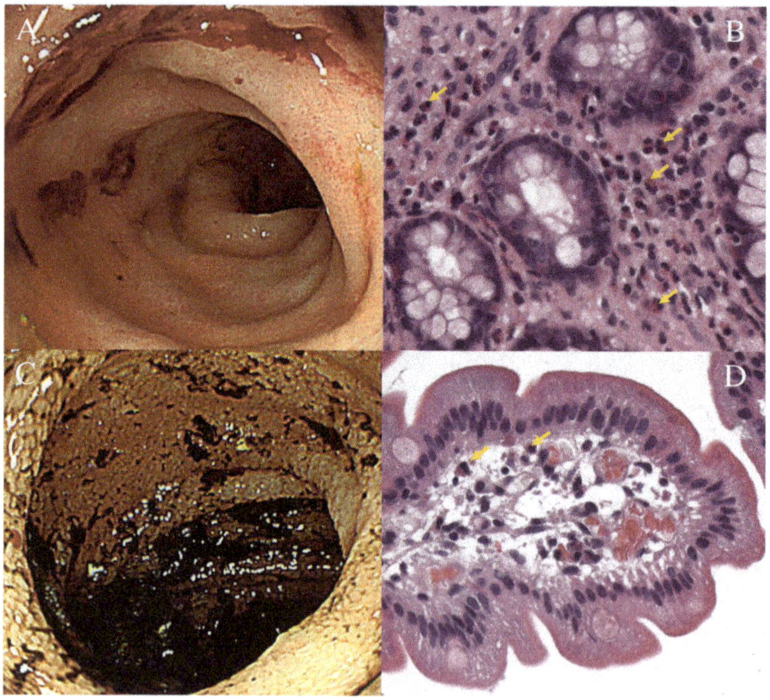

Fig. 3 The findings of endoscopy and biopsies. **a** Macroscopic finding of colonoscopy revealing colitis with bleeding. **b** Biopsy specimen of colonoscopy revealing massive infiltration of eosinophils (orange arrows) (periodic acid-Schiff, × 200), consistent with eosinophilic colitis. **c** Macroscopic finding of endoscopy revealing duodenitis with bleeding. **d** Biopsy specimen of colonoscopy revealing massive infiltration of eosinophils (yellow arrows) (periodic acid-Schiff, × 200), consistent with eosinophilic gastroenteritis

various pathological conditions previously identified as causes. This allows for early and prompt diagnosis with subsequent early intervention, which is needed for improving the prognosis of organ damage associated with HES. Now, HES is defined broadly as blood hypereosinophilia (HE) (AEC of ≥ 1500/μL) and includes clinical manifestations attributable to eosinophilia or tissue HE with blood eosinophilia (AEC above the upper limit of normal for the reference laboratory) (Table 2) [8]. As described previously (shown in Table 3), HE has many differential diagnoses [8].

At a 2005 international consensus conference on HES treatment, a classification scheme was proposed that subdivided patients with HES into six clinically defined groups to facilitate treatment decisions [9]. This classification was refined in 2010 [10] and continues to be updated as our understanding of the relationship between this condition's etiology and response to therapy evolves [11]. HES is divided into the following six clinical variants (Table 2) [8]. Overlap HES, one of the clinical variants of HES, is defined as eosinophilic disease restricted to a single organ system, accompanied by peripheral eosinophilia > 1500/μL [8]. Eosinophilic gastrointestinal disorders (EGIDs), a group of rare differential diagnoses of HE (shown in Table 3) [8], are often categorized as part of this group. Patients with EGID may present with nausea, vomiting, diarrhea, abdominal pain, dysmotility, and failure to thrive, depending on the degree and location of the eosinophilic infiltration. Our patient was considered as having overlap HES, because her clinical manifestations showed EGID presenting as eosinophilic gastroenteritis and colitis.

HES of any etiology can cause serious, potentially life-threatening, complications, including cardiac involvement, thromboembolism, and neurologic manifestations. Although clinical and laboratory findings associated with aggressive disease and poor prognosis include AEC > 100,000/μL, signs of congestive heart failure, and resistance to corticosteroid therapy, specific biomarkers of disease progression have not been identified [8]. Consequently, the decision to initiate urgent therapy depends on both the acuity and severity of the clinical presentation and the perceived risk of rapid progression [6].

When life-threatening manifestations are present or imminent, high-dose corticosteroid therapy should be initiated immediately [6, 8]. The recommended dosing ranges from 1 mg/kg PSL to 1 g methylprednisolone depending on the severity of the clinical manifestations [8]. Intravenous administration should be considered to ensure adequate absorption in patients who are acutely ill

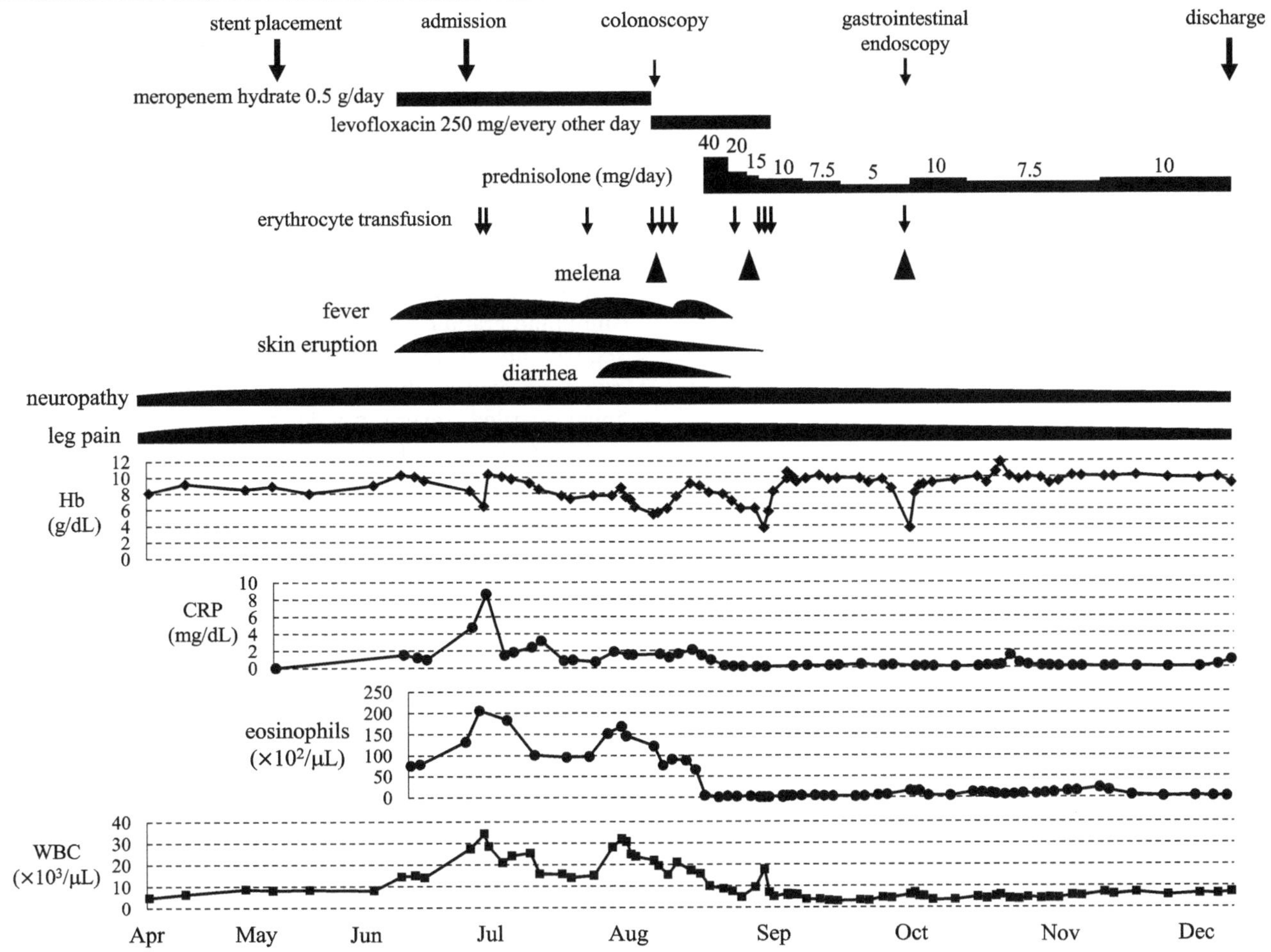

Fig. 4 The clinical course of our case

or have signs or symptoms of gastrointestinal involvement [8]. In a multicenter study including 188 HES patients, it was found that 81% had been initially treated with steroids. The median dose of PSL or an equivalent steroid was 40 mg daily. Nearly 75% were on maintenance steroids for an extended period, with an average dose of 10 mg PSL daily. The duration of therapy ranged from 2 months to 20 years. Eighty-five percent of the patients on steroid monotherapy had a partial or complete remission within 1 month of therapy initiation [12]. In our case, although steroid therapy was very effective, it was necessary to continue 10 mg of oral PSL to ensure complete resolution because bleeding recurred when oral PSL was reduced to a lower dosage.

To date, seven cases with eosinophilia and clinical symptoms due to nickel including our case had been described [13–18]. Gray reported the first case of a patient who developed eosinophilia due to ingestion of a nickel coin and presented with Loffler's syndrome, transient migratory infiltrates associated with peripheral eosinophilia [13]. Four cases of occupational asthma with HE associated with exposure to nickel dust have been previously reported [14–17]. These five cases had transient mild eosinophilic pneumonia [13, 14] or asthma [15–17] that could be treated with low-dose corticosteroid. Meanwhile, Fung et al. reported a case of fulminant HE and eosinophilic myocarditis triggered by the nickel in implantable cardioverter-defibrillator components superimposed on advanced non-ischemic dilated cardiomyopathy, who eventually needed cardiac transplantation [18]. Previous reports have suggested that organ complications of eosinophilia due to nickel cause damage to organs close to the exposure site and that the severity also correlates with the intensity of the exposure (Table 4). Although symptoms in the previous cases developed in a short period, the timing of the onset of eosinophilia was unknown and symptoms progressed slowly in our case. However, eosinophilia was confirmed under the mucosa of the stomach and colon, which is downstream of the stent position of the abdominal aorta. We suspected that eosinophils

Table 2 Definition and classification of eosinophilia [1–3] and hypereosinophilic syndrome (HES) [7]

Definition of eosinophilia	
• % eosinophils in the peripheral blood: 3–5%	
and/or	
• AEC: 350–500/μL	
Classification of the severity of eosinophilia	
• Mild	AEC: upper limit of normal to 1500/μL
• Moderate	AEC: 1500–5000/μL
• Severe	AEC: > 5000/μL
Definition of HES	
• AEC: ≥ 1500/μL	
and	
• Clinical manifestations attributable to eosinophilia or tissue HE with blood eosinophilia	
Classification of HES	
• Myeloproliferative HE/HES (M-HE/M-HES)	
• Lymphocytic variant HE/HES (L-HE/L-HES)	
• Overlap HES	
• Associated HE/HES	
• Familial HE/HES	

AEC absolute eosinophil count, *HE* hypereosinophilia

could be sprayed along the bloodstream, so the symptom onset might progress slowly. Likewise, in our case, deterioration of symptoms and increase of leukocytes accompanying a prominent eosinophilia increase were observed after insertion of an indwelling stent, and these symptoms were improved by steroid therapy. Thus, it was suspected that stent placement, in particular a reaction to nickel in the stent material, might have caused the HES in our case. Similar to the case reported by Fung et al. [18], we considered that, in our case, the degree of eosinophilia and the severity of its complication became severe because of the indwelling nickel stent. Unfortunately, removal of the stent was technically impossible, and the reaction to nickel could not be confirmed by an allergy test because the patient was undergoing steroid therapy.

In our case, the referral doctor initially diagnosed eosinophilic granulomatosis with polyangiitis (EGPA) from leg pain and eosinophilia. However, our patient had been receiving dialysis therapy for a long time, and CT findings revealed severe calcification of systemic arterial walls, consistent with PAD. Therefore, although subjective symptom progression was observed with systemic inflammation after stent placement, the leg pain was assumed to be a symptom mainly associated with PAD. Even after stent placement, the leg pain persisted mildly, especially during dialysis, and vasculitis was not proven histologically. Therefore, as mentioned above, the final diagnosis of our case was designated as overlap HES. Considering these facts, we suggest that, because elderly patients with underlying diseases usually have various complications, clinicians should be wary of ascribing a disease to a single pathological condition and consider the coexistence of multiple diseases, even when symptoms point to a single condition.

Conclusions

Here, we report an unusual case of HES that manifested as eosinophilic gastroenteritis and colitis caused by

Table 3 Differential diagnoses of hypereosinophilia [8]

Category	Examples
• Allergic disorders	Asthma, atopic dermatitis
• Drug hypersensitivity	Eosinophilia-myalgia syndrome, DRESS, interstitial nephritis, eosinophilic hepatitis
• Infection	
▪ Helminthic	Strongyloidiasis, trichinellosis, filariasis, schistosomiasis, hookworm
▪ Ectoparasitic	Scabies, myiasis
▪ Protozoan	Isosporiasis, sarcocystis myositis
▪ Fungal	Coccidiodomycosis, allergic bronchopulmonary aspergillosis, histoplasmosis
▪ Viral	HIV
• Neoplasia	Leukemia, lymphoma, adenocarcinoma
• Immunologic disorders	
▪ Immunodeficiency	DOCK8 deficiency, hyper-IgE syndrome, Omenn's syndrome
▪ Autoimmune and idiopathic	Sarcoidosis, inflammatory bowel disease, IgG4 disease, other connective tissue diseases
• Miscellaneous	Radiation exposure, cholesterol emboli, hypoadrenalism, IL-2 therapy
• Rare eosinophilic disorders	Idiopathic HES, EGPA, EGIDs

DRESS drug reaction with eosinophilia and systemic symptoms, *HIV* human immunodeficiency virus, *DOCK8* dedicator of cytokinesis 8, *IgE* immunoglobulin E, *IgG4* immunoglobulin G4, *IL-2* interleukin-2, *EGPA* eosinophilic granulomatosis with polyangiitis, *EGIDs* eosinophilic gastrointestinal disorders

Table 4 Previous reports of hypereosinophilia due to nickel [13–18]

No.	Author	Year	Age	Gender	Cause	Clinical manifestations	Treatment	Outcome	Ref.
1	Gray J (Canada)	1982	67	Female	Ingestion of nickel coin	Eosinophilic pneumonia	Coin removed	Improved	[13]
2	Toyoshima M (Japan)	1994	16	Male	Occupationally exposed	Eosinophilic pneumonia	Corticosteroid (i.v., oral)	Improved	[14]
3	De Hauteclocque C (France)	2002	40	Male	Occupationally exposed	Asthma	n.d.	n.d.	[15]
4	Marraccini P (Italy)	2008	43	Female	Occupationally exposed	Asthma	n.d.	n.d.	[16]
5	Song GW (Korea)	2013	34	Male	Occupationally exposed	Asthma	Corticosteroid (inhaled), job change	Improved	[17]
6	Fung E (USA)	2016	45	Male	ICD	Eosinophilic myocarditis	Corticosteroid (i.v., oral)	Not improved (C.T.)	[18]
7	Our case (Japan)	2018	65	Female	Nickel stent replacement	EGIDs	Corticosteroid (oral)	Improved	

ICD implantable cardioverter-defibrillator, *C.T.* cardiac transplantation, *EGIDs* eosinophilic gastrointestinal disorders, *i.v.* intravenous, *ref.* reference, *n.d.* not described

nickel stent replacement therapy in a patient undergoing hemodialysis. Early identification of and medical intervention for her HES resulted in a successful outcome. We conclude, therefore, that it is vital for clinicians to perform differential diagnoses considering the possibility of HES in order to effect timely and appropriate treatment. Moreover, it is important that data from similar cases be accumulated and future studies conducted to improve the prognoses of HES patients.

Abbreviations

AEC: Absolute eosinophil count; CRP: C-reactive protein; CT: Computed tomography; EGIDs: Eosinophilic gastrointestinal disorders; Hb: Hemoglobin; HE: Hypereosinophilia; HES: Hypereosinophilic syndrome; PAD: Peripheral arterial disease; PSL: Prednisolone; WBC: White blood cell count

Acknowledgements

The authors would like to express their sincere thanks to the medical staff of Kochi Medical School Hospital, Nankoku, Japan.

Authors' contributions

EA, TH, OI, SI, TM, KH-O, YS, KI, and YT provided information on the discussion and treatment of the patient. EA, TH, and OI collected the data and wrote the manuscript. All authors read and approved the final manuscript.

Competing interests

The authors declare that they have no competing interests.

Author details

[1]Department of Endocrinology, Metabolism and Nephrology, Kochi Medical School, Kochi University, Kohasu, Oko-cho, Nankoku, Kochi 783-8505, Japan. [2]Laboratory of Anatomy, Department of Biomedical Sciences, Graduate School of Veterinary Medicine, Hokkaido University, Kita 18, Nishi 9, Kita-Ku, Sapporo 060-0818, Japan.

References

1. Nayak-Rao S. A patient with hemodialysis intolerance and hypereosinophilia. Saudi J Kidney Dis Transpl. 2015;26:366–7.
2. Gotlib J. World Health Organization-defined eosinophilic disorders: 2014 update on diagnosis, risk stratification, and management. Am J Hematol. 2014;89:325–37.
3. Brigden M, Graydon C. Eosinophilia detected by automated blood cell counting in ambulatory North American outpatients. Incidence and clinical significance. Arch Pathol Lab Med. 1997;121:963–7.
4. Rothenberg ME. Eosinophilia. N Engl J Med. 1998;338:1592–600.
5. Hardy WR, Anderson RE. The hypereosinophilic syndromes. Ann Intern Med. 1968;68:1220–9.
6. Curtis C, Ogbogu P. Hypereosinophilic syndrome. Clin Rev Allergy Immunol. 2016;50:240–51.
7. Chusid MJ, Dale DC, West BC, Wolff SM. The hypereosinophilic syndrome: analysis of fourteen cases with review of the literature. Medicine (Baltimore). 1975;54:1–27.
8. Klion AD. How I treat hypereosinophilic syndromes. Blood. 2015;126: 1069–77.
9. Klion AD, Bochner BS, Gleich GJ, Nutman TB, Rothenberg ME, Simon HU, et al. The Hypereosinophilic Syndromes Working Group. Approaches to the treatment of hypereosinophilic syndromes: a workshop summary report. J Allergy Clin Immunol. 2006;117:1292–302.
10. Simon HU, Rothenberg ME, Bochner BS, Weller PF, Wardlaw AJ, Wechsler ME, et al. Refining the definition of hypereosinophilic syndrome. J Allergy Clin Immunol. 2010;126:45–9.
11. Valent P, Klion AD, Horny HP, Roufosse F, Gotlib J, Weller PF, et al. Contemporary consensus proposal on criteria and classification of eosinophilic disorders and related syndromes. J Allergy Clin Immunol. 2012; 130:607–12. e9
12. Ogbogu PU, Bochner BS, Butterfield JH, Gleich GJ, Huss-Marp J, Kahn JE, et al. Hypereosinophilic syndromes: a multicenter, retrospective analysis of clinical characteristics and response to therapy. J Allergy Clin Immunol. 2009;124:1319–25. e3
13. Gray J. Löffler's syndrome following ingestion of a coin. Can Med Assoc J. 1982;127:999–1000.
14. Toyoshima M, Sato A, Taniguchi M, Imokawa S, Nakazawa K, Hayakawa H, et al. A case of eosinophilic pneumonia caused by inhalation of nickel dusts. Nihon Kyobu Shikkan Gakkai Zasshi. 1994;32:480–4. Article in Japanese
15. De Hauteclocque C, Morisset M, Kanny G, Kohler C, Mouget B, Moneret-Vautrin DA. Occupational asthma due to hard metals hypersensitivity. Rev Mal Respir. 2002;19:363–5. Article in French
16. Marraccini P, Cantone L, Previdi M, Patrini L, Costamagna P. Respiratory allergy to nickel. Description of an atypical clinical case. G Ital Med Lav Ergon. 2008;30:139–41. Article in Italian
17. Song GW, Ban GY, Nam YH, Park HS, Ye YM. Case report of occupational asthma induced by polyvinyl chloride and nickel. J Korean Med Sci. 2013;28: 1540–2.

Comparison of intradialytic plasma volume change between online hemodiafiltration and standard hemodialysis

Masayuki Tanemoto[1,2*], Yu Ishimoto[2], Yukio Kosako[2] and Yukio Okazaki[2]

Abstract

Background: Intradialytic plasma volume change (IPVC) owing to ultrafiltration is a dominant cause of intradialytic hypotension (IDH). Lower occurrence of IDH in hemodiafiltration (HDF) than in standard hemodialysis (std-HD) indicates that HDF has preventive effect on IPVC. This study examined whether online HDF (ol-HDF) prevented IPVC compared with std-HD.

Methods: In 115 std-HD, 59 push-pull ol-HDF (pp-ol-HDF), 39 pre-dilution ol-HDF (pre-ol-HDF), and 33 post-dilution ol-HDF (post-ol-HDF) sessions, we calculated IPVC using intradialytic change of hemoglobin ($IPVC_{Hb}$) and also using the change of hematocrit ($IPVC_{Ht}$), and compared them in association with intradialytic body weight loss (IBWL) between the dialysis modes.

Results: Both $IPVC_{Hb}$ and $IPVC_{Ht}$ were not different between the modes; in std-HD, pp-ol-HDF, pre-ol-HDF, and post-ol-HDF, $IPVC_{Hb}$ were 0.10 ± 0.06, 0.11 ± 0.07, 0.10 ± 0.05, and 0.10 ± 0.06, respectively, and $IPVC_{Ht}$ were 0.10 ± 0.07, 0.11 ± 0.07, 0.10 ± 0.06, and 0.10 ± 0.06, respectively. IPVCs divided by relative IBWL to DW (IBWL/DW) were also not different between the modes; in std-HD, pp-ol-HDF, pre-ol-HDF, and post-ol-HDF, $IPVC_{Hb}$/IBWL/DW were 1.9 ± 2.0, 1.7 ± 4.6, 2.1 ± 0.9, and 2.1 ± 1.8, respectively, and $IPVC_{Ht}$/IBWL/DW were 1.9 ± 2.2, 1.9 ± 3.7, 2.1 ± 1.1, and 2.1 ± 2.0, respectively.

Conclusion: Irrespective of the modes, ol-HDF has the same level of IPVC as std-HD.

Keywords: Hemodiafiltration, Hemodialysis, Hypotension, Plasma volume, Ultrafiltration

Background

Hemodialysis is a renal replacement therapy for end-stage renal disease [1]. As an outpatient-based treatment, maintenance hemodialysis is performed intermittently (2–3 sessions per week) and for short duration (3–5 h) per session. The intermittent treatment inevitably leads to fluid accumulation between sessions, which needs to be removed by ultrafiltration during each session [2]. The removal induces intradialytic plasma volume change (IPVC), which is a dominant cause of intradialytic hypotension (IDH); the reduction in systolic blood pressure was related to the reduction in IPVC, and an individual threshold of IPVC was noted for IDH [3–5].

Hemodiafiltration (HDF) is a mode of hemodialysis performed by a combination of diffusive transport and convective transport where appropriate fluid balance is maintained by infusing substitution fluid [6]. Lower occurrence of IDH in HDF than in standard hemodialysis (std-HD), where only diffusive transport is performed, indicates that convective transport can provide preventive effect on IPVC [7–9]. Several different modes of HDF are available depending on the site of substitution fluid infusion; the fluid is infused upstream, downstream, and through the membrane of the dialyzer in pre-dilution mode (pre-HDF), post-dilution mode (post-HDF), and push-pull mode (pp-HDF), respectively [6]. Preparation of infusion fluid from non-pyrogenic dialysate further enabled an 'online' option for HDF (ol-HDF) [10]. The preventive effect of HDF on IPVC would differ depending on the modes. In the present report, we

* Correspondence: mtanemoto-tky@umin.ac.jp
[1]Division of Nephrology, Department of Internal Medicine, 418-1 Kamihayami, Kuki, Saitama 346-8530, Japan
[2]Dialysis Unit, Shin-Kuki General Hospital, 418-1 Kamihayami, Kuki, Saitama 346-8530, Japan

compared IPVC between std-HD and three different modes of online HDF.

Methods

Sessions and dialysis conditions

This study was a retrospective analysis of dialysis sessions at a single dialysis center. In addition to std-HD, three different modes of online HDF (pp-ol-HDF, pre-ol-HDF, post-ol-HDF) had been performed. Sessions after long dialysis interval in adult (> 18 years old) patients under maintenance dialysis (≥ 3.5 h/session, 2–3 sessions/week, > 6 months), where complete blood cell count tests were performed for blood samples at the start and end of sessions, were included. Sessions with blood transfusion or fluid infusion during dialysis treatment were excluded. The hospital ethics committee approved the study.

Dialysis sessions were performed using bicarbonate dialysate (Na^+ 140, K^+ 2.0, Ca^{2+} 1.5, Mg^{2+} 0.5, Cl^- 111, HCO_3^- 35, and glucose 8.3 mmol/L). The dialysate temperature and flow rate were set at 35–36 °C and 500 mL/min, respectively. Blood flow rates were individually prescribed to achieve a dialyzer clearance of urea to volume of distribution area (Kt/V) of > 1.2 [11], and ranged from 180 to 280 mL/min. For HDF, one of the following online modes, which are regularly performed in Japan using dialysate as substitution fluid, was selected; pre-ol-HDF with a constant replacement rate of 10 L/h, post-ol-HDF with a constant replacement rate of 2.5 L/h, and pp-ol-HDF with intermittent replacement of 0.2 L every 30 min [12].

Data collection and definitions

Pre-dialysis and post-dialysis blood samplings were performed just after the venipuncture at the start of the sessions and just before the wash-back at the end of the sessions, respectively. To avoid the influence of postural and food-intake effects on hemodynamics, the patients were placed in a supine position for > 20 min before the pre-dialysis sampling, kept lying on beds, and not allowed to eat or drink until the end-of-session [13, 14]. Pre-dialysis and post-dialysis body weight (BW) was measured before the start of the sessions and after the end of the sessions, respectively. Intradialytic BW loss (IBWL) was calculated as "IBWL = pre-dialysis BW − post-dialysis BW," and relative IBWL to DW was calculated as "IBWL/DW." IPVC was calculated by using the intradialytic change of hemoglobin concentration (Hb) as "$IPVC_{Hb}$ = 1 − (pre-dialysis Hb)/(post-dialysis Hb)" and by using the change of hematocrit (Ht) as "$IPVC_{Ht}$ = 1 − (pre-dialysis Ht)/(post-dialysis Ht)." To indicate IPVCs relative to IBWL, IPVCs divided by IBWL ($IPVC_{Hb}$/IBWL and $IPVC_{Ht}$/IBWL) were used.

Dry weight (DW) was adjusted for each patient to maintain cardio thoracic ratio < 52% and no pulmonary congestion on chest radiography. For the participants with valvular heart disease, vena cava diameter normalized for body surface area < 11.5 mm/m^2 and its respiratory fluctuation under the adjusted DW were confirmed on echocardiography. Relative post-dialysis BW to DW (post-dialysis BW/DW) was used as a measure of the fluid status. The plasma level of atrial natriuretic peptide (ANP) was measured at the end of dialysis sessions where the post-dialysis BW was <DW + 0.3 kg. Measurements of ANP with cardiac arrhythmia were excluded from the analysis.

Statistical analysis

Continuous variables were reported as the mean ± standard deviation. Comparisons were done by the one-way analysis of variance and then the Tukey's post hoc tests for patient characteristics and by a mixed-effects model analysis for intradialytic measures. Discrete variables were reported as counts, and comparisons were done by the Pearson's chi-square test. A correlation between parameters was analyzed by using the Pearson's correlation test, and R of the prediction model for linear regression was obtained. All statistical analyses were performed using the SPSS software package (Dr. SPSS II, SPSS Inc., Chicago, IL, USA). A probability value of $P < 0.001$ was considered statistically significant.

Results

At most, 5 sessions per patient from 75 patients were included in the study. Dialysis mode was changed in 31 patients, and 115 std-HD, 59 pp-ol-HDF, 39 pre-ol-HDF, and 33 post-ol-HDF sessions (a total of 246 sessions) were included in the analyses. Table 1 shows the summary of patient characteristics. None of the characteristics examined (age, gender proportion, dialysis lengths, diabetes mellitus prevalence, and the proportion of antihypertensives treatment) were significantly different between the modes.

Laboratory measures of pre-dialysis and post-dialysis blood samples and indicators of intradialytic body fluid status were compared between the modes (Table 2). None of the measures and the indicators examined were significantly different between the modes. While the levels of pre-dialysis Hb and Ht were generally lower in std-HD than in ol-HDFs, the levels of post-dialysis Hb and Ht were also generally lower in std-HD than in ol-HDFs, and the levels of $IPVC_{Hb}$ and $IPVC_{Ht}$ were not significantly different between the modes. The levels of post-dialysis ANP compared in 151 out of the 246 sessions were also not significantly different between the modes.

Table 1 Patient characteristics

Characteristic	std-HD (n = 55)	ol-HDF			P
		pp (n = 23)	pre (n = 24)	post (n = 27)	
Age (years)	67 ± 10	71 ± 11	65 ± 10	66 ± 10	0.25
Sex (% female)	18	26	17	15	0.76
Dialysis (months)	63 ± 67	52 ± 58	71 ± 71	71 ± 70	0.72
Diabetes mellitus (%)	53	39	46	44	0.71
Antihypertensives (%)					
RASI	36	22	33	30	0.64
CCB	33	35	29	30	0.97
β-blockers	15	4	17	15	0.58
Diuretics	38	35	38	41	0.98

Data are presented as either mean ± SD or % in each group
Abbreviations: CCB calcium channel blockers, *ol-HDF* online hemodiafiltration, *std-HD* standard hemodialysis, *post* post-dilution mode, *pp* push-pull mode, *pre* pre-dilution mode, *RASI* renin-angiotensin-system inhibitors

Table 2 Comparison between dialysis modes

Measure	std-HD (n = 115)	ol-HDF			P
		pp (n = 59)	pre (n = 39)	post (n = 33)	
Pre-dialysis					
Hb (g/dL)	10.5 ± 1.2	10.8 ± 0.9	10.7 ± 1.1	10.8 ± 1.2	0.19
Ht (%)	32.0 ± 3.7	33.0 ± 2.8	32.6 ± 3.3	33.2 ± 3.6	0.28
Alb (g/dL)	3.4 ± 0.3	3.4 ± 0.3	3.5 ± 0.3	3.5 ± 0.3	0.04
Na (mmol/L)	139 ± 3	139 ± 2	140 ± 3	140 ± 3	0.43
Post-dialysis					
Hb (g/dL)	11.7 ± 1.5	12.2 ± 1.2	11.9 ± 1.3	12.1 ± 1.5	0.14
Ht (%)	35.9 ± 4.7	37.3 ± 3.7	36.4 ± 3.9	37.1 ± 4.6	0.22
Alb (g/dL)	3.8 ± 0.4	3.9 ± 0.6	3.9 ± 0.3	3.9 ± 0.4	0.25
BW/DW	1.005 ± 0.020	1.007 ± 0.011	1.003 ± 0.008	1.002 ± 0.018	0.76
ANP (pg/mL)	66.0 ± 65.4 (n = 61)	69.3 ± 41.8 (n = 35)	63.8 ± 53.7 (n = 29)	90.2 ± 78.0 (n = 26)	0.41
DW (kg)	54.4 ± 10.3	51.5 ± 7.0	56.2 ± 9.9	56.6 ± 11.0	0.15
IBWL (kg)	2.5 ± 0.7	2.4 ± 0.9	2.6 ± 0.8	3.0 ± 0.8	0.19
IBWL/DW	0.048 ± 0.013	0.046 ± 0.016	0.047 ± 0.014	0.049 ± 0.013	0.16
UFR (L/h/kg)	0.013 ± 0.004	0.013 ± 0.004	0.013 ± 0.004	0.013 ± 0.003	0.16
IPVC					
Hb	0.10 ± 0.06	0.11 ± 0.07	0.10 ± 0.05	0.10 ± 0.06	0.73
Ht	0.10 ± 0.07	0.11 ± 0.07	0.10 ± 0.06	0.10 ± 0.06	0.48
IPVC/IBWL/DW					
Hb	1.9 ± 2.0	1.7 ± 4.6	2.1 ± 0.9	2.1 ± 1.8	0.95
Ht	1.9 ± 2.2	1.9 ± 3.7	2.1 ± 1.1	2.1 ± 2.0	0.99

Data are presented as mean ± standard deviation
Abbreviations: Alb serum albumin concentration, *ANP* plasma atrial natriuretic peptide concentration, *BW* body weight, *DW* dry weight, *Hb* hemoglobin, *Ht* hematocrit, *IBWL* intradialytic BW loss, *IPVC* intradialytic plasma volume change, *Na* serum sodium concentration, *ol-HDF* online hemodiafiltration, *post* post-dilution mode, *pp* push-pull mode, *pre* pre-dilution mode, *std-HD* standard hemodialysis, *UFR* ultrafiltration rate

Irrespective of the dialysis modes, $IPVC_{Hb}$ and $IPVC_{Ht}$ correlated well to each other (Fig. 1, $R = 0.97$, $P < 0.001$) and similarly correlated to IBWL/DW (Fig. 2). There were positive correlations between IBWL/DW and $IPVC_{Hb}$ (left panel, $R = 0.51$, $P < 0.001$) and between IBWL/DW and $IPVC_{Ht}$ (right panel, $R = 0.50$, $P < 0.001$). The slopes of the least squares line were 2.3 for both $IPVC_{Hb}$/IBWL/DW and $IPVC_{Ht}$/IBWL/DW, and the levels of IPVCs and IPVCs/IBWL/DW were similar between the modes (Table 2).

Discussion

The present findings revealed that ol-HDF in either push-pull, pre-dilution, or post-dilution mode did not prevent IPVC compared with std-HD; IPVC and IPVC/UFR in ol-HDFs were not different from those in std-HD.

In the present study, both $IPVC_{Hb}$ and $IPVC_{Ht}$ had positive correlations to IBWL/DW. The findings support the notion that intradialytic fluid removal by ultrafiltration induces IPVC and causes IDH [2–4]. However, there was wide variation in IPVCs, which indicated that factors other than ultrafiltration influenced IPVC [5, 14–16]. Vascular refilling by interstitial fluid, which occurs during dialysis sessions, would be a dominant factor among them, and its rate would differ owing to individual difference. Thus, patients' individual difference in the vascular refilling rate could have caused the variation in IPVCs.

Relative volume excess to DW could also facilitate the vascular refilling [3, 14, 15], and inappropriate DW might influence IPVC. However, inappropriate DW would not have influenced the present findings significantly, because not only the levels of post-dialysis BW/DW but also those of ANP, which reflect volume status, were not different between the modes. Furthermore, independency of the vascular refilling from the volume status relative to DW was reported previously [17].

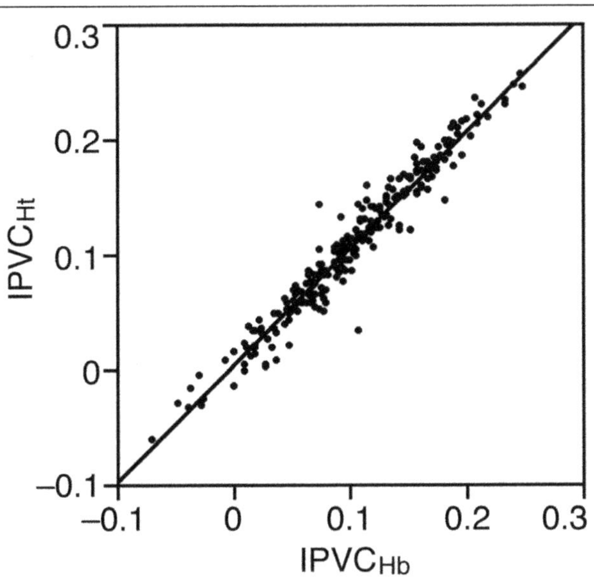

Fig. 1 Scatter plot comparing $IPVC_{Hb}$ with $IPVC_{Ht}$. There was a positive correlation between $IPVC_{Hb}$ and $IPVC_{Ht}$ with a linear approximation of $y = 1.02\,x - 0.0003$ ($R = 0.97$, $P < 0.001$). $IPVC_{Hb}$ intradialytic plasma volume change based on hemoglobin, $IPVC_{Ht}$ intradialytic plasma volume change based on hematocrit

Reduction of core-temperature by not-pre-warmed substitution fluid, i.e., thermal effect, was proposed to be a dominant factor preventing IDH in HDF [18, 19]. The present findings might support the proposal of thermal effect. Online HDFs, where pre-warmed dialysate was used as substitution fluid and thermal effect would not have occurred, had no preventive effect on IPVC compared with std-HD. However, factors other than thermal effect could contribute the IDH prevention by ol-HDF. Online HDF may increase the vascular tone or facilitate the vascular refilling between dialysis sessions, because it was reported to have increased pre-dialysis blood pressure compared with std-HDF [8].

Intradialytic loss of albumin can decrease the vascular refilling, which increases IPVC. Thus, the possible loss of albumin, which is larger in ol-HDF than in std-HD, will overestimate IPVC in ol-HDF than in std-HD [20]. The present findings that post-dialysis Alb levels were similar while pre-dialysis Alb levels were generally lower in std-HD than in ol-HDFs would indicate difference in intradialytic albumin loss between std-HD and ol-HDFs. Therefore, the present findings of same IPVCs levels between the modes might have indicated smaller IPVC in ol-HDFs than in std-HD. However, intradialytic albumin loss would not have influenced IPVC, because recent report showed that inward oncotic force had little effect on the vascular refilling [15].

Inducing intracellular-to-extracellular water movement, an increase in Na can facilitate the vascular refilling [21]. During dialysis session, Na is reaching the sodium concentration of dialysate. Thus, differences in pre-dialysis Na could have influenced IPVC. However, in the present study, the levels of pre-dialysis Na were not different between the modes. Additionally, recent data suggest that inward osmotic force has little effect on the vascular refilling [15]. Therefore, intradialytic Na change would not have influenced IPVCs significantly in the present study.

The convection volume, which indicates the effectiveness of convective transport in HDF, can influence IPVC [5, 22]. However, the convection volume would not have influenced the present findings significantly; in spite of differences in the convection volume, the levels of IPVCs were not different between the modes of HDF. Furthermore, in spite of inferiority in convective transport, std-HD had same levels of IPVCs as those of HDFs.

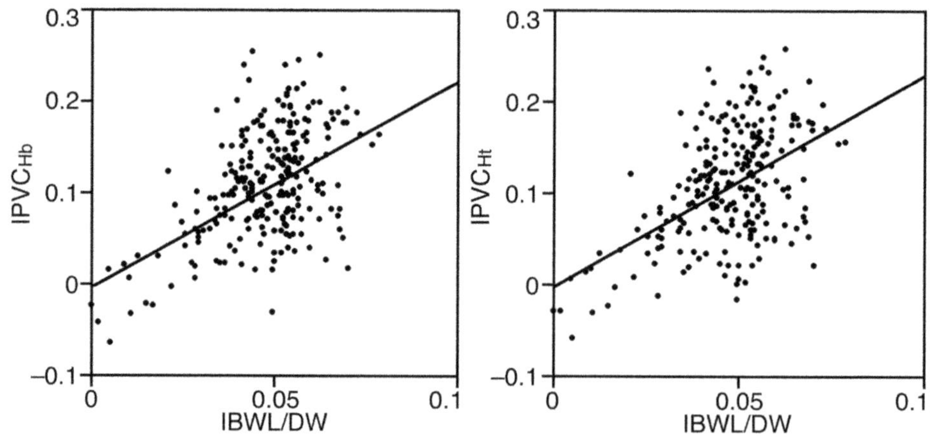

Fig. 2 Scatter plot comparing IBWL with IPVC. There was a positive correlation between IBWL/DW and $IPVC_{Hb}$ with a linear approximation of $y = 2.3\ x–0.003$ (left panel, $R = 0.51$, $P < 0.001$). There was a positive correlation between IBWL/DW and $IPVC_{Ht}$ with a linear approximation of $y = 2.3\ x–0003$ (right panel, $R = 0.50$, $P < 0.001$). *IBWL* intradialytic body weight loss, DW dry weight, $IPVC_{Hb}$ intradialytic plasma volume change based on hemoglobin, $IPVC_{Ht}$ intradialytic plasma volume change based on hematocrit

The present report has several limitations. Firstly, the small sample size is an important limitation. The sample is somewhat skewed, and the study may be limited by the possibility of selection bias. However, variation between the modes would not have affected the present findings significantly; despite the variation, IPVCs and UFR were at the same levels between the modes. Secondly, being a retrospective study, the method of IPVC evaluation was limited. Other methods such as a method using bioimpedance need to be evaluated. Thus, whether the present findings can be generalized needs to be confirmed in prospective studies of large sample sizes and in crossover studies with measurement of bioimpedance.

Conclusions

Online HDF in either push-pull, pre-dilution, or post-dilution mode had the same level of IPVC as std-HD. The findings indicate that ol-HDF has no preventive effect on IPVC irrespective of its modes.

Abbreviations

Alb: Serum albumin concentration; DW: Dry weight; IDH: Intradialytic hypotension; IPVC: Intradialytic plasma volume change; Na: Serum sodium concentration; ol-HDF: Online hemodiafiltration; post-ol-HDF: Post-dilution mode ol-HDF; pp-ol-HDF: Push-pull mode ol-HDF; pre-ol-HDF: Pre-dilution mode ol-HDF; std-HD: Standard hemodialysis

Acknowledgements

We thank Satoshi Ikenaga and Tensho Oka for the excellent technical assistance.

Funding

This study was not supported by any grants or funding.

Authors' contributions

MT designed the study, performed the data analysis, and wrote the manuscript. YI, YK, and YO collected the clinical data. All authors read and approved the final manuscript.

Competing interests

The authors declare that they have no competing interests.

References

1. Becker BN, Stone WJ. Options for renal replacement therapy: special considerations. Semin Nephrol. 1997;17:176–87.
2. Movilli E, Cancarini GC, Cassamali S, Camerini C, Brunori G, Maffei C, et al. Inter-dialytic variations in blood volume and total body water in uraemic patients treated by dialysis. Nephrol Dial Transplant. 2004;19:185–9.
3. Lins LE, Hedenborg G, Jacobson SH, Samuelson K, Tedner B, Zetterholm UB, et al. Blood pressure reduction during hemodialysis correlates to intradialytic changes in plasma volume. Clin Nephrol. 1992;37:308–13.
4. Sands JJ, Usvyat LA, Sullivan T, Segal JH, Zabetakis P, Kotanko P, et al. Intradialytic hypotension: frequency, sources of variation and correlation with clinical outcome. Hemodial Int. 2014;18:415–22.
5. Donauer J, Kolblin D, Bek M, Krause A, Bohler J. Ultrafiltration profiling and measurement of relative blood volume as strategies to reduce hemodialysis-related side effects. Am J Kidney Dis. 2000;36:115–23.
6. Colussi G, Frattini G. Quantitative analysis of convective dose in hemofiltration and hemodiafiltration: "predilution" vs. "postdilution" reinfusion. Hemodial Int. 2007;11:76–85.
7. Wang AY, Ninomiya T, Al-Kahwa A, Perkovic V, Gallagher MP, Hawley C, et al. Effect of hemodiafiltration or hemofiltration compared with hemodialysis on mortality and cardiovascular disease in chronic kidney failure: a systematic review and meta-analysis of randomized trials. Am J Kidney Dis. 2014;63:968–78.
8. Locatelli F, Altieri P, Andrulli S, Bolasco P, Sau G, Pedrini LA, et al. Hemofiltration and hemodiafiltration reduce intradialytic hypotension in ESRD. J Am Soc Nephrol. 2010;21:1798–807.
9. Altieri P, Sorba G, Bolasco P, Asproni E, Ledebo I, Cossu M, et al. Predilution haemofiltration—the second Sardinian multicentre study: comparisons between haemofiltration and haemodialysis during identical Kt/V and session times in a long-term cross-over study. Nephrol Dial Transplant. 2001;16:1207–13.
10. Tattersall JE, Ward RA. Online haemodiafiltration: definition, dose quantification and safety revisited. Nephrol Dial Transplant. 2013;28:542–50.

11. National Kidney Foundation. KDOQI Clinical Practice Guideline for Hemodialysis Adequacy: 2015 update. Am J Kidney Dis. 2015;66:884–930.
12. Masakane I, Nakai S, Ogata S, Kimata N, Hanafusa N, Hamano T, et al. An overview of regular dialysis treatment in Japan (as of 31 December 2013). Ther Apher Dial. 2015;19:540–74.
13. Inagaki H, Kuroda M, Watanabe S, Hamazaki T. Changes in major blood components after adopting the supine position during haemodialysis. Nephrol Dial Transplant. 2001;16:798–802.
14. Daugirdas JT. Dialysis hypotension: a hemodynamic analysis. Kidney Int. 1991;39:233–46.
15. Danziger J, Hoenig MP. The role of the kidney in disorders of volume: core curriculum 2016. Am J Kidney Dis. 2016;68:808–16.
16. Steuer RR, Leypoldt JK, Cheung AK, Harris DH, Conis JM. Hematocrit as an indicator of blood volume and a predictor of intradialytic morbid events. ASAIO J. 1994;40:M691–6.
17. Kron S, Schneditz D, Leimbach T, Aign S, Kron J. Vascular refilling is independent of volume overload in hemodialysis with moderate ultrafiltration requirements. Hemodial Int. 2016;20:484–91.
18. Donauer J, Schweiger C, Rumberger B, Krumme B, Bohler J. Reduction of hypotensive side effects during online-haemodiafiltration and low temperature haemodialysis. Nephrol Dial Transplant. 2003;18:1616–22.
19. Karamperis N, Sloth E, Jensen JD. Predilution hemodiafiltration displays no hemodynamic advantage over low-flux hemodialysis under matched conditions. Kidney Int. 2005;67:1601–8.
20. Jean G, Hurot JM, Deleaval P, Mayor B, Lorriaux C. Online-haemodiafiltration vs. conventional haemodialysis: a cross-over study. BMC Nephrol. 2015;16:70.
21. Santos SF, Peixoto AJ. Sodium balance in maintenance hemodialysis. Semin Dial. 2010;23:549–55.
22. Ok E, Asci G, Toz H, Ok ES, Kircelli F, Yilmaz M, et al. Mortality and cardiovascular events in online haemodiafiltration (OL-HDF) compared with high-flux dialysis: results from the Turkish OL-HDF study. Nephrol Dial Transplant. 2013;28:192–202.

Suction towards a vessel wall by hemodialysis catheters—the establishment of a new experimental extracorporeal circulation system using pig veins

Yoshimitsu Takahashi[1*], Junichiro J. Kazama[3], Suguru Yamamoto[2], Takashi Oite[1] and Ichiei Narita[2]

Abstract

Background: Hemodialysis catheters are commonly used for vascular access in patients undergoing blood purification therapies. However, the sudden dysfunction of catheters represents a serious problem, and while we know that the major causative factor is suction between the catheter and the vessel wall, it is very difficult to evaluate this in vivo. Therefore, we created a new experimental system to investigate this phenomenon ex vivo, using pig veins, which allowed us to quantitatively analyze the effect of suction.

Methods: We attempted to create a model system for quantitative evaluation using azygos veins from a pig. Four types of catheters were inserted into an extracted pig vein: true circle type 1, true circle type 2, semi-circle type 1, and semi-circle type 2. We then circulated 50% glycerol solution through the vein at a flow rate (Qv) from 100 to 1000 mL/min. Glycerol solution was also circulated within the catheters at a flow rate (Qb) from 100 to 200 mL/min. We measured the frequency of suction towards the vessel wall ten times, under each experimental schedule, at a Qb of both 100 and 200 mL/min. We then measured the pressure between the pre-Qb pump and the blood circuit, when the arterial side opening was positioned approximately in the center of the blood vessel to prevent catheter suction towards the vessel wall.

Results: Suction towards the vessel wall occurred 8/10 times with the true circle type 1 catheter and 10/10 times with the semi-circle type 2 catheter in the arterial pore of the catheter is only one, when Qb and Qv were 100 and 100 mL/min, respectively. Suction towards the vessel wall occurred 3/10 times with the semi-circle type 2 catheter, when Qb and Qv were 100 and 1000 mL/min, respectively. The true circle type 1 catheter showed a minimum pressure of -58.6 ± 0.516 mmHg when Qb and Qv were 100 and 300 mL/min, respectively, while the true circle type 2 catheter showed a minimum pressure of -137 ± 5.96 mmHg when Qb and Qv were 200 and 300 mL/min, respectively.

Conclusions: We successfully established a novel ex vivo evaluation system for catheters using a pig vein which allowed us to recreate the effect of suction from catheters towards a vessel wall in vivo.

Keywords: Hemodialysis catheters, Suction towards the vessel wall, Pig vein, Evaluation system

* Correspondence: yoshimitsu2003@gmail.com
[1]Department of Clinical Engineering and Medical Technology, Faculty Medical Technology, Niigata University of Health and Welfare, 1398 Shimami-cho, Kita-ku, Niigata 950-3198, Japan
Full list of author information is available at the end of the article

Background

Hemodialysis catheters (catheters) are commonly used to obtain adequate vascular access in patients who require blood purification therapies. It is highly preferable to begin treatment promptly after inserting a catheter into the femoral vein or internal jugular vein. Thus, catheters are used frequently in patients with acute kidney injury (AKI) [1]. However, catheters often fail during blood purification therapy, most commonly due to catheter suction towards the vessel wall [2], thrombotic occlusion [3], and the development of a fibrin sheath [4]. These issues represent serious problems because there is no suitable method available at present with which to detect and evaluate these phenomena.

Until now, only highly experienced medical staff can recognize catheter dysfunction by individual perception of manipulation alone. When catheter dysfunction occurs, the circulating blood cannot be sent to a blood purification machine, thus making it very difficult to continue with blood purification therapy. Negative pressure in a blood circuit results in a deterioration in dialysis efficiency. A range of factors can cause catheter dysfunction. In particular, end-hole type catheters for high flow are often associated with catheter suction towards the vessel wall. To the best of our knowledge, there are no reports in the published literature which address the issue of quantitatively analyzing catheter suction towards the vessel wall using an ex vivo model.

In the present study, we describe the development of a novel ex vivo model using pig veins which allows us to quantitatively analyze the effect of suctioning towards the vessel wall.

Methods

We used four different catheters in this study (Fig. 1): true circle type 1 (BARD, USA, Georgia), true circle type 2 (BARD, USA, Georgia), semi-circle type 1 (NIPRO, JPN, Osaka), and semi-circle type 2 (Baxter, JPN, Tokyo). The catheter banding patterns show arterial side opening area. The catheter vertically striped patterns show arterial side sectional area. A schematic of the experimental system is shown in Fig. 2. We attempted to develop a model system using azygos veins from a pig (hereafter referred to as "pig vein"). We extracted 10 pig veins, as a model for the human femoral vein, from a 6-month-old pig weighing 120 kg. We selected pig vein 10 ± 2 mm in diameter and no venous valve, and the pig vein was refrigerated and used within the 7 days. The pig vein was set into 50% glycerol solution. We then inserted the catheters into the pig vein, and 50% glycerol solution was circulated around the vein at a body temperature (36 °C) to act as artificial blood. Flow rate in the pig vein (Qv) was set at 100, 200, 300, 500, and 1000 mL/min, in accordance with an earlier publication in which blood flow was reported to be 100~ 1000 mL/min within a vein [5]. These conditions simulated blood flow in the lower human circulatory system. Each catheter was separately inserted into the same pig vein. The arterial end hole of the catheter was adjusted so that the tip of the catheter's position could meet the target position. Next, we perforated the arterial two side holes of a true circle type 1 catheter. The diameter of these holes was located symmetrically and the upper end hole was 1 mm in diameter. In other words, the end hole of the catheter was located at the tip and on the arterial side. A blood circuit NV-Y871P (NIKKISO, Tokyo, Japan) was the connected to the catheter and glycerol solution was circulated using a DCS-26 blood purification machine (NIKKISO, Tokyo, Japan). We judged that suction towards the vessel wall occurred when Qb changed to 0 mL/min within 10 s of the Qb pump starting. We measured the frequency of suction towards the vessel wall ten times, for each experimental schedule, at a Qb of both 100 and

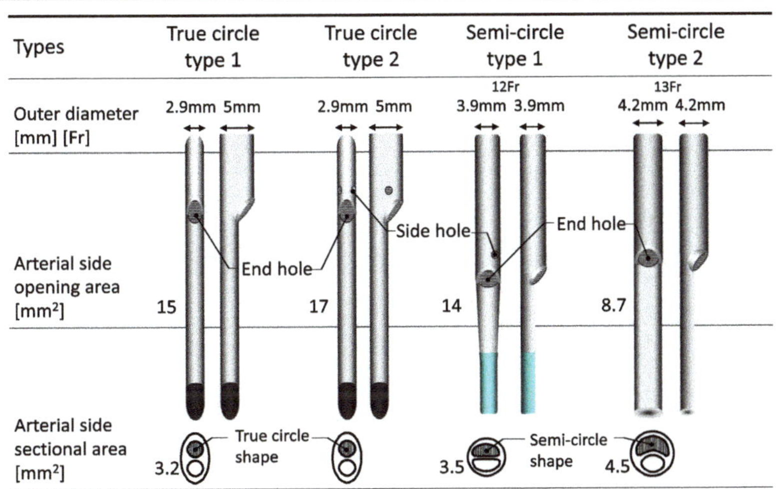

Fig. 1 Specification of the catheters

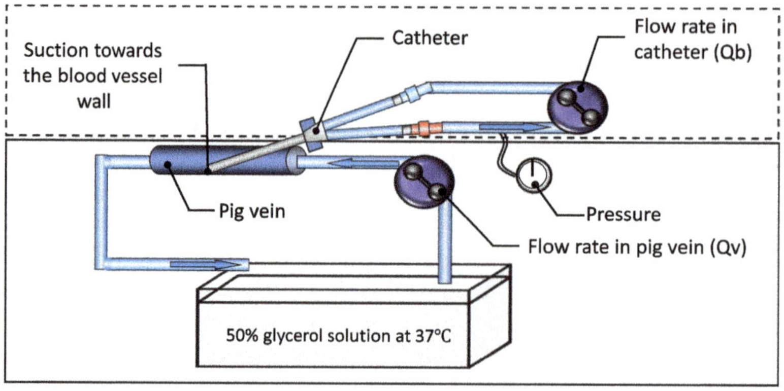

Fig. 2 Experimental system. Solid line shows the circuit of simulated blood vessel and dotted line shows the blood purification circuit

200 mL/min. A Handy Manometer PG-100 N/B (Copal Electronics, Tokyo, Japan) was connected to the blood circuit on the upstream side of the blood pump to measure the difference in negative pressure between the catheter and the pump. Next, we measured the pressure between the pre-Qb pump and the blood circuit when the arterial side opening was positioned in the center of blood vessel to prevent catheter suction towards the vessel wall. The data were analyzed with Scheffé's *F* test and an alpha level of 0.05 using Excel statistics 2012 for windows (Microsoft Corporation, Washington, USA).

Results

The frequency of suctioning towards the vessel wall by the catheters is shown in Fig. 3. Suction towards the vessel wall occurred 8/10 times with the true circle type 1 catheter and 10/10 times with the semi-circle type 2 catheter, when Qb and Qv were 100 and 100 mL/min, respectively (Fig. 3). However, no suction occurred via the side holes of the catheter. Suction towards the vessel wall occurred 10/10 times, with all catheters, when Qb and Qv were 200 and 100 mL/min, respectively (Fig. 3b). Suction towards the vessel wall occurred 2/10 times with the true circle type 1 catheter and 10/10 times with the semi-circle type 2 catheter, when Qb and Qv were 100 and 200 mL/min, respectively (Fig. 3c). Suction towards the vessel wall occurred 10/10 times with all catheters when Qb and Qv were 200 and 100 mL/min, respectively (Fig. 3d), while suction towards the vessel wall occurred 3/10 times with the true circle type 1 catheter, and 10/10 times with the semi-circle type 2 catheter, when Qb and Qv were 100 and 300 mL/min, respectively (Fig. 3e). Suction towards the vessel wall occurred 10/10 times with the true circle type 1 catheter, 2/10 times with the semi-circle type 1 catheter, and 10/10 times with the semi-circle type 2 catheter, when Qb and Qv were 200 and 300 mL/min, respectively (Fig. 3f).

Suction towards the vessel wall occurred 3/10 times with the true circle type 1 catheter, 2/10 times with the semi-circle type 1 catheter, and 5/10 times with the

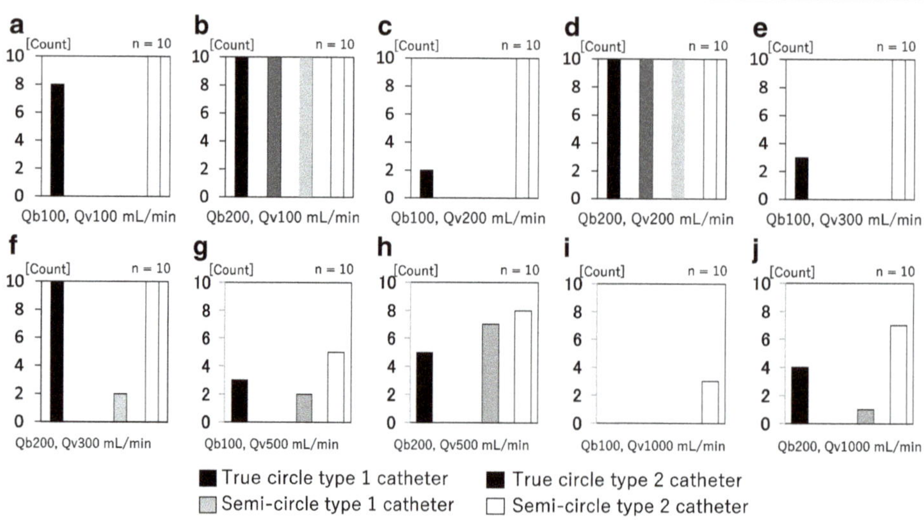

Fig. 3 a–j Frequency of suctioning towards the vessel wall

semi-circle type 2 catheter, when Qb and Qv were 100 and 500 mL/min, respectively (Fig. 3g). Suction towards the vessel wall occurred 5/10 times with the True circle type 1 catheter, 7/10 times with the semi-circle type 1 catheter, and 8/10 times with the semi-circle type 2 catheter, when Qb and Qv were 200 and 500 mL/min, respectively (Fig. 3h). Suction towards the vessel wall occurred 3/10 times with the semi-circle type 2 catheter, when Qb and Qv were 100 and 1000 mL/min, respectively (Fig. 3i). Finally, suction towards the vessel wall occurred 4/10 times with the true circle type 1 catheter, 1/10 times with the semi-circle type 1 catheter, and 7/10 times with the semi-circle type 2 catheter, when Qb and Qv were 200 and 1000 mL/min, respectively (Fig. 3j).

Arterial pressures are shown in Fig. 4. The true circle type 2 catheter showed a minimum pressure of − 80.3 ± 2.16 mmHg when Qb and Qv were 100 and 100 mL/min, respectively, (Fig. 4a) and a minimum pressure of − 165.3 ± 1.89 mmHg when Qb and Qv were 200 and 100 mL/min, respectively, (Fig. 4b). The true circle type 2 catheter showed a minimum pressure of − 69.5 ± 0.527 mmHg when Qb and Qv were 100 and 200 mL/min, respectively, (Fig. 4c) and a minimum pressure value of − 151 ± 0.919 mmHg when Qb and Qv were 200 and 200 mL/min, respectively (Fig. 4d). The true circle type 1 catheter showed a minimum pressure of − 58.6 ± 0.516 mmHg when Qb and Qv were 100 and 300 mL/min, respectively (Fig. 4e). The true circle type 2 catheter showed a minimum pressure of − 137 ± 5.96 mmHg when Qb and Qv were 200 and 300 mL/min, respectively (Fig. 4f). The true circle type 2 catheter showed a minimum pressure of − 57.4 ± 0.700 mmHg when Qb and Qv were 100 and 500 mL/min, respectively (Fig. 4g). The true circle type 2 catheter showed a minimum pressure of − 119 ± 0.990 mmHg when Qb and Qv were 200 and 500 mL/min, respectively (Fig. 4h). The true circle type 2 catheter showed a minimum pressure of − 46.6 ± 0.700 mmHg when Qb and Qv were 100 and 1000 mL/min, respectively (Fig. 4i), while the true circle type 2 catheter showed a minimum pressure of − 107 ± 0.630 mmHg when Qb and Qv were 200 and 1000 mL/min, respectively (Fig. 4j).

It is important to note that these catheters differ in their design; the true circle type 1 catheter arterial tip design features one end hole, while the true circle type 2 catheter arterial tip design features one end hole and two side holes. Pressure values were significantly lower for the true circle type 2 catheter than the true circle type 1 catheter ($P < 0.01$, Fig. 4a–j).

Discussion

Several studies have reported that polyvinyl chloride (PVC) and natural rubber tubes can be used as for evaluating catheters in experimental system [6]. However, we believe that these materials significantly influence the results of the evaluation because the Young's modulus is very different in PVC and natural rubber tubes compared to biomaterials. For example, Young's modulus has been reported to be 6.9–29 MPa in PVC, 3000–8000 kPa in natural rubber, but only 40–100 kPa

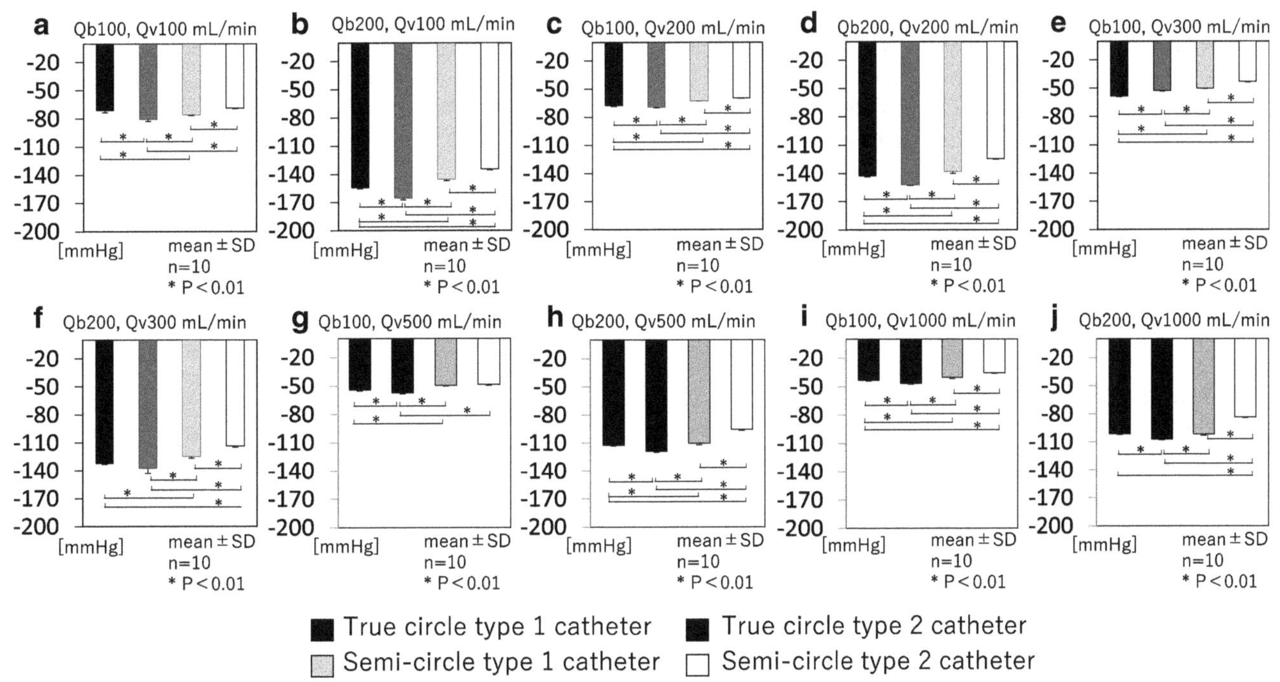

Fig. 4 a–j Pre-pump pressure

in the inferior vena cava. It is therefore highly evident that Young's modulus or PVC and natural rubber are low very different from that in the living body. Because of this, in the present study, we chose to use the azygos vein, harvested from a pig, to construct an experimental system for evaluating catheters in conditions which were similar to the living body.

The frequency of suctioning towards the vessel wall

The true circle type 2 catheter showed the lowest frequency of suction towards the vessel wall and was therefore very efficient at preventing suction towards the vessel wall. It is evident that the side holes on this type of catheter can carry blood to a dialyzer, even if the end hole has caused suction towards the vessel wall. In contrast, the true circle type 1 catheter, which does not have side holes, caused suction towards the vessel wall in all of the conditions we examined, although there were variations in the frequency of suction. It is reasonable to consider that the side holes of the True circle type 1 catheter were effective in preventing suction towards the vessel wall. The semi-circle type 1 catheter showed the second lowest frequency of suction towards the vessel wall; this type of catheter possesses not only an end hole but also one side hole of 1-mm diameter, while also featuring a different angle and shape to the opening on the arterial side compared to true circle type 2 catheters. We considered that the true circle type 1 catheter and the semi-circle type 2 catheter caused incidences of suction towards the vessel wall because of their lack of side holes. In addition, we believe that differences in frequency of suctioning towards the vessel wall between the true circle type 1 and semi-circle type 2 catheters were most likely caused by the angle and shape of the opening on the arterial side. The end hole of a catheter with a shallow opening angle can easily cause suction towards the vessel wall; in our case, the semi-circle type 2 catheters have a shallower opening angle than that of the true circle type 1 catheter. Consequently, the features of the arterial side opening on catheters can represent significant causative factors for suction against vessel walls.

Differences in arterial pressure

Against our expectation, the lowest arterial pressure observed in our experiments was with the true circle type 2 catheter, which also showed the lowest frequency of suctioning towards the vessel wall. In contrast, the highest arterial pressure was recorded with the semi-circle type 2 catheter, which also showed the largest frequency of suctioning towards the vessel wall.

We believe that the true circle type 2 catheter showed the lowest arterial pressure because it also had the smallest arterial side section area (3.2 mm^2). In our experiments, the arterial pressure of the true circle type 2 catheter was lower than that of the true circle type 1 catheter, despite these catheters exhibiting the same sectional area on the arterial side. At present, we cannot explain this difference and need to carry out further investigations. The highest arterial pressures were associated with the semi-circle type 2 catheter; this may be the result of this catheter exhibiting the thickest (13 Fr) outer diameter and the smoothest blood flow. Collectively, our present data suggest that we should measure arterial pressure in the proximity of the catheter opening area on the arterial side given that factors such as the shape and position of the opening area can exert affect.

Conclusions

We established a novel ex vivo catheter evaluation system using venous vessels from a pig. This system allowed us to reproduce catheter suction towards vessel walls in vivo. In addition, suctioning towards the vessel wall was easy to improve and was dependent upon the catheter structure with end hole and side hole.

Acknowledgements

Not applicable.

Funding

No funding.

Authors' contributions

YT participated in the design of this study and drafted the manuscript. JK and SY considered the experimental system. TO and IN kindly reviewed and revised the manuscript. All authors read and approved the final manuscript.

Competing interests

The authors declare that they have no competing interests.

Author details

[1]Department of Clinical Engineering and Medical Technology, Faculty Medical Technology, Niigata University of Health and Welfare, 1398 Shimami-cho, Kita-ku, Niigata 950-3198, Japan. [2]Division of Clinical Nephrology and Rheumatology, Niigata University Graduate School of Medical and Dental Sciences, Niigata, Japan. [3]Department of Nephrology and Hypertension, Fukushima Medical University, Fukushima 951-8520, Japan.

References

1. Canaud B, Desmeules S, Klouche K, Leray-Moragués H, Béraud JJ. Vascular access for dialysis in the intensive care unit. Prevention and treatment of acute. Ren Fail. 2004;18:159–74.

2. Canneyt K, Biesen W, Vanholder R, Segers P, Verdonck P, Eloot S. Evaluation of alternatives for dysfunctional double lumen central venous catheters using a two-compartmental mathematical model for different solutes. Int J Artif Organs. 2013;36:17–27.
3. Besarab A, Pandey R. Catheter management in hemodialysis patients: delivering adequate flow. Clin J Am Soc Nephrol. 2011;6:227–34.
4. Niyyar VD, Chan MR. Interventional nephrology. Catheter dysfunction-- prevention and troubleshooting. Clin J Am Soc Nephrol. 2013;8:1234–43.
5. Whitmore RL. Rheology of the circulation. Oxford:Pergamon Press; 1968.
6. Stroud CC, Meyer SL, Bawkon MC, Smith HG, Klein MD. Vascular access for extracorporeal circulation. Resistance in double lumen cannulas. ASAIO Trans. 1991;37:418–9.

22

Prevalence of nutritional risk and its impact on functional recovery in older inpatients on maintenance hemodialysis

Yoshitaka Shimizu*, Tatsu Fujiura and Hidetaka Wakabayashi

Abstract

Background: Poor nutritional status and functional impairment are common in patients with end-stage renal disease (ERSD) on maintenance hemodialysis (MHD). Although nutritional status is associated with functional dependence and rehabilitation outcome in several diseases, this association remains unclear in patients with ESRD. The aim of this study was to investigate nutritional risk and its impact on rehabilitation outcomes in MHD inpatients who required rehabilitation.

Methods: A retrospective cohort study was performed in 57 consecutive MHD inpatients aged 65 or older who had undergone rehabilitation. The Geriatric Nutritional Risk Index (GNRI) was used to assess nutritional risk and was calculated from height, dry body weight, and serum albumin level at the start of rehabilitation. Nutritional risk was defined as a GNRI < 91.2. The activities of daily living were used as a measure of rehabilitation outcome and were assessed by the Barthel Index (BI) at the start of rehabilitation and discharge. The Mann-Whitney *U* test and multiple regression analysis were performed. In the multiple regression analysis, BI gain was the dependent variable and age, sex, and GNRI were the independent variables.

Results: The study included 34 men and 23 women. Mean (± SD) GNRI was 79.8 ± 9.9. Of the 57 patients, 50 (87.7%) were identified as having a nutritional risk and 7 were not. The gain in BI was significantly higher in patients without nutritional risk (median 50 vs. 10, $p = 0.03$). Multiple regression analysis showed GNRI was associated independently with BI gain ($R^2 = 0.14$, $\beta = 0.29$, $p = 0.03$).

Conclusions: The majority of the MHD patients who underwent rehabilitation had a nutritional risk. Nutritional risk was associated independently with functional recovery.

Keywords: Hemodialysis, Geriatric Nutritional Risk Index, Activities of daily living, Rehabilitation

Background

Poor nutritional status and functional impairment are common in patients with end-stage renal disease (ESRD) on maintenance hemodialysis (MHD). In chronic kidney disease, poor nutritional status due to multiple factors is categorized as protein-energy wasting and is associated with adverse clinical outcomes especially in ERSD patients [1]. The reported prevalence of malnutrition in dialysis patients ranges between 18 and 75% [2, 3]. In addition, 19–26% of MHD patients have a functional impairment in activities of daily living (ADLs); that is, they cannot perform one or more tasks in ADLs without assistance such as bathing, dressing, toilet use, transfer, feeding, and continence [4, 5]. This is especially apparent in MHD patients aged 65 years or older, with 52% reported to have impaired ADLs [6]. Because ADL impairment is associated with mortality in MHD patients [4], it is important to prevent and minimize these impairments. Rehabilitation is one method for treating impaired ADLs, and there are some ADL measures that can be used to assess rehabilitation outcomes [7, 8]. Although

* Correspondence: shimizu198966@gmail.com
Department of Rehabilitation Medicine, Yokohama City University Medical Center, 4-57 Urafune-chou, Minami ward, Yokohama City 232-0024, Japan

rehabilitation is very important, there have only been a small number of published reports on rehabilitation outcomes in MHD patients with impaired ADLs [9].

Although nutritional status is associated with functional dependence and rehabilitation outcome in several diseases, this association remains unclear in patients with ESRD. A meta-analysis of 240 studies showed malnutrition, and related risks were associated directly with functional dependency [10]. It has also been reported that malnutrition is associated with poor rehabilitation outcomes in patients with stroke [11], chronic heart failure [12], or chronic obstructive pulmonary disease [12]. However, we are unaware of any previous reports on the association between nutritional status and rehabilitation outcomes in MHD patients.

The aim of this study was therefore to assess nutritional risk and its impact on rehabilitation outcomes in MHD inpatients who required rehabilitation.

Methods

A retrospective cohort study was performed in 57 inpatients who had been admitted consecutively to the Yokohama City University Medical Center and were subsequently referred by attending physicians to the Department of Rehabilitation Medicine between April 2015 and March 2017.

The study included patients aged 65 or older who had undergone both maintenance hemodialysis and rehabilitation during their hospital stay. Patients were excluded from the study if they had undergone new or temporary hemodialysis, had less than two rehabilitation sessions, or had died during their hospital stay.

All participants underwent hemodialysis three times a week and physical therapy five times a week. They underwent physical therapy of 20 or 40 min per session, while some participants received occupational therapy and/or speech therapy if required. Rehabilitation was performed mainly in an exercise room but sometimes was carried out at the bedside when patients could not come to the exercise room because of their physical condition. According to the disease, general condition, and ADLs of each patient, the doctors made a rehabilitation order that included the location, outline of the program, frequency, and length of each session. The therapist in charge of each patient decided the details of the rehabilitation program. Each program was designed with the purpose of improving or maintaining ADL. Each program mainly included a range of motion exercises, resistance training, and practice of ADLs. The practice of ADLs regarding moving such as sitting, standing up, walking, and going up and down stairs was performed as physical therapy. The practice of other activities such as feeding, grooming, and dressing was performed as occupational therapy and speech therapy. If the patient was fully independent for ADLs, resistance training and aerobic exercise were performed to achieve further improvement in physical function.

Nutritional status was assessed by the Geriatric Nutritional Risk Index (GNRI) [13]. This index has been reported to be an accurate tool for identifying MHD patients at nutritional risk [14] and is calculated as GNRI = {14.89 × serum albumin (g/dl)} + {41.7 × (body weight/ideal body weight)}. The ideal body weight was defined as the value calculated from height and a body mass index (BMI) of 22 kg/m^2. In cases with a (body weight/ideal body weight) > 1, this value was replaced by 1 [13]. For this study, GNRI was calculated from the serum albumin level and body weight measured at the hemodialysis session closest to the start of rehabilitation. Serum albumin level (g/dL) was measured by an improved bromocresol purple (BCP) method before hemodialysis, body weight (kg) after hemodialysis, and height (cm) at admission, with the values expressed to one decimal place. In accordance with a previous study [14], the risk of malnutrition in MHD patients was defined as a GNRI < 91.2.

ADLs were evaluated by physical therapists in charge of each patient at the start of rehabilitation and at discharge using the Barthel Index (BI). The BI consists of the following ten items: feeding, moving from bed to a wheelchair and back, grooming, toilet use, bathing, mobilization (level surface), going up and down stairs, dressing, bowel continence, and bladder continence. The BI score ranges from 0 to 100, with higher scores indicating greater functional independence of ADLs [8]. Age, sex, C-reactive protein (CRP, mg/dL), etiology of chronic kidney disease, causative disease for admission, and number of days from admission to the start of rehabilitation and from the start of rehabilitation to discharge were also recorded.

A previous study demonstrated that the minimal clinically important difference of the 20-point BI in stroke patients was 1.85 [15], equivalent to 9.25 in the 100-point BI scale. In patients with chronic kidney disease who were hospitalized and underwent physical therapy, the standard deviation of the BI was reported to be 13.4 [16]. Assuming the proportion of patients with or without nutritional risk was equal and using the values $\alpha = 0.05$, $\beta = 0.8$, $\delta = 9.25$, and $\sigma = 13.4$, we calculated that it was necessary to include 34 participants in each group in order to reject the null hypothesis that the gain in BI was equal. We therefore planned to recruit 68 patients in the study.

The statistical analyses were performed using JMP ® Pro 12.2 (SAS Institute Inc.; Cary, NC, USA). Fisher's exact test and the Mann-Whitney *U* test were used to determine whether or not there were differences in the characteristics of patients with or without a risk of malnutrition. A multiple regression analysis was performed to examine whether GNRI was associated independently with the gain in BI from the start of rehabilitation to discharge. In this analysis, the dependent variable was BI gain, and the independent variables were age, sex, and GNRI. Age and sex were selected as the regression factors because according to previous studies [17, 18], they have a strong probability of affecting rehabilitation outcome. A p value < 0.05 was considered statistically significant.

Results

A total of 100 patients underwent both hemodialysis and rehabilitation during the study period. Thirty-seven patients who underwent new or temporary hemodialysis during their hospital stay, 1 patient who underwent rehabilitation less than two times, and 5 patients who died were excluded from the analysis. The remaining 57 patients (34 men, 23 women) were included in the study; all underwent physical therapy, 14 had occupational therapy, and 13 received speech therapy.

Table 1 shows the results of the comparison of differences in clinical indices between patients with or without a risk of malnutrition. Mean GNRI (± SD) at the start of rehabilitation was 79.8 ± 9.9. Fifty patients (87.7%) were identified as being at risk of malnutrition and 7 patients (12.3%, all males) were not. Median BI at the start of rehabilitation was 35 with an interquartile range of 10–60. The gain in BI from the start of rehabilitation to discharge was significantly greater in patients not at risk of malnutrition than in patients at risk of malnutrition. There was no significant difference between the two groups in the number of days from either admission to the start of rehabilitation or the start of rehabilitation to discharge.

Table 2 shows the results of the multiple regression analysis of the gain in BI adjusted for age, sex, and GNRI. GNRI was the only factor associated independently with BI gain ($\beta = 0.268$, 95% confidence intervals 0.080, 1.494, $p = 0.030$). We estimated that CRP may affect serum albumin concentration. However, CRP could not be included in the multiple regression analysis because it correlated strongly with both serum albumin concentration ($r = -0.607$, $p < 0.001$) and GNRI ($r = -0.523$, $p < 0.001$).

Discussion

This study obtained two main findings regarding the prevalence of nutritional risk and its impact on rehabilitation outcome in older MHD inpatients who had undergone rehabilitation. Firstly, 87.7% of MHD patients who underwent rehabilitation were identified as having a nutritional risk, assessed by GNRI. Secondly, nutritional risk was associated independently with rehabilitation outcome.

The majority of MHD patients in our study who underwent rehabilitation were identified as having a nutritional risk. Yamada et al. reported a prevalence of 39.3% for nutritional risk in MHD patients [14], a value lower than that observed in our study. A possible reason for this difference may be variations in the characteristics of the subjects, as the Yamada et al. study was on outpatients and also included patients younger than 65 years. Evidence from a meta-analysis of 240 studies, including various healthcare settings, showed malnutrition, and its risks were associated directly with a setting-related level of dependence. The prevalence of malnutrition in rehabilitation/sub-acute care was also shown to be higher than in all other settings including the community, outpatients, home-care services, hospitals, nursing homes, and long-term care [10]. Granger et al. reported that a BI of 60 points appeared to be a pivotal score at which stroke patients moved from functional dependency to assisted independence [19]. In the present study, the upper quartile of BI at the start of rehabilitation was 60, and therefore, the majority of the patients were considered to be functionally dependent. It is possible this high rate of patients with functional dependency was the reason for the high prevalence of nutritional risk observed in our study. We therefore consider that nutritional assessment is very important in MHD patients who are undergoing rehabilitation.

Our data showed nutritional risk in MHD inpatients was associated independently with a gain in the BI and that patients without nutritional risk achieved greater gains in this index. Other studies have reported the impact of GNRI score in MHD patients on mortality [20], physical function [21], and quality of life [21]. Our study is the first to show an influence of GNRI on rehabilitation outcome in MHD patients. This result indicates that the GNRI may be useful for predicting rehabilitation outcomes in MHD inpatients. We consider a cutoff value of GNRI < 91.2 may be useful for predicting whether or not rehabilitation will be more effective.

The high prevalence of nutritional risk and its impact on rehabilitation outcomes indicate the importance of rehabilitation nutrition. Yoshimura et al. reported that nutritional intervention added to resistance training during convalescent rehabilitation improved ADLs in older patients with a decreased muscle mass [22]. There are only a small number of reports on the combination of nutritional intervention and exercise training in adult MHD patients, and the benefit of this combination therefore remains uncertain [23, 24]. In addition, there are no reports on this combination in older MHD patients or MHD patients with impaired ADLs. Nutritional intervention added to rehabilitation has the potential to improve both nutritional status and rehabilitation outcomes in MHD patients with impaired ADLs. There is also evidence in patients with stroke and hip fracture that nutritional improvement is associated with greater gains in ADLs [25–27]. The concept of rehabilitation nutrition involving rehabilitation and management of nutritional care is important in MHD patients with impaired ADLs [28].

This study had some limitations. First, the only subjects in the study were those referred to the Department of Rehabilitation Medicine and did not include patients admitted consecutively to the target hospital during the

Table 1 Characteristics and comparison of clinical indices in patients with or without a nutritional risk

	Total (*n* = 57)	With a nutritional risk (*n* = 50)	Without a nutritional risk (*n* = 7)	*P* value
Age (years), mean ± SD	73.8 ± 6.4	73.8 ± 6.5	70.5 ± 5.8	0.809
Sex, males/females	34/23	27/23	7/0	0.034
Albumin (g/dL), mean ± SD	2.8 ± 0.6	2.7 ± 0.4	3.65 ± 0.2	<.001
BMI (kg/m^2), mean ± SD	20.8 ± 3.1	20.6 ± 3.2	22.1 ± 2.4	0.016
GNRI, mean ± SD	79.8 ± 9.9	77.6 ± 8.3	96.0 ± 1.9	<.001
CRP (mg/dL), median (IQR)	3.365 (0.98–7.742)	3.797 (1.621–9.847)	0.441 (0.235–1.863)	0.014
BI at baseline, median (IQR)	35 (10–60)	35 (11.25–60)	30 (7.5–45)	0.750
BI at discharge, median (IQR)	70 (30–90)	65 (25–90)	85 (77.5–92.5)	0.121
BI gain, median (IQR)	15 (0–30)	10 (0–30)	50 (25–85)	0.027
Length of stay (days), median (IQR)	37 (22–52)	38.5 (23.25–51.25)	29 (19.5–44)	0.436
Days from A to R (days), median (IQR)	8 (5–14)	9 (6–14)	7 (3–8.5)	0.065
Duration of rehabilitation (days), median (IQR)	27 (15–36)	27 (15–36)	25 (15–35.5)	0.855
Duration of hemodialysis (years), median (IQR)	7 (6–12)	7 (3–13)	6 (1–7)	0.200
Causative disease for admission (*n*)				
Ischemic heart disease	10	9	1	
Aortic disease	4	4		
Valvular disease of the heart	4	4		
Congestive heart failure	3	3		
Cerebral infarction	7	3	4	
Parkinson's disease	1		1	
Lumbar disease	6	6		
Fracture	3	3		
Osteoarthritis	3	3		
Psychiatric disease	3	2	1	
Perforation of the digestive tract	2	2		
Pneumonia	2	2		
Shunt complication	2	2		
Other	7	7		
Etiology of chronic kidney disease (*n*)				
Diabetic nephropathy	30	27	3	
Nephrosclerosis	9	6	3	
Chronic glomerulonephritis;	6	6		
Multiple renal cysts	3	2	1	
Rapidly progressive glomerulonephritis	1	1		
SLE nephritis	1	1		
Nephronophthisis	1	1		
Chronic pyelonephritis	1	1		
Drug-induced kidney injury	1	1		
Renal infarction	1	1		
Unknown	3	3		

BMI body mass index, *GNRI* Geriatric Nutritional Risk Index, *BI* Barthel Index, *Days from A to R* days from admission to start of rehabilitation, *IQR* interquartile range, *SLE* systemic lupus erythematosus

Table 2 Results of the multiple regression analysis with gain in the Barthel Index as the dependent variable

	B	β	95% confidence interval of B	*P* value
Age	− 0.997	− 0.234	− 2.098, 0.1046	0.075
Sex	2.686	0.098	− 4.421, 9.794	0.452
GNRI	0.787	0.268	0.080, 1.494	0.030

$R^2 = 0.139$
GNRI Geriatric Nutritional Risk Index

study period. The results of this study can therefore not be applied to the general population of hospitalized MHD patients. Second, the nutritional risk was assessed using only the GNRI and did not include other more reliable and detailed measures. Third, the requisite sample size was not reached. Fourth, we used serum albumin level measured by an improved BCP method that has been used widely over the past decade, replacing the bromocresol green (BCG) method. It has been reported that the percentage of malnourished patients assessed by controlling nutritional status (CONNUT) differs depending on whether the BCP or BCG method is used to measure albumen level [29]. The Japanese Society of Laboratory Medicine recommends that if the serum albumin level measured by the BCP method is ≤ 3.5 g/L, the cutoff value should be modified from the value developed for the BCG method [30]. Because the BCG method was the main test used in the past, the GNRI would have been developed using the serum albumin level measured by that method. Therefore, it is possible that the serum albumin level needs to be modified in our study. Furthermore, we were not able to consider factors in the multiple regression analysis that were likely to affect the gain in BI, such as causative disease for admission because of the small number of the participants, and CRP because of its multicollinearity with the GNRI. Further studies investigating the association between nutritional status and rehabilitation outcome in MHD patients should perform a more detailed nutritional assessment in order to diagnose malnutrition and protein-energy wasting.

Conclusion

The majority of the MHD patients who underwent rehabilitation had a nutritional risk. Nutritional risk was associated independently with rehabilitation outcome. The GNRI has potential as a predictor of rehabilitation outcome in MHD patients.

Abbreviations

ADLs: Activities of daily living; BI: Barthel Index; BMI: Body mass index; ERSD: End-stage renal disease; GNRI: Geriatric Nutritional Risk Index; MHD: Maintenance hemodialysis

Acknowledgements

We are grateful to all the staff in the Department of Rehabilitation Medicine, Yokohama University Medical Center.

Funding

We have no financial support.

Authors' contributions

YS conceived the study and drafted the manuscript. YS, TF, and HW interpreted the data and revised the manuscript. All authors read and approved the final manuscript.

Competing interests

The authors declare that they have no competing interests.

References

1. Fouque D, Kalantar-Zadeh K, Kopple J, Cano N, Chauveau P, Cuppari L, et al. A proposed nomenclature and diagnostic criteria for protein-energy wasting in acute and chronic kidney disease. Kidney Int. 2008;73(3):391–8.
2. Kopple JD. McCollum Award Lecture, 1996: protein-energy malnutrition in maintenance dialysis patients. Am J Clin Nutr. 1997;65(5):1544–57.
3. Kalantar-Zadeh K, Ikizler TA, Block G, Avram MM, Kopple JD. Malnutrition-inflammation complex syndrome in dialysis patients: causes and consequences. Am J Kidney Dis. 2003;42(5):864–81.
4. Bossola M, Di Stasio E, Antocicco M, Pepe G, Tazza L, Zuccalà G, et al. Functional impairment is associated with an increased risk of mortality in patients on chronic hemodialysis. BMC Nephrol. 2016;17(1):72. https://doi.org/10.1186/s12882-016-0302-y.
5. Jassal SV, Karaboyas A, Comment LA, Bieber BA, Morgenstern H, Sen A, et al. Functional dependence and mortality in the international dialysis outcomes and practice patterns study (DOPPS). Am J Kidney Dis. 2016;67(2):283–92.
6. Cook WL, Jassal SV. Functional dependencies among the elderly on hemodialysis. Kidney Int. 2008;73(11):1289–95.
7. Katz S, Ford Ford AB, Moskowitz RW, Jackson BA, Jaffe MW. Studies of illness in the aged. The index of ADL: a standardized measure of biological and psychosocial function. JAMA. 1963;185:914–9.
8. Mahoney FI, Barthel DW. Functional evaluation: the Barthel Index. Md State Med J. 1965;14:61–5.
9. Endo M, Nakamura Y, Murakami T, Tsukahara H, Watanabe Y, et al. Rehabilitation improves prognosis and activities of daily living in hemodialysis patients with low activities of daily living. Phys Ther Res. 2017;20(1):9–15.
10. Cereda E, Pedrolli C, Klersy C, Bonardi C, Quarleri L, Cappello S, et al. Nutritional status in older persons according to healthcare setting: a systematic review and meta-analysis of prevalence data using MNA. Clin Nutr. 2016;35(6):1282–90.
11. Davis JP, Wong AA, Schluter PJ, Henderson RD, O'Sullivan JD, Read SJ. Impact of premorbid undernutrition on outcome in stroke patients. Stroke. 2004;35(8):1930–4.
12. Anker SD, John M, Pedersen PU, Raguso C, Cicoira M, Dardai E, et al. ESPEN guidelines on enteral nutrition: cardiology and pulmonology. Clin Nutr. 2006;25(2):311–8.
13. Bouillanne O, Morineau G, Dupont C, Coulombel I, Vincent JP, Nicolis I, et al. Geriatric nutritional risk index: a new index for evaluating at-risk elderly medical patients. Am J Clin Nutr. 2005;82(4):777–83.
14. Yamada K, Furuya R, Takita T, Maruyama Y, Yamaguchi Y, Ohkawa S, et al. Simplified nutritional screening tools for patients on maintenance hemodialysis. Am J Clin Nutr. 2008;87(1):106–13.
15. Hsieh YW, Wang CH, Wu SC, Chen PC, Sheu CF, Hsieh CL. Establishing the minimal clinically important difference of the Barthel Index in stroke patients. Neurorehabil Neural Repair. 2007;21(3):233–8.
16. Sarmento LA, Pinto JS, da Silva AP, Cabral CM, Chiavegato LD. Effect of conventional physical therapy and Pilates in functionality, respiratory muscle strength and ability to exercise in hospitalized chronic renal patients: a randomized controlled trial. Clin Rehabil. 2017;31(4):508–20.
17. Inouye M, Kishi K, Ikeda Y, Takada M, Katoh J, Iwahashi M, et al. Prediction of functional outcome after stroke rehabilitation. Am J Phys Med Rehabil. 2000;79(6):513–8.
18. Reeves MJ, Bushnell CD, Howard G, Gargano JW, Duncan PW, Lynch G, et al. Sex differences in stroke: epidemiology, clinical presentation, medical care, and outcomes. Lancet Neurol. 2008;7(10):915–26.

19. Granger CV, Dewis LS, Peters NC, Sherwood CC, Barrett JE. Stroke rehabilitation: analysis of repeated Barthel index measures. Arch Phys Med Rehabil. 1979;60(1):145–54.
20. Kobayashi I, Ishimura E, Kato Y, Okuno S, Yamamoto T, Yamakawa T, et al. Geriatric Nutritional Risk Index, a simplified nutritional screening index, is a significant predictor of mortality in chronic dialysis patients. Nephrol Dial Transplant. 2010;25(10):3361–5.
21. Beberashvili I, Azar A, Sinuani I, Shapiro G, Feldman L, Sandbank J, et al. Geriatric nutritional risk index, muscle function, quality of life and clinical outcome in hemodialysis patients. Clin Nutr. 2016;35(6):1522–9.
22. Yoshimura Y, Uchida K, Jeong S, Yamaga M. Effects of nutritional supplements on muscle mass and activities of daily living in elderly rehabilitation patients with decreased muscle mass: a randomized controlled trial. J Nutr Health Aging. 2016;20(2):185–91.
23. Dong J, Sundell MB, Pupim LB, Wu P, Shintani A, Ikizler TA. The effect of resistance exercise to augment long-term benefits of intradialytic oral nutritional supplementation in chronic hemodialysis patients. J Ren Nutr. 2011;21(2):149–59.
24. Martin-Alemañy G, Valdez-Ortiz R, Olvera-Soto G, Gomez-Guerrero I, Aguire-Esquivel G, Cantu-Quintanilla G, et al. The effects of resistance exercise and oral nutritional supplementation during hemodialysis on indicators of nutritional status and quality of life. Nephrol Dial Transplant. 2016;31(10):1712–20.
25. Nii M, Maeda K, Wakabayashi H, Nishioka S, Tanaka A. Nutritional improvement and energy intake are associated with functional recovery in patients after cerebrovascular disorders. J Stroke Cerebrovasc Dis. 2016;25(1):57–62.
26. Nishioka S, Wakabayashi H, Nishioka E, Yoshida T, Mori N, Watanabe R. Nutritional improvement correlates with recovery of activities of daily living among malnourished elderly stroke patients in the convalescent stage: a cross-sectional study. J Acad Nutr Diet. 2016;116:837–43.
27. Nishioka S, Wakabayashi H, Momosaki R. Nutritional status changes and activities of daily living after hip fracture in convalescent rehabilitation wards: a retrospective observational cohort study from the Japan Rehabilitation Nutrition Database. J Acad Nutr Diet. 2018. https://doi.org/10.1016/j.jand.2018.02.012.
28. Uno C, Wakabayashi H, Maeda K, Nishioka S. Rehabilitation nutrition support for a hemodialysis patient with protein-energy wasting and sarcopenic dysphagia: a case report. Ren Replace Ther. 2018;4:18.
29. Alcorta MD, Alvarez PC, Cabetas RN, Martín MA, Valero M, Candela CG. The importance of serum albumin determination method to classify patients based on nutritional status. Clin Nutr ESPEN. 2018;25:110–3.
30. Maekawa M, Muramoto Y, Seimiya M, Kariyone K. Recommendation on measurement of serum albumin - how to handle the difference between measured values by BCG method and improved BCP method. Rinsho Byori. 2014;62(1):5–9 (in Japanese).

23

A case of vertebral arteriovenous fistula in a patient undergoing maintenance hemodialysis

Kinuko Dote[1*], Nobuyuki Takahashi[1], Tomoko Niki[2], Tomoya Ishiguro[3] and Ichiro Shiojima[4]

Abstract

Background: Vertebral arteriovenous fistula (AVF) is an uncommon vascular disorder and defined as abnormal connections of the extracranial vertebral artery or its branches into the neighboring vein or deep venous plexus. This can be spontaneous or traumatic in origin. Spontaneous cases may be congenital or associated with dysplasia of vascular wall. Traumatic cases are due either to blunt or penetrating trauma, or iatrogenic trauma.

Case presentation: A vertebral AVF was detected by carotid duplex ultrasonography, and an endovascular treatment was successfully performed in a 72-year-old woman with 1 year history of hemodialysis.

Conclusion: An extensive observation by carotid duplex ultrasonography is needed to detect vertebral AVF in patients who have a history of dialysis catheter insertion to internal jugular vein.

Keywords: Vertebral arteriovenous fistula, Hemodialysis, Carotid duplex ultrasonography

Background

Vertebral arteriovenous fistula (AVF) is defined as abnormal connections of the extracranial vertebral artery or its branches into the neighboring vein or deep venous plexus [1]. Spontaneous cases may be congenital or associated with dysplasia of vascular wall [2]. On the other hand, traumatic cases are due either to blunt or penetrating trauma, or iatrogenic trauma [3].

The diagnosis of vertebral AVF relied on catheter angiography, but recent advances in non-invasive imaging modalities make the diagnosis much easier [4].

For the treatment of vertebral AVF, preservation of the parental artery is important and must be attempted. Endovascular treatment is a minimally invasive treatment modality and does not have the disadvantages of open surgery [5–7]. Different types of endovascular approaches, transvenous, transarterial or both with coil or balloon embolization are reported [6, 8]. We report a case of vertebral AVF in a hemodialysis patient, first detected by the carotid duplex ultrasonography and successfully treated with endovascular therapy.

Case presentation

A 72-year-old woman with established end-stage renal disease secondary to hypertension who was on hemodialysis for 1 year using a left upper-extremity dialysis access fistula. She had a history of dialysis catheter insertion into the right internal jugular vein at the initiation of hemodialysis. On physical examination, blood pressure was 155/89 mmHg and regular heart rhythm of 75 bpm. Auscultation revealed no abnormal heart sounds and lung crepitations. A neck bruit might be the only presenting sign, and there was a thrill over her right neck. Laboratory data obtained before dialysis were hemoglobin 11.8 g/dl, blood urea nitrogen 70 mg/dl, creatinine 10.03 mg/dl, calcium 9.6 mg/dl, inorganic phosphorus 4.0 mg/dl, N-terminal pro-brain natriuretic peptide 1840 pg/ml. Human atrial natriuretic peptide was 68.5 pg/ml after dialysis. Chest X-ray showed neither pulmonary congestion nor cardiomegaly, with a cardiothoracic ratio

* Correspondence: doteki@kouri.kmu.ac.jp
[1]Department of Medicine, Kori Hospital, Kansai Medical University, 8-45 Korihondori-cho, Neyagawa City, Osaka 572-8551, Japan
Full list of author information is available at the end of the article

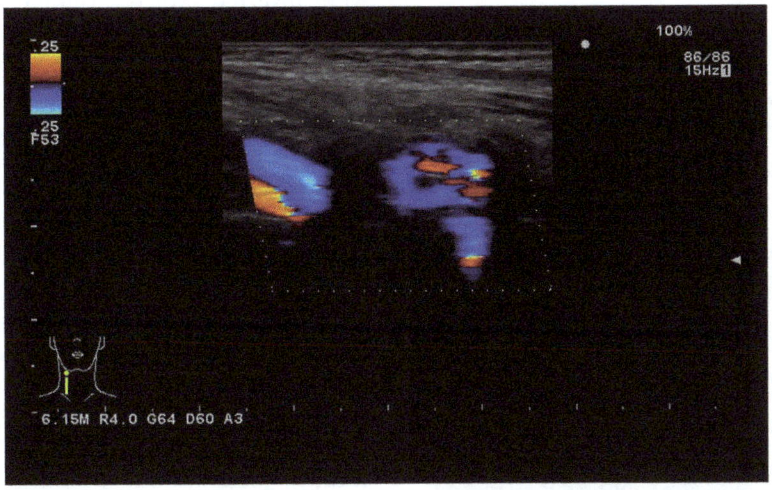

Fig. 1 Carotid duplex ultrasonography. The mosaic pattern of bloodstream in the right vertebral artery

of 54%. Medications included ezomeprazole magnesium 20 mg/day, nifedipine CR 40 mg/day, doxazosin 4 mg/day, olmesartan 40 mg/day, azosemide 60 mg/day, carvedilol 2.5 mg/day, lanthanum carbonate 1500 mg/day, sevelamer hydrochloride 750 mg/day, and atorvastatin 10 mg/every other day. Low molecular-weight heparin was used for anticoagulation during dialysis session. The carotid duplex ultrasonography was performed for the screening of vascular wall thickness and luminal stenosis of carotid and vertebral arteries, which detected a mosaic pattern of bloodstream in the right vertebral artery with a high peak systolic velocity of 89.6 cm/s at the right C6/7 level and a slow peak systolic velocity of 30 cm/s at the right C4/5 level (Figs. 1 and 2). Cervical magnetic resonance angiography (MRA) revealed a right-sided mass lesion at C5/6 level next to the right epidural venous plexus (Fig. 3). Distal right vertebral artery was not detected. Cone beam computed tomography (CT) revealed a fistulous communication between the ventromedial part of the right C5/6 level vertebral artery and the vertebral venous plexus (Fig. 4). The patient underwent a digital subtraction angiography examination to clear up the architect of the AVF and to plan treatment strategy. Injection of contrast agent to the right vertebral artery showed a single high flow side-to-side fistula at the right C5/6 level; vertebral artery flowed into the neighboring vertebral venous plexus, then drained to epidural venous plexus in the spinal canal and finally to the vertebral venous plexus outside the spinal canal via intervertebral vein, or directly drained to the subclavian vein (Fig. 5). Although diagnosis of vertebral AVF and its accurate localization were obtained by catheter

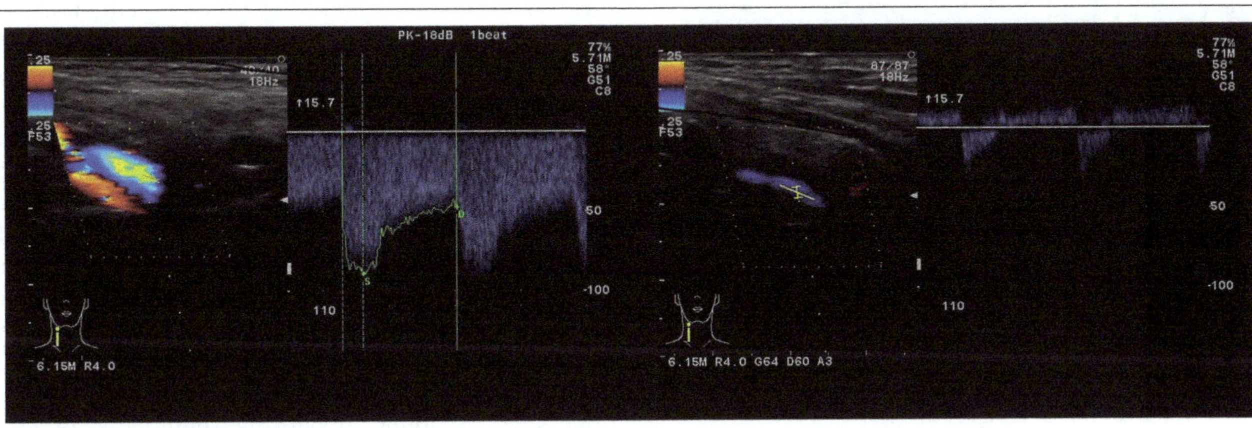

Fig. 2 Carotid duplex ultrasonography. The high peak systolic velocity of 89.6 cm/s at the right C6/7 level (left) and the slow peak systolic velocity of 30 cm/s at the right C4/5 level (right)

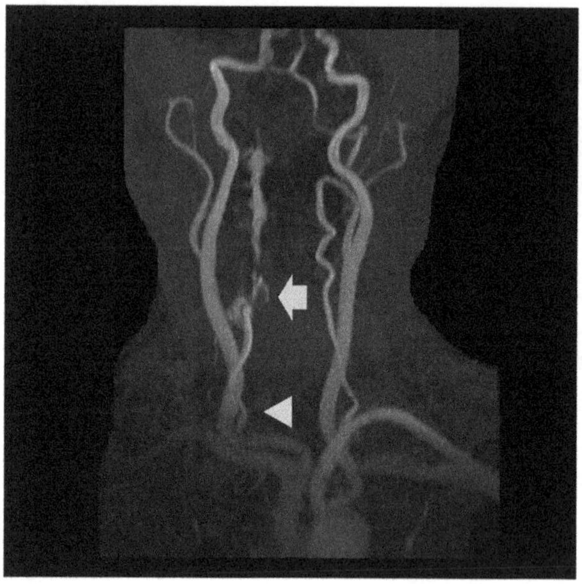

Fig. 3 Cervical magnetic resonance angiography imaging at the right C5/6 level revealed insufficient filling of the distal right vertebral artery (headed arrow) and detection of the right epidural venous plexus (arrow)

angiography, non-invasive imaging modalities such as color duplex ultrasonography, CT, and MRA can also reveal correct localization of fistula, especially duplex scan is the simplest and least invasive method. Under local anesthesia, after microcatheters were inserted into the right vertebral artery and vein, the fistula was completely occluded by 18 coils from arterial side and 3 coils from venous side. The final angiogram showed no residual filling of the fistula and a normal filling of distal vertebral artery (Fig. 5). The neck thrill disappeared immediately after the procedure.

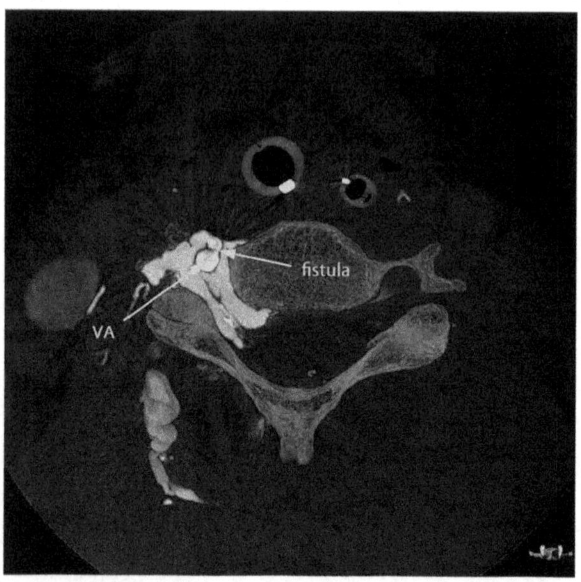

Fig. 4 Cone beam computed tomography revealed the fistulous communication (arrow) between the right C5/6 level vertebral artery (arrow) and the neighboring right vertebral venous plexus. VA, vertebral artery

Discussion

Vertebral AVF is a rare vascular disorder and can be spontaneous or traumatic in origin [2]. Spontaneous ones are complicated by primary vascular pathologies like neurofibromatosis, fibromuscular dysplasia, Marfan's syndrome, or Ehlers-Danlos syndrome [9, 10]. The causes of traumatic fistulas are penetrating trauma (stab wounds), blunt trauma (whiplash injury), gunshot wounds, surgical events, hyperextension injury following car accident, after nerve block injection, or by catheter insertion [2, 3]. Most traumatic vertebral AVFs involve the long second portion (intraforaminal) of vertebral artery, whereas spontaneous AVFs usually involve the third portion where the artery leaves the foramen of the atlas and enters the foramen magnum [11]. Although a spontaneous nature cannot be fully denied, fistula might have been caused by injury to the vertebral artery at the time of dialysis catheter insertion to the right neck in our case. We have investigated literatures from 1969 to 2018 by PubMed and found 31 cases describing the details of vertebral AVF that were related to catheter insertion; two of them were dialysis catheter [2, 3, 8, 12–16] (Table 1). Catheter-related iatrogenic cause is not uncommon among traumatic vertebral AVF. According to the report by Vinchon et al., 18 of 28 cases were caused by iatrogenic trauma; 14 occurred after arterial puncture during venous catheterization, 2 after direct percutaneous carotid angiography, and 2 after jugular vein puncture for Greenfield filter insertion [2]. Other causes included surgery (two), penetrating cervical trauma (three), and blunt trauma (five) [2]. The risk of arterial puncture during percutaneous internal jugular vein puncture has been markedly reduced using ultrasound guidance. Even if it does occur, development of vertebral AVF is a rare complication because vertebral artery runs posteriorly through inside of transverse foramen of cervical vertebra. However, as shown in ultrasonography obtained from a normal volunteer, vertebral artery runs quite close to internal jugular vein (Fig. 6), so that an erroneous puncture may accidentally occur. Anatomical variations such as goiter, ankylosing spondylitis, or even obesity might increase the risk of erroneous puncture [13]. In addition, it is sometimes difficult to

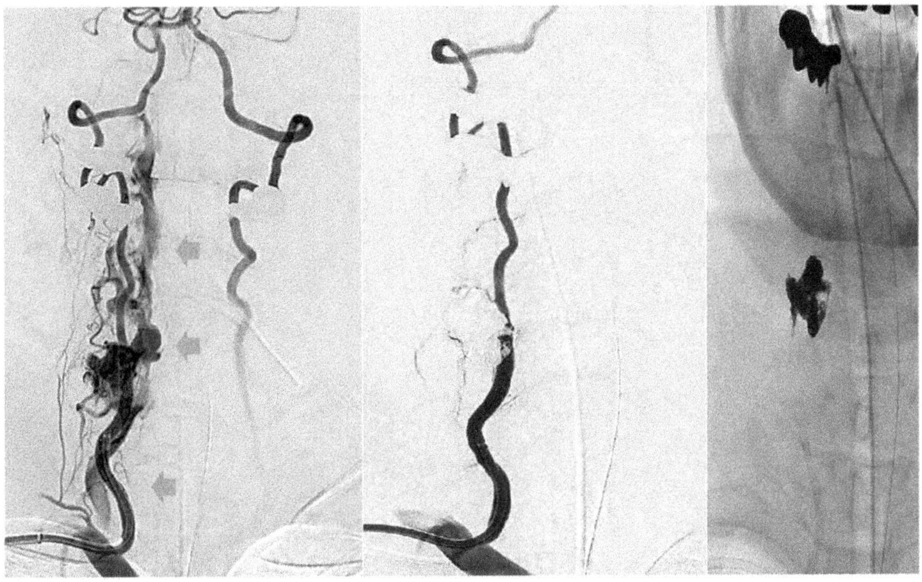

Fig. 5 Digital subtraction angiography of the right vertebral artery (anterior-posterior view) revealed a single high flow side-to-side fistula (middle arrow) between the right vertebral artery (lower arrow) and the neighboring right vertebral venous plexus and the right epidural venous plexus (upper arrow) (left). Complete obliteration of fistula (middle). Coils in the right vertebral arteriovenous fistula (right)

visualize whether the tip of the needle or catheter is remaining inside the vein even under the use of ultrasound guidance.

Symptomatology depends on the site of the vertebral AVF and the flow pattern. Most of the patients are asymptomatic, and the fistula is found after systematic auscultation [3]. Tinnitus, the most frequent symptom, is enhanced by exertion, straining, elevated blood pressure, pregnancy, and diminished or abolished by percutaneous compression or turning the head [17, 18]. Vertebrobasilar insufficiency is also common including headache and vertigo [19]. Very rarely there are symptoms of cervical radiculopathy [20]. Although the mechanism of cervical radiculopathy is often unclear, direct compression by dilated draining veins or a false aneurysm penetrating the vertebral canal are reported especially in Recklinghausen patients [21, 22]. AVF sometimes causes high-cardiac output state due to increasing venous return [23]. This is very important especially in hemodialysis patients. Because they already have AVF for hemodialysis, additional presence of AVF may cause a congestive heart failure. Fortunately, she had never suffered from heart failure because AVF was so small and cardiac output was 5 L/min.

Carotid duplex ultrasonography, MRA and CT are non-invasive and useful methods to diagnose vertebral AVF. Although ultrasound is limited by operator's ability, it is useful as the first line investigation. We found fistula incidentally by regular checkup for vascular wall thickness and luminal stenosis of carotid and vertebral arteries. The vertebral AVF was detected by a mosaic pattern of blood flow and the change in peak systolic velocity in the vertebral artery at C5/6 level, which was further confirmed by MRA and CT. The use of MRA in imaging the vertebral artery is well established [24]. Contrast enhanced MRA was not performed in our case to avoid exposure to gadolinium contrast agent in dialysis patients, but MRA clearly demonstrated fistulous connection of arterial flow to vertebral and epidural venous plexus.

The goal of the treatment is occlusion of the fistula site and preservation of the patency of vertebral artery. Open surgical repair of vertebral artery injuries is extremely challenging because of multiple factors; the most significant one is obtaining adequate exposure with proximal and distal vascular control [24]. Surgical treatment of extracranial vertebral artery has greatly evolved in recent years, now primarily involves endovascular transcatheter therapies including coil or balloon occlusion of the fistula and stent-assisted arterial reconstruction [24]. Intravascular coils with smaller diameters than the balloon may be used when the orifice of the fistula is too small to allow safe inflation of the detachable balloon [9]. In our case, the embolic materials were placed both proximal and distal to the fistula via both vertebral artery and vein for the complete elimination of the fistula.

Table 1 Review of the literature on vertebral AVF caused by jugular catheter insertion

Case no.	Sex	Age (years)	Clinical presentation	Cause	Side	Level	Treatment	Clinical outcome	Reference no.
1	F	72	Murmur	Jugular dialysis catheter	R	C5/6	coil	Asymptomatic	Present
2	M	53	Symptom-free	Jugular catheter	R	C5/6	balloon occlusion	Asymptomatic	3
3	M	34	Tinnitus	Jugular catheter	L	C5/6	Balloon occlusion	Asymptomatic	3
4	M	71	Symptom-free	Jugular catheter	L	C5	Balloon occlusion	Asymptomatic	3
5	M	51	Symptom-free	Jugular catheter	R	C6	Balloon occlusion	Asymptomatic	3
6	F	66	Vertigo	Jugular catheter	R	C6	Balloon occlusion	Asymptomatic	3
7	F	57	Symptom-free	Jugular catheter	L	C6	Balloon occlusion	Asymptomatic	3
8	M	68	Neurological	Jugular catheter	L	C6	Balloon occlusion	Asymptomatic	3
9	F	35	Tinnitus	Jugular catheter	R	C5	Balloon occlusion	Asymptomatic	2
10	M	37	Symptom-free	Jugular catheter	R	C5/6	Abstention	Not occluded	2
11	M	38	Symptom-free	Jugular catheter	R	C3	Surgical repair	Asymptomatic	2
12	M	45	Vertebral ischemia	Jugular catheter	R	C5/6	Surgical repair/balloon occlusion	Asymptomatic	2
13	M	47	Tinnitus	Jugular catheter	R	C6	Abstention	Not occluded	2
14	M	49	Symptom-free	Jugular catheter	R	C6	Abstention	Not occluded	2
15	M	51	Tinnitus	Jugular catheter	R	C6	Surgical repair/balloon occlusion	Asymptomatic	2
16	M	53	Symptom-free	Jugular catheter	R	C5/6	Surgical repair/balloon occlusion	Asymptomatic	2
17	M	55	Symptom-free	Jugular catheter	R	C5/6	Balloon occlusion	Asymptomatic	2
18	F	56	Symptom-free	Jugular catheter	R	C3	Balloon occlusion	Asymptomatic	2
19	F	57	Symptom-free	Jugular catheter	L	C5/6	Abstention	Asymptomatic	2
20	F	57	Symptom-free	Jugular catheter	L	C6	Balloon occlusion	Asymptomatic	2
21	F	61	Tinnitus	Jugular catheter	R	C5/6	Surgical repair/balloon occlusion	Asymptomatic	2
22	M	61	Tinnitus	Jugular catheter	R	C6	Surgical repair	Asymptomatic	2
23	F	66	Vertebral ischemia	Jugular catheter	R	C6	Balloon occlusion	Asymptomatic	2
24	M	70	Neurological	Jugular catheter	R	C5/6	Balloon occlusion	Asymptomatic	2
25	M	71	Symptom-free	Jugular catheter	L	C4/5	Balloon occlusion	Not occluded	2
26	F	77	Symptom-free	Jugular catheter	R	C6	Surgical repair	Asymptomatic	2
27	M	66	Murmur	Swan-Ganz's catheter	R		Balloon occlusion	Asymptomatic	8
28	F	11	Radiculopathy	Jugular catheter	R	C2–5	Balloon occlusion	Asymptomatic	12
29	F	69	Murmur	Jugular catheter	R	Unknown	Surgical repair	Asymptomatic	13
30	M	72	Blood gas analysis consistent with arterial blood	Jugular dialysis catheter	L	C5	Balloon occlusion	Asymptomatic	14
31	M	57	Murmur	Jugular catheter	R	Unknown	Surgical repair	Asymptomatic	23
32	F	42	Dizziness, nausea, headache	Jugular catheter	R	Unknown	Surgical repair	Asymptomatic	24

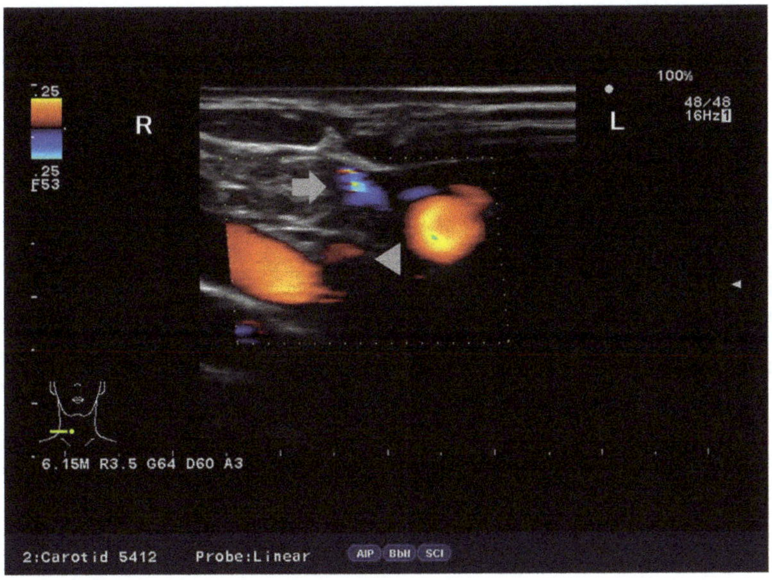

Fig. 6 Carotid ultrasonography of the right vertebral artery (headed arrow) and the right internal jugular vein (arrow) obtained from a normal volunteer

Conclusion

A case of vertebral AVF was first confirmed by systemic auscultation and carotid duplex ultrasonography. We should be aware of vertebral AVF in patients undergoing hemodialysis who had a history of dialysis catheter insertion to the neck.

Abbreviations

AVF: Arteriovenous fistula; CT: computed tomography; MRA: magnetic resonance angiography

Authors` contributions

KD, TN, and TI performed acquisition and interpretation of the data. KD drafted the manuscript and is responsible for the final version of the manuscript. NT and SI supported the entire process of preparing the manuscript. All authors read and approved the final manuscript.

Authors` information

Department of Medicine, Kori Hospital, Kansai Medical University.

Competing interests

The authors declare that they have no competing interests.

Author details

[1]Department of Medicine, Kori Hospital, Kansai Medical University, 8-45 Korihondori-cho, Neyagawa City, Osaka 572-8551, Japan. [2]Department of Laboratory Medicine, Kori Hospital, Kansai Medical University, Neyagawa City, Osaka, Japan. [3]Department of Neurointervention, Osaka City General Hospital, Osaka City, Osaka, Japan. [4]Second Department of Internal Medicine, Kansai Medical University, Hirakata City, Osaka, Japan.

References

1. Halbach VV, Higashida RT, Hieshima GB. Treatment of vertebral arteriovenous fistulas. AJR Am J Roentgenol. 1988;150:405–12.
2. Vinchon M, Laurian C, George B, et al. Vertebral arteriovenous fistulas: a study of 49 cases and review of the literature. Cardiovasc Surg. 1994;2: 359–69.
3. Beaujeux RL, Reizine DC, Casasco A, et al. Endovascular treatment of vertebral arteriovenous fistula. Radiology. 1992;183:361–7.
4. Mortimer A, Stubbs E, Cookson D, et al. Delayed presentation of a vertebral arterio-venous fistula secondary to penetrating cervical trauma: endovascular management using coil embolisation - a case report. J Radiol Case Rep. 2009;3:9–15.
5. Hauck EF, Nauta HJ. Spontaneous spinal epidural arteriovenous fistulae in neurofibromatosis type-1. Surg Neurol. 2006;66:215–21.
6. Barkhordarian S. Stent graft repair of traumatic vertebral pseudoaneurysm with arteriovenous fistula. Vasc Endovasc Surg. 2007;41:153–7.
7. Geraci AR, Upson JF, Greene DG. Congenital vertebral arteriovenous fistula. JAMA. 1969;210:727–8.
8. Guglielmi G, Viñuela F, Duckwiler G, et al. High-flow, small-hole arteriovenous fistulas: treatment with electrodetachable coils. AJNR Am J Neuroradiol. 1995;16:325–8.
9. Bahar S, Chiras J, Carpena JP, et al. Spontaneous vertebro-vertebral arterio-venous fistula associated with fibro-muscular dysplasia. Report of two cases. Neuroradiology. 1984;26:45–9.
10. Kähärä V, Lehto U, Ryymin P, et al. Vertebral epidural arteriovenous fistula and radicular pain in neurofibromatosis type I. Acta Neurochir. 2002;144: 493–6.
11. de Bray JM, Bertrand P, Bertrand F, Jeanvoine H. Spontaneous arteriovenous fistulas of the vertebral artery. Apropos of a case--review of the literature. Rev Med Interne. 1986;7:133–9.
12. Herrera DA, Vargas SA, Dublin AB. Endovascular treatment of traumatic injuries of the vertebral artery. Am J Neuroradiol. 2008;29(8):1585–9.
13. Stock U, Link J, Dutschke P. Iatrogenic vertebrojugular arteriovenous fistula. Anaesthesia. 1996;51(7):687–8.
14. Yamamoto A, Suzuki K, Sakaida H, et al. Management of inadvertent vertebral artery injury due to central venous catheterization in a coagulopathic patient. Acute Med Surg. 2015;3(3):265–7.
15. Varga ZA, Gyori-Molnar I, Kollar L, et al. A surgically treated arteriovenous fistula between the vertebral artery and internal jugular vein after insertion of a central venous catheter for mitral valve replacement. J Thorac Cardiovasc Surg. 2002;123(3):575–7.

16. Surber R, Werner GS, Cohnert TU, et al. Recurrent vertebral arteriovenous fitula after surgical repair: treatment with a self-expanding stent-graft. J Endovasc Ther. 2003;10:49–53.
17. Kim YH, Gildenberg PL, Duchesneau PM. Angiographic evidence of spontaneous closure of nontraumatic arteriovenous fistula of the vertebral artery. Case report J Neurosurg. 1973;38:658–61.
18. Goodman SJ, Hasso A, Kirkpatrick D. Treatment of vertebrojugular fistula by balloon occlusion. Case report. J Neurosurg. 1975;43:362–7.
19. Gobin YP, Duckwiler GR, Viñuela F. Direct arteriovenous fistulas (carotid-cavernous and vertebral-venous). Diagnosis and intervention. Neuroimaging Clin N Am. 1998;8:425–43.
20. Tenjin H, Kimura S, Sugawa N. Coil embolization of vertebro-vertebral arteriovenous fistula: a case report. Surg Neurol. 2005;63:80–3.
21. Deans WR, Bloch S, Leibrock L, et al. Arteriovenous fistula in patients with neurofibromatosis. Radiology. 1982;144:103–7.
22. Peeters FL. Endovascular treatment of spontaneous vertebro-vertebral fistulas. Rofo. 1990;153:724–5.
23. Tay KY, U-King-Im JM, Trivedi RA, et al. Imaging the vertebral artery. Eur Radiol. 2005;15:1329–43.
24. O'Shaughnessy BA, Bendok BR, Parkinson RJ, et al. Transarterial coil embolization of a high-flow vertebrojugular fistula due to penetrating craniocervical trauma: case report. Surg Neurol. 2005;64:335–40.

24

Glecaprevir and pibrentasvir combination therapy for hepatitis C virus-infected Japanese patients on hemodialysis

Yoshiaki Tanaka[1*], Takanori Masaki[2], Haruki Uojima[1,3], Takayasu Ohtake[4], Tomoaki Fujikawa[5], Yasuhiro Yamanouchi[6], Naohisa Wada[1], Kousuke Kubota[1], Hisashi Hidaka[1], Takahide Nakazawa[1], Akitaka Shibuya[7], Togo Aoyama[2], Ji Hyun Sung[3], Makoto Kako[3], Shuzo Kobayashi[4], Yasuo Takeuchi[2] and Wasaburo Koizumi[1]

Abstract

Background: It remains unclear whether hepatitis C virus (HCV)-infected Japanese patients on hemodialysis (HD) have an altered viral response to glecaprevir (GLE) and pibrentasvir (PIB) combination therapy and whether this treatment is safe for this patient group. Therefore, we investigated the characteristics associated with virological response to GLE and PIB combination therapy for HCV in Japanese patients undergoing HD. This study aimed to evaluate the safety and efficacy of GLE and PIB combination therapy in HCV-infected Japanese patients on HD.

Methods: This multicenter, single-arm, open-label, and prospective study was conducted at four centers in Japan and enrolled Japanese patients with chronic HCV genotype 1b, 2a, and 2b infections. Enrolled patients received 300 mg GLE in combination with 120 mg PIB once daily for either 8 or 12 weeks. The primary endpoint of this trial was the rate of sustained virological response at 12 weeks after treatment (SVR12). Furthermore, pharmacological effects and adverse events associated with combination therapy were evaluated.

Results: A total of 18 HD patients with HCV infection were enrolled in this study. Of these patients, 17 (94.4%) achieved SVR12. Among patients receiving combination therapy for 8 weeks, only one experienced a virological relapse at week 12 after the end of treatment. Despite the absence of treatment-related deaths, adverse events were observed in 9 patients (50.0%) during treatment. The most frequent adverse event was pruritus, which occurred in 7 patients (38.9%).

Conclusions: GLE and PIB combination therapy was effective and tolerable in Japanese HD patients with chronic HCV genotype 1b, 2a, and 2b infections.

Keywords: Glecaprevir, Pibrentasvir, Chronic kidney disease, Hepatitis C virus, Hemodialysis

Background

The introduction of direct-acting antivirals (DAAs), which refer to small-molecule inhibitors of different viral proteins, has improved both the sustained virological response (SVR) rates and the tolerability of prolonged treatment in comparison with interferon (IFN)-based medicine [1, 2]. As treatment-related toxicity associated with IFN and ribavirin (RBV) is common, an IFN-free regimen with DAAs can be particularly effective for patients with end-stage renal disease, including those on hemodialysis (HD) [3–5].

In Japan, several combined regimens, including daclatasvir (DCV)/asunaprevir (ASV), ombitasvir/paritaprevir/ritonavir, and elbasvir/grazoprevir, which are primarily eliminated by hepatic metabolism, are available for the effective treatment of HD patients with hepatitis C virus (HCV) genotype 1b infections [6–8]. Despite the remarkable success of IFN-free regimens for patients with HCV

* Correspondence: tanakay@kitasato-u.ac.jp
[1]Department of Gastroenterology, Internal Medicine, Kitasato University School of Medicine, Sagamihara, Kanagawa, Japan
Full list of author information is available at the end of the article

genotype 1 infections, currently available regimens without RBV provide insufficient SVR rates in patients with genotype 2 infections.

Glecaprevir (GLE) is a nonstructural protein (NS) 3/4A protease inhibitor coformulated with pibrentasvir (PIB), an NS5A inhibitor, and is currently being investigated as a regimen with potential efficacy against all HCV genotypes [9–11]. The pharmacokinetics of GLE and PIB, which are primarily eliminated by hepatic metabolism, have been assessed in patients with end-stage renal disease. In addition, GLE and PIB are not removed from plasma by HD [12]. Recently, the EXPEDITION-4 trial in patients with HCV genotype 1–5 or 6 infection has reported the safety and efficacy of 12-week GLE and PIB combination therapy as treatment for chronic HCV in patients undergoing HD, showing dramatically improved rates of SVR at 12 weeks after treatment (SVR12) [12]. Therefore, this regimen is expected to yield beneficial results in specific populations, such as HCV genotype 2-infected Japanese patients with insufficient renal function. However, it remains unclear whether HCV-infected Japanese patients on HD experience positive outcomes with respect to SVR and safety following GLE and PIB combination therapy. Furthermore, the treatment duration of GLE and PIB combination therapy was 8 weeks for patients who neither had compensated liver cirrhosis nor had received previous DAA therapy in Japan. To the best of our knowledge, there are no data on the efficacy of 8-week GLE and PIB combination therapy in patients undergoing HD. Accordingly, this study aimed to evaluate the safety and efficacy of GLE and PIB combination therapy in HCV-infected Japanese patients on HD.

Methods

Ethics

This study was approved by the institutional review board (IRB)/ethics committee of Kitasato University School of Medicine (IRB number: C17-237) and Tokushukai Medical Group (IRB number: TGE00926-024) and is registered in the University Hospital Medical Information Network (UMIN) Clinical Trials Registry as UMIN000029781.

Study design and patients

This multicenter, single-arm, open-label, and prospective study was conducted at four centers in Japan. The enrollment commenced in November 2017, and the study was completed in July 2018. Patients with chronic HCV genotype 1b, 2a, and 2b infections who were undergoing HD received GLE and PIB. All enrolled patients received 300 mg GLE in combination with 120 mg PIB once daily for either 8 or 12 weeks. According to the manufacturer's prescribing information for both medications, treatment duration should be 12 weeks for patients who had compensated liver cirrhosis and/or received previous DAA therapy. Diagnosis of liver cirrhosis was based on laboratory results, ultrasonography, and computed tomography revealing a hepatic cirrhotic appearance and/or splenomegaly. Liver biopsy was not performed for all patients because of the high risk of life-threatening complications. The discontinuation criteria for the enrolled patients were as follows: (1) occurrence of viral breakthrough (increase in plasma HCV-RNA levels exceeding 1 $\log_{10}$ IU/mL compared with the lowest recorded on-treatment value), (2) occurrence of severe adverse events according the National Cancer Institute's Common Terminology Criteria for Adverse Events (CTCAE) version 4.0, and (3) patient's desire to terminate.

Eligibility criteria

This study enrolled Japanese patients with chronic HCV genotype 1b, 2a, and 2b infections for at least 6 months and plasma HCV-RNA levels ≥ 2 $\log_{10}$ IU/mL. Treatment-naïve or treatment-experienced patients (previously treated with IFN-based therapy and/or IFN-free therapy) aged ≥ 20 years who were currently undergoing HD were included in the study. Conversely, patients with (1) decompensated liver cirrhosis (Child–Pugh classes B and C), (2) hepatocellular carcinoma, (3) resistance-associated variants of NS5A-P32 deletion among those with HCV genotype 1b, (4) infection/coinfection with hepatitis B virus or human immunodeficiency virus, (5) previous exposure to IFN-based therapy or DAA inhibitors within 1 month before drug administration, and (6) alanine aminotransferase (ALT) levels greater than five times the upper limit of the normal range, platelet and white blood cell (WBC) counts lower than 50,000 and 4000/mm^3, respectively, and hemoglobin (Hb) levels less than 8.5 g/dL were excluded from the study.

Clinical parameters

The clinical characteristics of enrolled patients were evaluated. Data on demographics, plasma HCV-RNA levels, and baseline laboratory results before study drug administration were collected. Blood samples were obtained at each study visit before dialysis, and plasma HCV-RNA levels were quantified using Cobas TaqMan version 2.0 assay (Roche Diagnostics, Tokyo, Japan). The lower limit of quantification was 1.2 $\log_{10}$ IU/mL. HCV-RNA levels were measured at baseline; at treatment weeks 4, 8, and 12 (in patients in the 12-week treatment duration group); and at post-treatment weeks 4, 8, and 12.

We analyzed baseline resistance-associated variants at signature amino acid positions associated with resistance for genotype 1b using direct sequencing, such as NS5A-Y93, L31, P32, and NS3/4 D168 [13]. With respect to the laboratory tests performed, WBC, neutrophil, and platelet counts and levels of Hb, total protein, serum albumin, blood urea nitrogen (BUN), serum creatinine, total bilirubin, aspartate aminotransferase (AST), ALT, Mac-2-binding protein glycan isomer (M2BPGi), and α-fetoprotein were analyzed.

Efficacy

The primary endpoint of this trial was the SVR rate in the cohort (HCV-RNA level below the lower level of quantification) at 12 weeks after the end of treatment (SVR12) according to intention-to-treat analysis. We also investigated the mean decrease in plasma HCV-RNA levels between baseline and week 4 after combination therapy administration and the proportion of patients showing SVR at week 4.

Safety assessment

To evaluate safety and tolerability, we assessed the pharmacological effects and adverse events that occurred after the initiation of combination therapy during each study visit from the first day of study drug administration to 30 days after the last dose. The severity of any adverse events was graded using CTCAE version 4.0.

Statistical evaluation

Data were analyzed using the SPSS v.24.0 software package (IBM Corp., Armonk, NY, USA). All data were expressed as minimum, maximum, and median values. To assess the pharmacological effects of study treatment, Wilcoxon signed-rank test was used for the analysis of paired data. All differences with a p value < 0.05 were considered significant.

Results

Characteristics of patients

Among 1022 HD patients who were serologically tested in 16 dialysis facilities using third-generation enzyme-linked immunosorbent assay, 56 (5.5%) and 20 (2.0%) patients tested positive for hepatitis C antibody and HCV RNA, respectively. Of these 20 patients, two dropped out during the run-in period owing to failure to meet the criteria for commencing treatment, whereas the remaining 18 patients received combination therapy. Among these patients, two did not complete the study owing to clinical events (Fig. 1). Thirteen patients received combination therapy for 8 weeks, and five patients who had compensated liver cirrhosis and/or underwent previous DAA therapy received combination therapy for 12 weeks. The demographics and other baseline clinical characteristics of enrolled patients are summarized in Table 1.

The median age of patients was 67.5 years (range, 48–84 years), and 14 patients (77.8%) were male. Furthermore, four patients (22.2%) had liver cirrhosis, and four (22.2%) were previously treated with IFN-based and/or DAA-based therapy. Nine, six, and three patients were infected with genotypes 1b, 2a, and 2b, respectively. The HCV level was 6.55 $\log_{10}$ IU/mL (range, 4.1–7.3 $\log_{10}$ IU/mL). NS5A-Y93H, L31 M/V, and D168E in genotype 1b were detected in three patients (11.7%) who had a history of DAA therapy (DCV and ASV combination

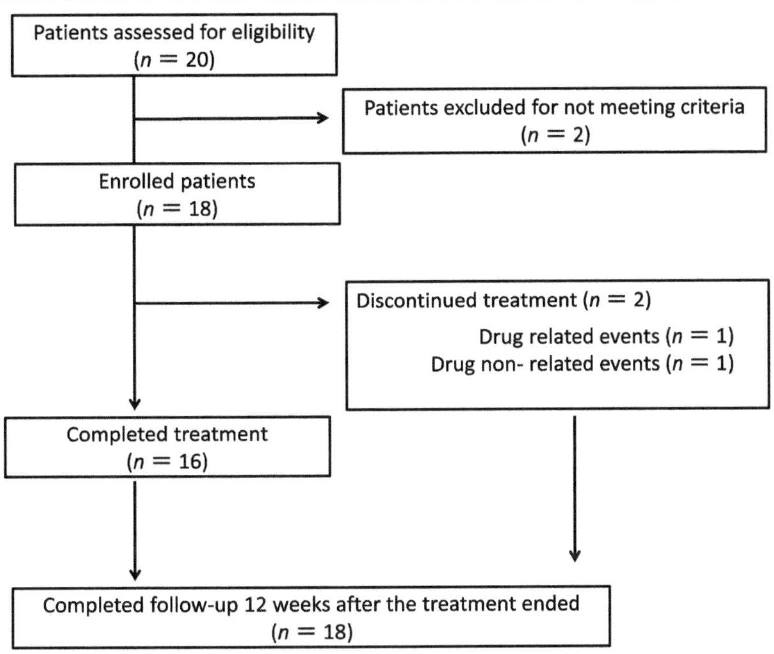

Fig. 1 Study flow diagram

Table 1 Patient baseline clinical characteristics

Characteristics		All patients
N		18
Age	Years	67.5 (48–84)
Sex, male	*n* (%)	14 (77.8)
Duration of hemodialysis	Years	2.7 (0.3–30)
Etiology of end-stage renal disease	*n* (%)	
Diabetic nephropathy		9 (50.0)
Hypertensive kidney disease		5 (27.8)
Glomerulonephritis		2 (11.1)
Others		2 (11.1)
Weight	kg	65.5 (46.0–81.5)
HCV genotype	*n* (%)	
1b		9 (50.0)
2a		6 (33.3)
2b		3 (16.7)
HCV treatment history	*n* (%)	
Naïve		14 (77.8)
Interferon-based therapy		3 (18.8)
Interferon-free therapy: daclatasvir and asunaprevir		3 (18.8)
Liver cirrhosis	*n* (%)	4 (22.2)
Serum HCV-RNA levels	Log_{10}IU/ml	6.55 (4.1–7.3)
Baseline polymorphisms	*n* (%)	
NS3/4 only		0
NS5A only		0
Both NS3 and NS5A		3 (16.7)
Laboratory data		
Hemoglobin	g/dL	11.8 (9.9–14.5)
White blood cell	/μl	5650 (3300–8000)
Platelets	$\times 10^4$/μl	17.4 (6.2–27.8)
Aspartate aminotransferase	IU/L	20 (9–162)
Alanine aminotransferase	IU/L	16 (5.0–168)
Total protein	g/dL	7.3 (6.0–8.7)
Serum albumin	g/dL	4.0 (2.4–4.5)
Blood urea nitrogen	mg/dL	41.0 (19.9–63.0)
Creatinine	mg/dL	8.6 (4.4–13.0)
Total bilirubin	mg/dL	0.4 (0.2–0.9)
Hemoglobin A1c	%	5.7 (4.3–8.8)
Alpha-fetoprotein	ng/ml	2.0 (1–4.8)
M2BPGi	C.O.I	1.9 (0.52–19)

Data are expressed as median, *n* (%), min-max
RNA ribonucleic acid, *M2BPGi* Mac-2 binding protein glycan isomer

therapy). The duration of HD was 2.7 years (range, 0.3–30 years), and the cause of end-stage renal disease was diabetic nephropathy, hypertensive kidney disease, and glomerulonephritis in nine, five, and two patients, respectively. The serum albumin, serum creatinine, and ALT levels were 4.0 g/dL (range, 2.4–4.5 g/dL), 8.6 mg/dL (range, 4.4–13.0 mg/dL), and 16 IU/L (range, 5–168 IU/L), respectively.

Virological response

The results of the primary endpoint analysis indicated an SVR12 rate of 94.4% (17/18). The SVR12 rates in patients with genotype 1b, 2a, and 2b infections were 9/9, 6/6, and 2/3, respectively. The median decrease in plasma HCV-RNA levels between baseline and week 4 in all patients after combination therapy administration was 5.5 log_{10} IU/mL.

Patients receiving combination therapy for 8 weeks vs. 12 weeks

Among patients treated with combination therapy for 8 weeks, only one patient experienced virological relapse at week 12 after the end of treatment. The proportions of patients with undetectable HCV-RNA levels at treatment weeks 4 and 8 and at post-treatment week 12 were 100% (13/13), 100% (13/13), and 92.3% (12/13), respectively.

In patients treated with combination therapy for 12 weeks, including those with liver cirrhosis and/or previous DAA exposure, two clinical events led to the discontinuation of combination therapy. The proportions of patients with undetectable HCV-RNA levels at treatment weeks 4 and 8 and at post-treatment week 12 were 100% (5/5), 100% (4/4), and 100% (5/5), respectively.

Treatment response for previous DAA treatment failure

The demographics of patients with previous DAA treatment failure and other baseline clinical characteristics are summarized in Table 2. The previous DAA treatments for all patients were DCV and ASV combination therapy. All patients who experienced previous virological failure following DAA treatment substantially had variants within the HCV NS 3/4 and NS5A region. The SVR12 rate for patients who had previous DAA treatment failure was 100% (3/3).

Virological failure

Virological failure was observed in only one patient. After combination therapy administration for 8 weeks, virological relapse occurred at week 12 after the end of treatment. The patient was a 63-year-old man who had HCV genotype 2b and HCV-RNA level of 6.5 log_{10} IU/mL without a history of previous DAA exposure. The duration of HD was 6.5 years, and the cause of end-stage renal disease was diabetic nephropathy. Ultrasonography revealed chronic liver disease. The M2BPGi level was 0.6 C.O.I.; the AST to platelet ratio index and FIB-4 index were 1.667 and 1.03, respectively.

Table 2 The demographics of patients with previous DAA treatment failure and other baseline clinical characteristics

Case	Duration span (weeks)	Genotype	Liver cirrhosis	Previous DAA treatment	L31	Y93	D168	SVR 12	Discontinuation therapy	Adverse events
1	8	2a						+		
2	12	1b	+	DCV+ASV	L31 V>M>L	Y93 H	D168 E	+		Pruritus
3	8	2a						+		Pruritus
4	8	1b			Wild	Wild	Wild	+		
5	8	2b						+		
6	8	1b			Wild	Wild	Wild	+		Pruritus
7	12	2a	+					+		Pruritus, fatigue
8	8	2a						+		
9	8	2b						+		
10	12	1b	+	DCV+ASV	L31 M	Y93 H	D168 D>E	+		
11	8	1b			Wild	Wild	Wild	+		
12	12	1b	+		Wild	Wild	Wild	+	Weeks 8 (pruritus)	Bloating, pruritus
13	12	1b		DCV+ASV	L31 M	Y93 H	D168E	+	Weeks 6 (cellulitis)	Cellulitis
14	8	1b			Wild	Wild	Wild	+		
15	8	2a						+		Pruritus
16	8	2b						Relapse		
17	8	2a						+		Headache
18	8	1b			Wild	Wild	Wild	+		Pruritus

DCV daclatasvir, *ASV* asunaprevir

Pharmacological effects

Following drug administration, a decrease in the median ALT level from 16 to 8 IU/L and in the mean M2BPGi level from 1.8 to 1.5 C.O.I. was observed at the end of treatment ($p < 0.001$, 0.075, respectively). The baseline and post-treatment Hb levels were indistinguishable (11.8 vs. 11.6 g/dL, $p = 0.757$). There were no significant differences in WBC, neutrophil, and platelet counts and levels of total protein, serum albumin, BUN, serum creatinine, total bilirubin, and α-fetoprotein between baseline and post-treatment.

Safety assessment

The incidences of drug-related adverse events and adverse drug reactions are shown in Table 3. Adverse events were observed in nine patients (50.0%) during treatment. The most frequent adverse event was pruritus, which was noted in seven patients (38.9%). Specifically, pruritus occurred in 4 of 14 (28.6%) cases with chronic hepatitis and 3 of 4 (75%) cases with compensated liver cirrhosis. Pruritus occurred more frequently in patients with compensated liver cirrhosis. There were no grade 2 or higher abnormalities in AST, ALT, and total bilirubin levels, and grade 3 or higher anemia was not observed. Although there were no treatment-related deaths, two clinical events led to the discontinuation of combination therapy. One patient with a history of HCV treatment with DAA was hospitalized because of right leg cellulitis (grade 3) at treatment week 6. Cellulitis was not considered by the trial investigators to be drug-related. Another patient who had compensated liver cirrhosis exhibited grade 2 pruritus at week 2, and treatment with GLE and PIB was scheduled for 12 weeks. Although antihistamine and nalfurafine hydrochloride were administered, the patient opted to discontinue the treatment with these drugs at week 8.

Table 3 Adverse events and laboratory abnormalities during the treatment period

	Chronic hepatitis ($n = 14$) (%)		Compensated cirrhosis ($n = 4$) (%)	
	< Grade 3	≥ Grade 3	< Grade 3	≥ Grade 3
Pruritus	4 (28.6)	0	3 (75.0)	0
Headache	1 (7.1)	0	0	0
Bloating	0	0	1 (25.0)	0
Fatigue	0	0	1 (25.0)	0
Cellulitis	0	0	0	1 (25.0)

Discussion

In a meta-analysis, Fabrizi et al. reported that the estimated adjusted relative risk of all-cause mortality was 1.34 times (95% confidence interval, 1.13–1.59) higher in anti-HCV-positive patients on HD than in anti-HCV-negative patients [14]. Söderholm et al. showed that IFN-based therapy improved the survival (odds ratio, 3.90) of patients with chronic hepatitis C infection before and during HD compared with that of untreated patients

[15]. Therefore, the high therapeutic effect of DAAs may further improve the outcomes of HD patients.

A phase III trial has reported the efficacy and safety of GLE and PIB for HCV in 332 Japanese patients. Of these patients, 320 did not have renal impairment, and the SVR12 rate for patients without renal impairment was 97.8% (313/320) [16]. In this study, GLE and PIB combination therapy yielded an SVR rate of 94.4% for Japanese HD patients infected with HCV genotypes 1, 2a, and 2b. The present study showed that the SVR rate for patients with or without renal impairment was equivalent.

Until the introduction of GLE and PIB combination therapy, no IFN-free treatment without RBV for HCV genotype 2 infections was approved in Japan. DAA regimens with RBV for patients with stage 4 or 5 chronic kidney disease, including patients on HD, showed low tolerability and high rates of treatment discontinuation due to adverse events, such as reduced Hb level and elevated indirect bilirubin level [17–19]. GLE and PIB combination therapy, which can be provided regardless of baseline genotype, is often chosen because the drugs are cleared by the biliary system, and dose adjustment is not required for patients with severe renal impairment, including those on HD [20, 21]. This treatment regimen could contribute to the clinical practice in Japan, in which treatment options for patients with HCV genotype 2 infections who are undergoing HD remain few.

Our findings indicated that GLE and PIB combination therapy was effective in HD patients, including those with a history of DAA therapy and/or compensated liver cirrhosis. Phase I, II, and III trials on GLE and PIB combination therapy over an 8-week duration showed that a history of DAA therapy, genotype, and liver cirrhosis were independent factors affecting treatment response [22, 23]. In the present study, a treatment duration of 12 weeks led to positive outcomes in HD patients with liver cirrhosis and previous DAA treatment failure, suggesting that a sufficient treatment duration is viable in this patient group.

However, only one patient who received combination therapy for 8 weeks was reported to have had virological failure in this study. He had HCV genotype 2b without liver cirrhosis and a history of previous DAA therapy. The EXPEDITION-4 trial reported that no patients experienced virological failure with 12-week GLE and PIB combination therapy [12]. Although this patient had no risk factor for virological failure, to our knowledge, laboratory results and imaging examinations may have led to the underestimation of fibrosis stage. A treatment duration of 8 weeks may have been insufficient for this patient because of the extent and progression of liver fibrosis.

In this study, there were no treatment-related deaths or severe adverse events. A phase III trial also reported that GLE and PIB combination therapy was well tolerated by patients with no serious drug-related adverse events. A phase III trial in Japan reported a frequency rate of 6.9% (22/320) for pruritus in patients without renal impairment [16]. The frequency rate for pruritus (38.9%) in the present study was considerably higher than the rates in previous reports. Pruritus is a frequent side effect of these drugs, regardless of compensated liver cirrhosis. The mechanism for this remains unclear owing to limited available data. Moreover, pruritus is a symptom frequently observed in patients on HD, affecting 53.8% of patients on HD; however, its etiology is not completely understood [24]. Therefore, the incidence of pruritus may have increased because of the additive effect of GLE and PIB administration in patients undergoing dialysis.

In the present study, two patients who showed SVR12 had clinical events that led to the discontinuation of combination therapy. One patient with compensated liver cirrhosis chose to terminate treatment because of pruritus. Pruritus occurs more frequently in patients with compensated liver cirrhosis and can be more severe. Another patient with chronic cardiac disease was hospitalized owing to right leg cellulitis at treatment week 6. As such, cellulitis was likely due to edema resulting from the patient's poor cardiac function. We determined that this clinical event was not caused by combination therapy. It is well known that HCV patients on dialysis are at an increased risk of treatment discontinuation owing to adverse events unrelated to HCV treatment, such as infection and/or cardiac disease. Therefore, a shorter treatment duration is often more beneficial in this patient group.

The present study has three limitations. First, the study was performed on a small sample of patients; therefore, there might have been some selection bias. Second, it is unclear whether DAAs improve the long-term prognoses of these patients. Finally, as previously mentioned, more detailed in vivo pharmacokinetic studies on GLE and PIB combination therapy should be performed to determine whether HD affects serum concentrations and drug activity in patients.

Conclusions

The results of this single-arm, open-label study indicated that an RBV-free coformulation of GLE and PIB is effective as treatment for chronic HCV genotype 1b, 2a, and 2b infections in Japanese patients undergoing HD.

Abbreviations

ALT: Alanine aminotransferase; AST: Aspartate aminotransferase; ASV: Asunaprevir; BUN: Blood urea nitrogen; CTCAE: Common Terminology Criteria for Adverse Events; DAAs: Direct-acting antivirals; DCV: Daclatasvir; GLE: Glecaprevir; Hb: Hemoglobin; HCV: Hepatitis C virus; HD: Hemodialysis; IFN: Interferon; M2BPGi: Mac-2-binding protein glycan isomer; NS: Nonstructural protein; PIB: Pibrentasvir; RBV: Ribavirin; SVR: Sustained virological response; SVR12: Sustained virological response at 12 weeks after treatment; UMIN: University Hospital Medical Information Network; WBC: White blood cells

Acknowledgements
We thank Robert E. Brandt, Founder, CEO, and CME of MedEd Japan, for editing and formatting the manuscript. We also express our gratitude to Atsuko Takeuchi and Horio Kazue, laboratory technicians of Kitasato University School of Medicine, for analyzing resistance-associated variants.

Funding
This research received no funding.

Authors' contributions
YT and HU contributed equally to this work. YT, TM, YT, and WK designed the research. TO, TF, YY, NW, KK, HH, TN, AS, TA, JS, and MM performed the research. HU analyzed the data. YT and HU wrote the manuscript. All authors read and approved the final version of the manuscript.

Competing interests
The authors declare that they have no competing interests.

Author details
[1]Department of Gastroenterology, Internal Medicine, Kitasato University School of Medicine, Sagamihara, Kanagawa, Japan. [2]Department of Nephrology, Internal Medicine, Kitasato University School of Medicine, Sagamihara, Kanagawa, Japan. [3]Department of Gastroenterology, Shonan Kamakura General Hospital, Kamakura, Kanagawa, Japan. [4]Department of Kidney Disease and Transplant Center, Shonan Kamakura General Hospital, Kamakura, Kanagawa, Japan. [5]Department of Gastroenterology, Shonan Fujisawa Tokushukai Hospital, Fujisawa, Kanagawa, Japan. [6]Department of Kidney Disease, Shinfuji Hospital, Fuji, Shizuoka, Japan. [7]Department of Healthcare Administration, Kitasato University School of Medicine, Sagamihara, Kanagawa, Japan.

References

1. Toyoda H, Atsukawa M, Takaguchi K, Senoh T, Michitaka K, Hiraoka A, et al. Real-world virological efficacy and safety of elbasvir and grazoprevir in patients with chronic hepatitis C virus genotype 1 infection in Japan. J Gastroenterol. 2018. https://doi.org/10.1007/s00535-018-1473-z.
2. Okubo T, Atsukawa M, Tsubota A, Toyoda H, Shimada N, Abe H, et al. Efficacy and safety of ledipasvir/sofosbuvir for genotype 1b chronic hepatitis C patients with moderate renal impairment. Hepatol Int. 2018;12:133–42.
3. Pol S, Jadoul M, Vallet-Pichard A. An update on the management of hepatitis C virus-infected patients with stage 4-5 chronic kidney disease while awaiting the revised KDIGO guidelines. Nephrol Dial Transplant. 2017;32:32–5.
4. Arai T, Atsukawa M, Tsubota A, Ikegami T, Shimada N, Kato K, et al. Efficacy and safety of ombitasvir/paritaprevir/ritonavir combination therapy for genotype 1b chronic hepatitis C patients complicated with chronic kidney disease. Hepatol Res. 2018;48:549–55.
5. Alseiari M, Meyer KB, Wong JB. Evidence underlying KDIGO (kidney disease: improving global outcomes) guideline recommendations: a systematic review. Am J Kidney Dis. 2016;67:417–22.
6. Uojima H, Kobayashi S, Hidaka H, Shuichi M, Takayasu O, Takeshi K, et al. Virological response to daclatasvir and asunaprevir combination therapy for chronic hepatitis C virus genotype 1b infection in dialysis patients: a prospective, multicenter study. Ren Replace Ther. 2017;3:7.
7. Morisawa N, Koshima Y, Kuriyama S, Matsuyama M, Hayashi N, Satoh JI, et al. Effectiveness of a fixed combination formula of ombitasvir/paritaprevir/ritonavir for hepatitis C virus infection in patients on maintenance haemodialysis. Nephrology. 2017;22:562–5.
8. Maunoury F, Clément A, Nwankwo C, Levy-Bachelot L, Abergel A, Di Martino V, et al. Cost-effectiveness analysis of elbasvir-grazoprevir regimen for treating hepatitis C virus genotype 1 infection in stage 4-5 chronic kidney disease patients in France. PLoS One. 2018;13:e0194329.
9. Kosloski MP, Zhao W, Marbury TC, Preston RA, Collins MG, Pugatch D, et al. Effects of renal impairment and hemodialysis on the pharmacokinetics and safety of the glecaprevir and pibrentasvir combination in hepatitis C virus-negative subjects. Antimicrob Agents Chemother. 2018;62:e01990–17.
10. Krishnan P, Schnell G, Tripathi R, Beyer J, Reisch T, Dekhtyar T, et al. Integrated resistance analysis of CERTAIN-1 and CERTAIN-2 studies in hepatitis C virus-infected patients receiving glecaprevir and pibrentasvir in Japan. Antimicrob Agents Chemother. 2018;62:e02217 17.
11. Poordad F, Pol S, Asatryan A, Buti M, Shaw D, Hézode C, et al. Glecaprevir/pibrentasvir in patients with hepatitis C virus genotype 1 or 4 and past direct-acting antiviral treatment failure. Hepatology. 2018;67:1253–60.
12. Gane E, Lawitz E, Pugatch D, Papatheodoridis G, Bräu N, Brown A, et al. Glecaprevir and pibrentasvir in patients with HCV and severe renal impairment. N Engl J Med. 2017;377:1448–55.
13. Uchida Y, Kouyama J, Naiki K, Mochida S. A novel simple assay system to quantify the percent HCV-RNA levels of NS5A Y93H mutant strains and Y93 wild-type strains relative to the total HCV-RNA levels to determine the indication for antiviral therapy with NS5A inhibitors. PLoS One. 2014;9:e112647.
14. Fabrizi F, Takkouche B, Lunghi G, Dixit V, Messa P, Martin P. The impact of hepatitis C virus infection on survival in dialysis patients: meta-analysis of observational studies. J Viral Hepat. 2007;14:697–703.
15. Söderholm J, Millbourn C, Büsch K, Kövamees J, Schvarcz R, Lindahl K, et al. Higher risk of renal disease in chronic hepatitis C patients: antiviral therapy survival benefit in patients on hemodialysis. J Hepatol. 2018;68:904–11.
16. Atsukawa M, Chayama K, Suzuki F, Sato K, Karino Y, Atarashi T, et al. Efficacy and safety of glecaprevir/pibrentasvir in patients infected with HCV GT1 - 3 by renal impairment status: a pooled analysis of two phase 3 Japanese trials. Hepatology. 2017;66:634A–5A.
17. Ozer Etik D, Ocal S, Boyacioglu AS. Hepatitis C infection in hemodialysis patients: a review. World J Hepatol. 2015;7:885–95.
18. Abad S, Vega A, Hernández E, Mérida E, de Sequera P, Albalate M, et al. Universal sustained viral response to the combination of ombitasvir/paritaprevir/ritonavir and dasabuvir with/without ribavirin in patients on hemodialysis infected with hepatitis C virus genotypes 1 and 4. Am J Nephrol. 2017;45:267–72.
19. Liu CH, Liu CJ, Huang CF, Lin JW, Dai CY, Liang CC, et al. Peginterferon alfa-2a with or without low-dose ribavirin for treatment-naive patients with hepatitis C virus genotype 2 receiving haemodialysis: a randomised trial. Gut. 2015;64:303–11.
20. Franczyk-Skóra B, Gluba-Brzózka A, Wranicz JK, Banach M, Olszewski R, Rysz J. Sudden cardiac death in CKD patients. Int Urol Nephrol. 2015;47:971–82.
21. Pockros PJ, Reddy KR, Mantry PS, Cohen E, Bennett M, Sulkowski MS, et al. Efficacy of direct-acting antiviral combination for patients with hepatitis C virus genotype 1 infection and severe renal impairment or end-stage renal disease. Gastroenterology. 2016;150:1590–8.
22. Puoti M, Foster GR, Wang S, Mutimer D, Gane E, Moreno C, et al. High SVR12 with 8-week and 12-week glecaprevir/pibrentasvir therapy: an integrated analysis of HCV genotype 1-6 patients without cirrhosis. J Hepatol. 2018;69:293–300. https://doi.org/10.1016/j.jhep.2018.03.007.
23. Gane E, Poordad F, Wang S, Asatryan A, Kwo PY, Lalezari J, et al. High efficacy of ABT-493 and ABT-530 treatment in patients with HCV genotype 1 or 3 infection and compensated cirrhosis. Gastroenterology. 2016;151:651–9.
24. Peres LAB, Passarini SR, Branco MFBT, Kruger LA. Skin lesions in chronic renal dialysis. J Bras Nefrol. 2014;36:42–7.

25

Low serum albumin as a risk factor for infection-related in-hospital death among hemodialysis patients hospitalized on suspicion of infectious disease

Shun Minatoguchi[1,2*], Atsushi Nomura[1], Takahiro Imaizumi[1,2], Sho Sasaki[3], Takaya Ozeki[2,4], Daisuke Uchida[5], Hiroo Kawarazaki[6], Fumihiko Sasai[7], Keigo Tomita[8], Hideaki Shimizu[1] and Yoshiro Fujita[1]

Abstract

Background: Serum albumin is a marker of nourishment and inflammation. Although hypoalbuminemia in hemodialysis patients is reported as a risk factor for poor prognosis, few studies describe its effects on infectious diseases specifically. This study aimed to examine the relationship between the serum albumin level on admission and infection-related in-hospital death among hemodialysis patients.

Methods: This was a multicenter retrospective observational study that was undertaken in Japan. We reviewed the medical records of 507 hemodialysis patients aged > 18 years, whose blood cultures were obtained based on suspicion of infectious disease, and who were managed at seven Japanese tertiary dialysis units from August 2011 to July 2013. The outcome measure was infection-related in-hospital death. Multivariate logistic regression models adjusted for age, sex, the dialysis vintage, diabetes mellitus, bacteremia, and log C-reactive protein levels were used for the statistical analysis.

Results: Four hundred patients were analyzed and allocated to three groups based on their serum albumin levels: marked hypoalbuminemia (< 2.5 mg/dL), mild hypoalbuminemia (≤ 2.5–< 3.5 mg/dL), and normal albumin levels (≤ 3.5 mg/dL). The infection-related in-hospital death rates were 22.9% ($n = 11$), 12.5% ($n = 25$), and 4.6% ($n = 7$), respectively. The multivariate logistic regression models determined that a low serum albumin level was an independent risk factor for infection-related in-hospital death (odds ratio 0.35, 95% confidence interval 0.18–0.66).

Conclusions: A low serum albumin level strongly predicts infection-related in-hospital death in hemodialysis patients hospitalized on suspicion of infection. Like those with bacteremia or diabetes mellitus, hemodialysis patients with hypoalbuminemia require careful management of their infections.

Keywords: Albumin, Dialysis, Hypoalbuminemia, Infection, Mortality

* Correspondence: shunminatoguchi@gmail.com
[1]Department of Nephrology, Chubu Rosai Hospital, Nagoya, Japan
[2]Department of Nephrology, Nagoya University Graduate School of Medicine, 65 Tsurumai-cho, Showa-ku, Nagoya 466-8550, Japan
Full list of author information is available at the end of the article

Background

Infectious disease is one of the most important causes of morbidity and mortality among patients with end-stage renal disease (ESRD) [1–3]. According to the United States Renal Data System, infection is the second leading cause of death among patients with ESRD, and it comprises almost 9% of all deaths [4]. Similarly, almost 6000 hemodialysis patients in Japan die of infectious diseases annually, which amounts to approximately 20% of all-cause mortality of hemodialysis patients, and this rate is increasing every year [5, 6]. Given the high prevalence of infectious disease, early predictions of infection-related mortality could improve the outcome for hemodialysis patients.

Reports from previous studies have described diabetes, cancer, multisystem disease, vascular access type, serum albumin level, and being female as risk factors for infection-related mortality in patients who undergo renal replacement therapy [1, 7–9]. In this study, our focus was on serum albumin levels. Serum albumin is a known marker of nourishment, and it is also recognized as a marker of inflammation because it is an acute phase reactant [10–12]. Hypoalbuminemia in hemodialysis patients has been described as a risk factor for poor prognosis such as all-cause and cardiovascular-related mortality [8, 13–17]. However, infection-related mortality has been discussed in only two articles. Wang et al. [17] showed an association between serum albumin levels and bacteremia-related mortality, but did not discuss non-bacteremic infectious disease. Mehrotra et al. [8] discussed baseline and time-averaged serum albumin levels and changes in serum albumin levels, but they did not mention serum albumin levels at the onset of infectious disease.

In the general population, hypoalbuminemia has been described as a risk factor that is associated with poor clinical outcomes in acute illness [18], and it has been reported that the serum albumin level on admission is an independent risk factor associated with death, length of stay, and re-admission [19].

Although demonstrated in the general population, there has been insufficient evidence to support an association between hypoalbuminemia on admission and short-term mortality among hemodialysis patients who are usually more prone to develop hypoalbuminemia than the general population [10].

Therefore, we hypothesized that a low serum albumin level on admission is an important prognostic factor that is associated with short-term mortality, such as infection-related in-hospital death, among hemodialysis patients, as is the case within the general population. This study aimed to examine the influence of the serum albumin level on infection-related in-hospital death among chronic dialysis patients from whom blood cultures were obtained and who were hospitalized on suspicion of infectious disease.

Methods

Study population

This was a Japanese, multicenter, retrospective, observational study that involved hemodialysis patients who were managed at seven Japanese tertiary dialysis units from August 2011 to July 2013. We reviewed the medical records of consecutive hemodialysis patients who were over 18 years of age and from whom blood cultures were obtained at least twice based on the suspicion of infectious disease in an outpatient setting or within 48 h after admission. The dialysis units involved were participants in the Japanese Investigators with Innovative Network about Kidney Disease group (JOINT-KD group), which includes Chubu Rosai Hospital, Toyohashi Municipal Hospital, St. Marianna University School of Medicine Hospital, Kawasaki Municipal Tama Hospital, Inagi Municipal Hospital, Showa University Fujigaoka Hospital, and Iizuka Hospital. A total of 507 patients who were undergoing hemodialysis were enrolled to participate in this study. Patients who were not hospitalized or whose serum albumin level data were missing were excluded from the study.

Data collection

The patients' demographic, clinical, and laboratory data were extracted from their medical records. The laboratory data, including the serum albumin levels, were extracted from the results of the blood tests that were undertaken on admission.

Outcome measures

The study's primary outcome measure was infection-related in-hospital death. The definition of infection-related in-hospital death was death during hospitalization with a final diagnosis of an infectious disease. The final diagnoses were determined by the attending physicians in each hospital.

Statistical analyses

We allocated the patients to three groups based on their serum albumin levels: marked hypoalbuminemia (group 1 < 2.5 mg/dL), mild hypoalbuminemia (group 2 ≤ 2.5–< 3.5 mg/dL), and normal albumin levels (group 3 ≤ 3.5 mg/dL) and then the groups were evaluated by their baseline characteristics. The cutoff values were based on those of a previous study of hypoalbuminemia [20]. The continuous variables are expressed as the medians and interquartile ranges, and the categorical variables are expressed as numbers and percentages.

A logistic regression model was used to calculate the odds ratios (ORs) for infection-related in-hospital death, using group 3 as the reference category. This model was adjusted for age, sex, the dialysis vintage, diabetes mellitus, and bacteremia. These covariates were selected based on previous reports that describe the risk factors for infection-related mortality among hemodialysis patients [1, 21, 22]. We also calculated the ORs using the serum albumin levels as continuous variables in four models. Model 1 was unadjusted; model 2 was adjusted for age, sex, and present bacteremia; model 3 was adjusted for age, sex, present bacteremia, diabetes mellitus, and the dialysis vintage; and model 4 was adjusted for age, sex, present bacteremia, diabetes mellitus, the dialysis vintage, and the logarithmic (log) C-reactive protein (CRP) levels. A log transformation was applied to the CRP levels because of positive skewness (1.5). Multicollinearity among all of the covariates was evaluated using the variance inflation factor (VIF). A VIF > 10 indicates serious multicollinearity, and VIF values > 4 may be causes for concern.

In addition, we carried out a sensitivity analysis. We calculated the ORs using logistic regression models that incorporated all of the in-hospital cases, which included the cases for whom the serum albumin data were missing. The cases in which serum albumin data were missing were included after multiple imputation.

All of the analyses, with the exception of the sensitivity analysis, were performed using IBM SPSS Statistics, version 24.0 (IBM Corporation, Armonk, NY, USA). The sensitivity analysis was performed using R software, version 3.3.1 (The Comprehensive R Archive Network: https://cran.r-project.org). The multiple imputation was performed using the "mice" package [23]. A P value of < 0.05 was considered statistically significant.

Results

Baseline characteristics

A total of 507 hemodialysis patients were included in this study, and 400 patients were analyzed after excluding the patients who were not hospitalized and those whose serum albumin data were missing (Fig. 1). Table 1 shows the patients' baseline characteristics categorized according to the serum albumin groups. Mean age was 74 years. Table 2 presents the outcomes after admission, including bacteremia, infectious diseases, and mortality. The proportions of hemodialysis patients with final infectious disease diagnoses were 68.8% ($n = 33$), 62.0% ($n = 124$), and 56.6% ($n = 86$), in group 1, group 2, and group 3, respectively. The infection-related in-hospital death rates were 22.9% ($n = 11$), 12.5% ($n = 25$), and 4.6% ($n = 7$), and the proportions of patients with bacteremia were 18.8% ($n = 9$), 16.5% ($n = 33$), and 13.8% ($n = 21$) in group 1, group 2, and group 3, respectively.

Multivariate analysis of the risk factors for infection-related in-hospital death

Figure 2 presents the logistic regression model of infection-related in-hospital deaths that used group 3 as the reference category. The ORs for infection-related in-hospital deaths were 8.17 (95% CI 2.45–29.96) for group 1 and 3.03 (95% CI 1.13–8.12) for group 2. The logistic regression models in which the serum albumin levels were used as continuous variables are shown in Tables 3 and 4. The serum albumin level, diabetes mellitus, and bacteremia were significant risk factors for poor clinical outcomes in hemodialysis patients (Table 3). The four models used to analyze the serum albumin levels (Table 4) all showed significant associations between the serum albumin level on admission and infection-related in-hospital death. We assessed the covariates'

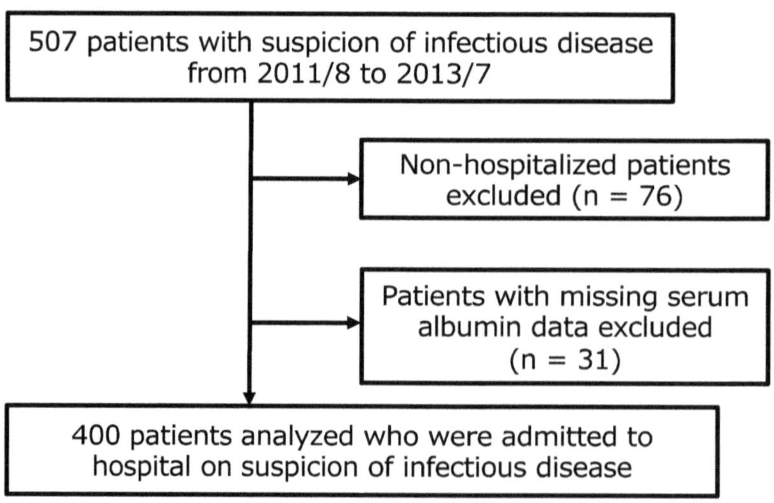

Fig. 1 Study flow chart

Table 1 Baseline characteristics ($N = 400$)

	Alb < 2.5 $n = 48$	2.5 ≤ Alb < 3.5 $n = 200$	3.5 ≤ Alb $n = 152$	Total $n = 400$	P value
Albumin (g/dL)	2.2 (2.0, 2.4)	3.1 (2.9, 3.3)	3.8 (3.6, 4.0)	3.3 (2.9, 3.7)	< 0.01*
Age (years)	72 (66, 80)	75 (69, 81)	71 (62, 79)	74 (66, 81)	< 0.01*
Sex (male)	25 (52.1)	125 (62.5)	110 (72.4)	260 (65.0)	0.021*
Dialysis vintage (month)	54 (25, 130)	63 (24, 119)	62 (24, 108)	62 (24, 116)	0.924
BMI (kg/m^2)	19.7 (17.2, 21.6)	19.5 (17.5, 22.0)	21.5 (19.0, 23.7)	20.1 (17.9, 22.8)	< 0.01*
Diabetes mellitus	19 (40.4)	84 (42.0)	74 (48.7)	177 (44.4)	0.387
Malignancy	7 (14.6)	27 (13.5)	16 (10.5)	50 (12.5)	0.633
Artificial devices	10 (20.8)	77 (38.5)	36 (23.7)	123 (30.8)	< 0.01*
Creatinine (mg/dL)	4.8 (4.0, 6.9)	6.2 (4.5, 8.3)	7.3 (5.4, 9.8)	6.4 (4.6, 8.6)	< 0.01*
Potassium (mEq/L)	3.8 (3.4, 4.4)	4.3 (3.7, 4.8)	4.3 (4.1, 5.2)	4.3 (3.8, 4.8)	< 0.01*
CRP (mg/dL)	10.1 (4.5, 21.5)	7.7 (3.4, 14.4)	4.0 (0.7, 9.7)	6.6 (1.9, 12.9)	< 0.01*
Hemoglobin (g/dL)	9.7 (8.4, 11.5)	10.6 (9.5, 11.5)	11.3 (10.2, 12.4)	10.7 (9.5, 11.9)	< 0.01*

BMI body mass index; *CRP* C-reactive protein
Continuous data are medians (IQR). Categorical data are *n* values (%)
Differences among groups were evaluated by a chi-square test for categorical variables and a Kruskall-Wallis test for continuous variables
*$P < 0.05$

multicollinearity using the VIF in this analysis, and all of the VIFs were < 4.0.

Table 5 shows the results of the sensitivity analysis that comprised multivariate logistic regression analysis after multiple imputation, which determined that a low serum albumin level was an independent risk factor for infection-related in-hospital death, consistent with the results from the multivariate analysis without multiple imputation.

Discussion

The results from the present study showed that the serum albumin level on admission was a significant risk factor for in-hospital infection-related death among hemodialysis patients from whom blood cultures were obtained and who had been hospitalized on suspicion of infectious disease. Hemodialysis patients who are hospitalized with infectious diseases have high infection-related mortality and readmission rates [24]. Indeed, infection-related mortality is significantly higher in ESRD patients with bacteremia compared with patients without bacteremia [21]. In our study, the bacteremia-related in-hospital death rate was 6.3%, which represented 58.1% of all of the infection-related in-hospital deaths. However, mortality in patients with infectious diseases in the absence of bacteremia is not negligible. Dalrymple et al. [24] reported that the in-hospital mortality rates for infection-related hospitalization without bloodstream infections or sepsis were between 2 and 16%, which concurs with the findings from our study that showed that the rate of infection-related in-hospital death without bacteremia was 4.5%. In addition, although there is a strong association between bacteremia and poor clinical outcomes, it is difficult to determine whether or not patients have bacteremia on admission. In contrast, the serum albumin levels are assessable on admission; hence, our study's findings suggest that the serum albumin levels

Table 2 Outcomes after admissions ($N = 400$)

	Alb < 2.5 $n = 48$	2.5 ≤ Alb < 3.5 $n = 200$	3.5 ≤ Alb $n = 152$	Total $n = 400$	P value
Bacteremia	9 (18.8)	33 (16.5)	21 (13.8)	63 (15.8)	0.657
Final diagnosis of infectious disease	33 (68.8)	124 (62.0)	86 (56.6)	243 (60.8)	0.282
Duration of hospitalization (days)	22 (9, 52)	19 (11, 37)	13 (7, 25)	16 (9, 35)	< 0.01*
In-hospital death (infection related)	11 (22.9)	25 (12.5)	7 (4.6)	43 (10.8)	< 0.01*
Duration from admission to infection-related death (days)	9 (5, 29)	15 (6, 25)	11 (2, 45)	14 (6, 28)	0.913
In-hospital death (infection related, with bacteremia)	5 (10.4)	15 (7.5)	5 (3.3)	25 (6.3)	0.121
In-hospital death (infection related, without bacteremia)	6 (12.5)	10 (5.0)	2 (1.3)	18 (4.5)	< 0.01*
In-hospital death (all cause)	15 (31.3)	40 (20.0)	12 (7.9)	67 (16.8)	< 0.01*

Continuous data are medians (IQR). Categorical data are n values (%)
Differences among groups were evaluated by a chi-square test for categorical variables and a Kruskall-Wallis test for continuous variables
*$P < 0.05$

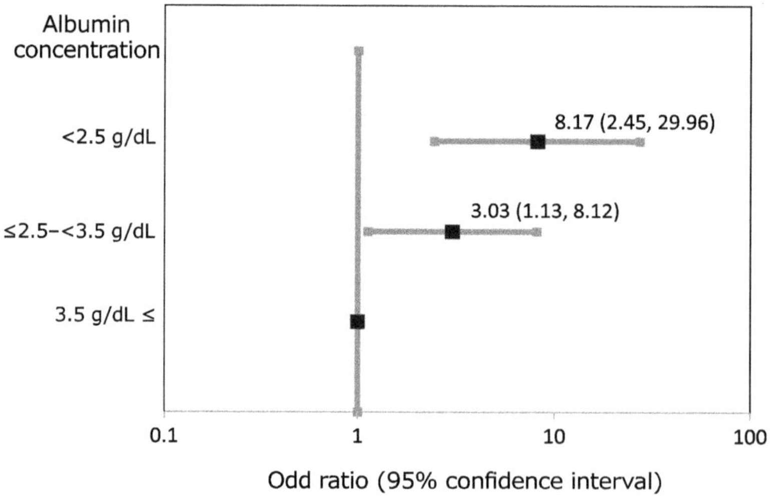

Fig. 2 Adjusted odds ratios (95% confidence intervals) for infection-related in-hospital death according to the albumin groups. The odds ratios were adjusted simultaneously for age, sex, the dialysis vintage, diabetes mellitus, and current bacteremia. Alb, albumin

may provide earlier prognostic predictions among patients who are suspected of carrying infectious diseases.

There are several strengths associated with our study that include its multicenter design. Several studies have assessed the relationship between hemodialysis and serum albumin levels, but few multicenter cohort studies that have specifically investigated infectious diseases among hemodialysis patients have been undertaken. This study focused on infectious diseases specifically, which enabled us to assess the data that were derived from the onset of the infectious diseases and their effects on the patients' prognoses. Additionally, the mean age of this cohort, which was 74 years, was important. The mean age in previous studies that assessed the relationship between hypoalbuminemia and infection-related mortalities were around 60 years [8, 17]. This is not applicable to the increased age of dialysis patients in recent years [5]. Although it has been shown that elderly patients are prone to hypoalbuminemia [25], we suggest that hypoalbuminemia is still a strong prognostic factor of infectious disease in elderly dialysis patients.

Our study has some limitations. First, the study's sample size was small compared with previous studies. This might have lowered our study's statistical power, but the findings from the multivariate analysis suggested a strong association between a low serum albumin level and poor outcomes. In addition, this was a multicenter study; hence, its external validity was high. The infection-related in-hospital death rate in our study was 10.8%, which concurs with that reported previously [24]. Second, there were no data that described the patients' courses after discharge and there was no information

Table 3 Univariate and multivariate logistic regression analysis of in-hospital infection related death

	Univariate analysis			Multivariate analysis¶		
	OR	[95% CI]	*P*	OR	[95% CI]	*P*
Sex (reference: female)	1.27	[0.64, 2.53]	0.49	1.68	[0.74, 3.83]	0.22
Age (per year increase)	1.01	[0.98, 1.04]	0.42	1.01	[0.97, 1.05]	0.53
Dialysis vintage (per month increase)	1.00	[1.00, 1.01]	0.09	1.00	[1.00, 1.01]	0.14
Diabetes mellitus (reference: without DM)	1.22	[0.65, 2.31]	0.53	2.35	[1.03, 5.35]	0.041*
Bacteremia (reference: without bacteremia)	11.66	[5.83, 23.32]	< 0.01*	11.47	[5.04, 26.01]	< 0.01*
log CRP (per point increase)	2.04	[1.44, 2.90]	< 0.01*	1.36	[0.94, 1.99]	0.11
Serum albumin (per g/dl increase)	0.38	[0.23, 0.63]	< 0.01*	0.35	[0.18, 0.66]	< 0.01*

¶Adjusted for age (years), sex, bacteremia, diabetes mellitus, dialysis vintage (months), and log CRP
*$P < 0.05$

Table 4 Odd's ratio for association of serum albumin (per g/dl increase) with infection related in-hospital death

Model	OR	[95% CI]	*P*
1[a]	0.38	[0.23, 0.63]	< 0.01*
2[b]	0.32	[0.18, 0.57]	< 0.01*
3[c]	0.30	[0.16, 0.55]	< 0.01*
4[d]	0.35	[0.18, 0.66]	< 0.01*

[a]Unadjusted
[b]Adjusted for age (years), sex, and bacteremia
[c]Adjusted for age (years), sex, bacteremia, diabetes mellitus, and dialysis vintage(months)
[d]Adjusted for age (years), sex, bacteremia, diabetes mellitus, dialysis vintage (months), and log CRP
*$P < 0.05$

regarding the patients' courses when they changed hospitals. In this study, 67 patients died during hospitalization, 265 patients were discharged from hospital, 64 patients were transferred to different hospitals, and 4 patients' courses were unknown. There were no data that described the mortality of the patients who were transferred. Third, the inclusion criteria were not very clear. Suspicion of infectious disease was subjectively assessed by each physician thereby creating a sampling bias. However, this does reflect the actual clinical management of dialysis patients. Fourth, we did not have data regarding other malnutrition and inflammation markers such as prealbumin, cholesterol, other rapid turnover proteins, and liver enzymes. Although low albumin levels are linked to a poor prognosis in this study, reasons for the hypoalbuminemia were not clear. There are many factors that affect serum albumin levels and our data showed that body mass index (BMI), CRP, and creatinine levels in the three albumin groups were statistically different. This means that the reasons for hypoalbuminemia in each case could be different. We could not estimate how malnutrition and inflammation impacted hypoalbuminemia due to the lack of data regarding other more specific markers, which could be a limitation. However, serum albumin levels are commonly assessed by clinicians and are very useful regardless of what causes the hypoalbuminemia. Fifth, as mentioned above, CRP levels in group 1 were negligible. This suggests high CRP levels are linked to poor prognosis, and the OR in the logistic regression model with CRP levels (Table 4, model 4) increased compared with the model without CRP levels (Table 4, model 3). The effect of hypoalbuminemia was attenuated by CRP due to the common causal pathway of inflammation. However, CRP has not been identified as a prognosis factor for infectious disease in past studies despite its predictive association with bacteremia and elevated inflammatory conditions [26, 27]. Finally, the timing of the serum albumin measurements was an important limitation. The serum albumin levels were only measured on admission in this study. Although we discussed serum albumin levels as an acute inflammatory reactant rather than a nutrient marker, single measurement of albumin levels was not enough to judge whether the hypoalbuminemia was chronic, whether it had occurred as a result of acute illness, or both. So, we assessed the multicollinearity between serum albumin levels and BMI, a known nutritional marker, and the VIF was < 4.0. This suggests that hypoalbuminemia in this study reflected not only malnutrition, which could be chronic hypoalbuminemia, but also acute reaction from inflammation. We did not evaluate the nutritional status of the participants other than BMI, so this could be a limitation. Furthermore, the serum albumin levels of hemodialysis patients fluctuate depending on the volume status; therefore, compared with the pre-dialysis levels, the post-dialysis serum albumin levels are higher, and the degrees of fluctuation correlate with the intra-dialysis volume loss. Kubrusly et al. [28] reported a comparative analysis of the pre- and post-dialysis albumin levels, and the mean albumin levels were 3.45 ± 0.55 g/dL and 3.90 ± 0.73 g/dL, respectively. Although these findings indicated that the intra-dialysis albumin fluctuations are not large, the timing of the serum albumin measurements could be a study limitation as we did not have any data that described the relationship between the timing of the blood tests and dialysis.

Table 5 Sensitivity analysis: multivariate logistic regression analysis of in-hospital infection-related death after multiple imputation

	Multivariate analysis (MI data)		
	OR	[95% CI]	*P*
Sex (reference: female)	1.68	[0.75, 3.75]	0.20
Age (per year increase)	1.02	[0.98, 1.06]	0.38
Dialysis vintage (per month increase)	1.00	[1.00, 1.01]	0.14
Diabetes mellitus (reference: without DM)	2.16	[0.98, 4.73]	0.06
Bacteremia (reference: without bacteremia)	10.88	[4.91, 24.11]	< 0.01*
log CRP (per point increase)	1.42	[0.98, 2.07]	0.07
Serum albumin (per g/dl increase)	0.34	[0.18, 0.64]	< 0.01*

Adjusted for age (years), sex, bacteremia, diabetes mellitus, dialysis vintage (months), and log CRP
*$P < 0.05$

Conclusions

The present study's findings showed that the serum albumin level was a significant risk factor for infection-related in-hospital death among hemodialysis patients who had been hospitalized on suspicion of infectious disease. Like those with bacteremia or diabetes mellitus, hemodialysis patients with hypoalbuminemia and infections should be carefully managed.

Abbreviations
BMI: Body mass index; CRP: C-reactive protein; ESRD: End-stage renal disease; ORs: Odds ratios; VIF: Variance inflation factor

Acknowledgements
The authors would particularly like to thank Dr. Yugo Shibagaki (St. Marianna University School of Medicine Hospital, Kawasaki, Japan) for the helpful discussions. We are also grateful for the time and efforts of the nephrologists, clinical research assistants, and patients of St. Marianna University School of Medicine, Toyohashi Municipal Hospital, Inagi Municipal Hospital, Kawasaki Municipal Tama Hospital, St. Marianna University School of Medicine Hospital, Showa University Fujigaoka Hospital, Iizuka Hospital, and Chubu Rosai Hospital.

Authors' contributions
SM and AN designed the study. SM performed the statistical analysis and wrote the manuscript. All other authors contributed to the study design, data collection, analysis, and writing of the manuscript. All authors read and approved the final manuscript.

Competing interests
The authors declare that they have no competing interests.

Author details
[1]Department of Nephrology, Chubu Rosai Hospital, Nagoya, Japan. [2]Department of Nephrology, Nagoya University Graduate School of Medicine, 65 Tsurumai-cho, Showa-ku, Nagoya 466-8550, Japan. [3]Division of Nephrology and Hypertension, St. Marianna University School of Medicine Hospital, Kawasaki, Japan. [4]Department of Nephrology, Toyohashi Municipal Hospital, Toyohashi, Japan. [5]Department of Nephrology and Hypertension, Kawasaki Municipal Tama Hospital, Kawasaki, Japan. [6]Department of Nephrology, Inagi Municipal Hospital, Tokyo, Japan. [7]Department of Nephrology, Showa University Fujigaoka Hospital, Yokohama, Japan. [8]Department of Nephrology, Iizuka Hospital, Iizuka, Japan.

References

1. Vogelzang JL, van Stralen KJ, Noordzij M, Diez JA, Carrero JJ, Couchoud C, et al. Mortality from infections and malignancies in patients treated with renal replacement therapy: data from the ERA-EDTA registry. Nephrol Dial Transplant. 2015;30:1028–37.
2. Masakane I, Nakai S, Ogata S, Kimata N, Hanafusa N, Hamano T, et al. An overview of regular dialysis treatment in Japan (as of 31 December 2013). Ther Apher Dial. 2015;19:540–74.
3. Jaber BL. Bacterial infections in hemodialysis patients: pathogenesis and prevention. Kidney Int. 2005;67:2508–19.
4. Saran R, Li Y, Robinson B, Abbott KC, Agodoa LY, Ayanian J, et al. US Renal Data System 2015 Annual Data Report: epidemiology of kidney disease in the United States. Am J Kidney Dis. 2016;67:Svii–Sviii.
5. Masakane I, Nakai S, Ogata S, Kimata N, Hanafusa N, Hamano T, et al. Annual Dialysis Data Report 2014, JSDT Renal Data Registry (JRDR). Renal Replace Ther. 2017;3:1–43.
6. Wakasugi M, Kazama JJ, Narita I. Mortality trends among Japanese dialysis patients, 1988–2013: a joinpoint regression analysis. Nephrol Dial Transplant. 2016;31:1501–7.
7. Ros S, Remon C, Qureshi AR, Quiros P, Lindholm B, Carrero JJ. Increased risk of fatal infections in women starting peritoneal dialysis. Perit Dial Int. 2013; 33:487–94.
8. Mehrotra R, Duong U, Jiwakanon S, Kovesdy CP, Moran J, Kopple JD, et al. Serum albumin as a predictor of mortality in peritoneal dialysis: comparisons with hemodialysis. Am J Kidney Dis. 2011;58:418–28.
9. Dhingra RK, Young EW, Hulbert-Shearon TE, Leavey SF, Port FK. Type of vascular access and mortality in U.S. hemodialysis patients. Kidney Int. 2001; 60:1443–51.
10. Friedman AN, Fadem SZ. Reassessment of albumin as a nutritional marker in kidney disease. J Am Soc Nephrol. 2010;21:223–30.
11. Kaysen GA, Stevenson FT, Depner TA. Determinants of albumin concentration in hemodialysis patients. Am J Kidney Dis. 1997;29:658–68.
12. Don BR, Kaysen G. Serum albumin: relationship to inflammation and nutrition. Semin Dial. 2004;17:432–7.
13. Owen WF, Lew NL, Liu Y, Lowrie EG, Lazarus JM. The urea reduction ratio and serum albumin concentration as predictors of mortality in patients undergoing hemodialysis. N Engl J Med. 1993;329:1001–6.
14. Kalantar-Zadeh K, Kilpatrick RD, Kuwae N, McAllister CJ, Alcorn H Jr, Kopple JD, et al. Revisiting mortality predictability of serum albumin in the dialysis population: time dependency, longitudinal changes and population-attributable fraction. Nephrol Dial Transplant. 2005;20:1880–8.
15. Honda H, Qureshi AR, Heimbürger O, Barany P, Wang K, Pecoits-Filho R, et al. Serum albumin, C-reactive protein, interleukin 6, and fetuin A as predictors of malnutrition, cardiovascular disease, and mortality in patients with ESRD. Am J Kidney Dis. 2006;47:139–48.
16. Chiu P-F, Tsai C-C, Wu C-L, Yang T-Y, Liou H-H, Chen H-L, et al. Trajectories of serum albumin predict survival of peritoneal dialysis patients. Medicine. 2016;95:e3202.
17. Wang I-K, Chang Y-C, Liang C-C, Chuang F-R, Chang C-T, Lin H-H, et al. Bacteremia in hemodialysis and peritoneal dialysis patients. Intern Med. 2012;51:1015–21.
18. Vincent J-L, Dubois M-J, Navickis RJ, Wilkes MM. Hypoalbuminemia in acute illness: is there a rationale for intervention? Ann Surg. 2003;237:319–34.
19. Herrmann FR, Safran C, Levkoff SE, Minaker KL. Serum albumin level on admission as a predictor of death, length of stay, and readmission. Arch Intern Med. 1992;152:125–6.
20. Akirov A, Iraqi HM, Atamna A, Shimon I. Low albumin levels are associated with mortality risk in hospitalized patients. Am J Med. 2017;130:1465.e11–9.
21. Sarnak MJ, Jaber BL. Mortality caused by sepsis in patients with end-stage renal disease compared with the general population. Kidney Int. 2000;58: 1758–64.
22. Sumida K, Yamagata K, Iseki K, Tsubakihara Y. Different impact of hemodialysis vintage on cause-specific mortality in long-term hemodialysis patients. Nephrol Dial Transplant. 2016;31:298–305.
23. van Buuren S, Groothuis-Oudshoorn K. mice: Multivariate Imputation by Chained Equations in R. J Stat Softw. 2011;45:1–67.
24. Dalrymple LS, Mu Y, Romano PS, Nguyen DV, Chertow GM, Delgado C, et al. Outcomes of infection-related hospitalization in Medicare beneficiaries receiving in-center hemodialysis. Am J Kidney Dis. 2015;65:754–62.
25. Hanafusa N, Sakurai S, Nangaku M. Heterogeneity of clinical indices among the older dialysis population—a study on Japanese dialysis population. Renal Replac Ther. 2016;3:1–9.
26. Simon L, Gauvin F, Amre DK, Saint-Louis P, Lacroix J. Serum procalcitonin and C-reactive protein levels as markers of bacterial infection: a systematic review and meta-analysis. Clin Infect Dis. 2004;39:206–17. https://doi.org/10.1086/421997.
27. Hedlund J, Hansson LO. Procalcitonin and C-reactive protein levels in community-acquired pneumonia: correlation with etiology and prognosis. Infection. 2000;28:68–73.
28. Kubrusly M, de Oliveira CMC, de Oliveira Santos DC, Mota RS, Pereira ML. Comparative analysis of pre- and post-dialysis albumin levels as indicators of nutritional and morbidity and mortality risk in hemodialysis patients. J Bras Nefrol. 2012;34:27–35.

Rehabilitation nutrition support for a hemodialysis patient with protein-energy wasting and sarcopenic dysphagia

Chiharu Uno[1*], Hidetaka Wakabayashi[2], Keisuke Maeda[3] and Shinta Nishioka[4]

Abstract

Background: Patients with end-stage renal failure may exhibit sarcopenia and protein-energy wasting (PEW). We report a case of improvement in physical function, muscle mass, and muscle strength by management of rehabilitation nutrition in a maintenance hemodialysis patient with PEW and sarcopenia.

Case presentation: A 60-year-old man with an 8-year history of dialysis was admitted for pneumococcal meningitis. When he was transferred for rehabilitation 36 days following the onset, he was transferred to our hospital for rehabilitation and hemodialysis. On admission, energy intake was 1200 kcal/day, via a nasogastric tube, due to sarcopenic dysphagia. He was diagnosed with PEW, based on results from a biochemical examination, physical examination, and his low dietary intake. His height, dry weight, body mass index, Mini Nutritional Assessment-Short Form, albumin, C-reactive protein, and Geriatric Nutritional Risk Index were 166 cm, 46.5 kg, 16.9 kg/m^2, 1 point, 2.1 g/dL, 0.22 mg/dL, and 63, respectively, indicating malnutrition. He was also diagnosed with sarcopenia because of low muscle mass, muscle strength, and physical function. Functional Independence Measure (FIM) was 58 points (motor 27, cognition 31). He was improved by a combination of rehabilitation including activities of daily living training, swallowing training, and nutrition management. Nutritional requirement was 1752 kcal/day of energy and 55.5 g/day (1.2 g/kg/day) of protein. Energy intake was added energy accumulation (300 kcal/day) to improve muscle mass and strength. On day 108, he was discharged to go home, he could walk outdoors, and his sarcopenic dysphagia improved.

Conclusion: Aggressive management of rehabilitation nutrition to increase dry weight may improve PEW and sarcopenic dysphagia in patients undergoing maintenance hemodialysis.

Keywords: Chronic kidney disease, Dry weight, Meningitis, Physical function, Sarcopenia

Background

Hemodialysis patients often have renal anemia, protein-energy wasting (PEW), skeletal muscle loss, muscle weakness, skeletal muscle dysfunction, exercise intolerance, fatigue, decreased activity of daily living, and ultimately, declined quality of life (QOL) [1]. In addition to these consequences, hemodialysis patients tend to decrease their dietary intake, which causes sarcopenia [2]. Furthermore, metabolic and endocrine abnormalities (such as nonspecific inflammation; catabolism; metabolic acidosis; insulin resistance; and loss of amino acids, water-soluble vitamins, and trace elements associated with dialysis treatment) can lead to sarcopenia. It has been shown that declining physical function and malnutrition in dialysis patients are risk factors for cardiovascular events and poor prognosis. Sarcopenic dysphagia is caused by muscle mass reduction and muscle weakness of swallow-related muscles accompanying sarcopenia in the whole body. There is no obvious disease causing swallowing disorder, and it is thought that swallowing disorder while eating is caused by the addition of elements

* Correspondence: chiharu83724@gmail.com
[1]Department of Nutrition, Sugiyama Hospital, 3-10 Yashirodai, Meito Ward, Nagoya, Aichi Prefecture 465-0092, Japan
Full list of author information is available at the end of the article

Table 1 Studies regarding nutritional interventions in hemodialysis patients with protein-energy wasting

Case number	Author	Reported year	Reference	Subjects	Design	Period	Results and clinical nutrition significance
1	Fouque et al.	2008	[4]	86 HD patients	Randomized controlled trial: ONS vs control groups	90 days	↑ DEI, DPI, SGA, QOL
2	Scott et al.	2009	[5]	88 HD patients	Randomized controlled trial: ONS vs control groups	90 days	↑ albumin, QOL
3	Moretti et al.	2009	[6]	49 HD patients	Randomized controlled trial: ONS vs control groups	1- year	↑ nPCR, albumin
4	Malgorzewia et al.	2011	[7]	55 HD patients: PEW (30) Control (25)	Randomized controlled trial: ONS vs control groups	90 days	↑ albumin, prealbumin in 30 PEW patients ↓ CRP, levels in both group
5	Magnard J et al.	2013	[8]	50 HD patients	Randomized controlled trial: exercise vs control group (energy intake 30–40 kcal/kg of ideal weight/day, and protein intake > 1.1 g/kg of ideal weight/day)	180 days	↑ walk function, albumin and prealbumin, body composition (LTI, FTI), muscle strength, postural stability, QOL (SF-36)
6	Ravel VA et al.	2013	[9]	98,489 HD patients	Prospective cohort study: reference level (60 to < 70 g/d), low protein nitrogen appearance (PNA) levels	8-years	↑ risk of death
7	Rattanasompattikul M et al.	2013	[10]	84 HD patients	Pilot-feasibility, double-blind, randomized, placebo-controlled trial: ONS、PTX、ONS + PTX、control groups	16 weeks	↑ albumin (ONS、PTX、ONS + PTX groups)
8	Pasian C et al.	2014	[11]	48 HD patients	Means of a dietetic intervention	28 days	↑ prealbumin, physical autonomy, grip strength
9	Mpio I et al.	2015	[12]	49 HD patients	Prospective study: optimization of protein and energy intake in the daily meals	1- year	↑ QOL ↓ mortality
10	Hristea D et al.	2016	[13]	21 HD patients	Pilot randomized controlled trial: nutrition-exercise group vs Nutrition group	6 months	↑ physical function (6MWT, balance), QOL(SF-36) No change albumin, prealbumin, CRP, BMI, lean- and fat-tissue index, or quadriceps force. Not to have the potential to reverse PEW.
11	Sohrabi Z et al.	2016	[14]	92 HD patients	A randomized, controlled, nonblinded, parallel trial: vitamin E–fortified Whey beverage vs whey beverage vs vitamin E vs control	8 weeks	Whey protein in the form of a new fermented whey beverage and vitamin E supplementation may improve SGA score and MIS in the short term.
12	Martin-Alemañy G et al.	2016	[15]	36 HD patients	Randomized controlled trial: ONS + resistance exercise (RE) vs control groups	90 days	↑ BW, BMI, AMC, TSF, fat mass percentage, grip strength, phase angle and albumin in both group ↓ prevalence of PEW
13	Jo IY et al.	2017	[16]	42 HD patients	Intervention study: personalized nutritional counseling	1- year	↑ DPI, albumin, and cholesterol levels ↓ body cell mass, fat free mass
14	Hajira B et al.	2017	[17]	100 HD patients	Intervention study: dietary counseling	60 days	↑ DEI, DPI, AC, TSF, cholesterol
15	Hosojima M et al.	2017	[18]	50 HD patients	Randomized, double-blind, cross-over pilot trial: endosperm protein vs soy and casein proteins	4 weeks	↑ nPCR

Abbreviations: *AC* arm circumference, *AMC* midarm muscle circumference, *BCM* body cell mass, *BMI* body mass index, *CRP* C-reactive protein, *DEI* dietary energy intake, *DPI* dietary protein intake, *FFM* fat free mass, *HD* hemodialysis, *MIS* malnutrition-inflammation score, *nPCR* normalized protein catabolic rate, *ONS* oral nutritional supplements, *PEW* protein-energy wasting, *PTX* pentoxifylline, *QOL* quality of life, *SF-36* 36-Item Short-Form Health Survey, *SGA* subject global assessment, *TSF* triceps skinfold thickness, *6MWT* 6-min walk test

Table 2 Summary of previous reports regarding protein-energy wasting and sarcopenic dysphagia

Case number	Author	Reported year	Reference	Age	Sex	Primary disease	Description of nutrition therapy	Evaluation of sarcopenia
1	Mamo Y et al.	2003	[19]	18 years	Man	Fibrocalcific pancreatic diabetes	Unknown	None
2	Kalantar-Zadeh K et al.	2009	[20]	54 years	Man	Type 2 diabetes and CKD	Unknown	None
3	Ikizler TA et al.	2013	[21]	74 years	Woman	Gastrointestinal viral disease, type 2 diabetes and CKD	Intravenous fluids and renal specific oral nutritional supplement	None
4	Wakabayashi et al.	2016	[22]	71 years	Man	Lung cancer	Rehabilitation nutrition	Yes
5	Maeda et al.	2016	[23]	80 years	Woman	Age-related functional decline	Rehabilitation nutrition	Yes
6	Hashida et al.	2017	[24]	76 years	Woman	Tongue cancer	Rehabilitation nutrition	Yes

Abbreviations: *CKD* chronic kidney disease

that accelerate sarcopenia, such as malnutrition, invasion, and waste for Elder of Flail [3]. Therefore, evaluation and treatment of PEW and sarcopenic dysphagia are very important issues in maintenance hemodialysis patients.

Nutritional therapies such as enteral nutrition, parenteral nutrition, and oral nutritional supplementation can be used to treat PEW [1]. A list of these studies, along with their reported nutritional outcomes, is provided in Table 1 [4–18]. The studies designed to establish the benefits of nutritional supplementation on the long-term improvements in overall nutritional status in hemodialysis patients with PEW have yielded encouraging results. The types of oral supplementations included regular meals, oral supplementation taken at home or during dialysis, and oral amino acid tablets. The duration of the treatment ranged from 1 month to over a year. The nutritional effects of these supplements are reported to improve nutritional indicators and body composition. In addition, reduction of mortality and improvement of PEW, physical function, and QOL have been reported. Also, exercise interventions for dialysis patients are recommended because they improve exercise tolerance and ameliorate PEW, increase skeletal muscle mass and muscle strength, suppress protein catabolism, and, therefore, increase QOL. Previous studies have reported that PEW and sarcopenic dysphagia, which is characterized by a loss of swallowing function and generalized muscle mass, could be improved by rehabilitation and nutritional support. However, to our knowledge, there are few case reports on rehabilitation nutrition management for hemodialysis patients with PEW and sarcopenic dysphagia. The case reports of PEW and sarcopenic dysphagia to date are listed in Table 2 [19–24]. It is unknown whether rehabilitation nutrition management is effective in improving sarcopenic dysphagia in hemodialysis patients with PEW and sarcopenia.

We report a case of a maintenance hemodialysis patient with PEW and sarcopenic dysphagia, showing improvement in physical function, muscle mass, and strength as a result of rehabilitation nutrition management [25].

Table 3 Hospitalization present condition

Hospitalization present condition		Sarcopenia index		Nutrition index	
Body height	166 cm	Physical function	Walking was impossible	MNA-SF	1 point
Dry weight	46.5 kg	CC	28 cm	GNRI	63
BMI	16.9 kg/m^2	Grip strength	Right 15 kg	MIS	21 points
HDS-R	27/30		Left 18 kg	Biochemical test	
MMSE	25/30	Swallowing function		Potassium	3.5 mEq/L
Dialysis condition		MWST	2 points	Phosphorus	3.3 mg/dL
Dialysis therapy	Hemodialysis	RSST	2/30 s	Blood urea nitrogen	41.6 mg/dL
Dialysis time	4 h	FILS	3	Creatinine	7.38 mg/dL
Dialyzer	VPS-18HA	Body function		CRP	0.22 mg/dL
Blood flow rate	200 ml/min	FIM	58 points	Albumin	2.1 g/dL

Abbreviations: *CC* calf circumference, *CRP* C-reactive protein, *FIM* Functional Independence Measure, *FILS* Food Intake LEVEL Scale, *GNRI* Geriatric Nutritional Risk Index, *MIS* malnutrition-inflammation score, *MMSE* Mini Mental State Examination, *MWST* modified water swallow test Nutritional Risk Index, *MNA-SF* Mini Nutritional Assessment Short Form, *RSST* repetitive saliva swallowing test

Case presentation

A 60-year-old man with an 8-year dialysis history as a result of immunoglobulin A nephropathy was admitted to an acute care hospital for generalized seizures due to pneumococcal meningitis and required mechanical ventilation. Before admission, he independently performed basic activities of daily living (ADL) and had neither central nervous system disease nor dysphagia. He was treated with antibiotic agents and was extubated after 10 days. After 36 days following the onset of symptoms, he was transferred to a long-term care hospital for rehabilitation and hemodialysis.

Nutrition and physical assessment

The condition observed at admission is shown in Table 3. Anthropometric measurement revealed the following: the body height was 166 cm, dry body weight was 46.5 kg, and body mass index (BMI) was 16.9 kg/m^2. The dry weight before onset was 49.5 kg, with a weight loss of 6. 1%/month. He had severe dysphagia, and Food Intake Level Scale (FILS) [26] was level 3 (swallowing training using a small quantity of food was performed). His score on the Mini Nutritional Assessment Short Form (MNA-SF) was 1-point, Geriatric Nutritional Risk Index (GNRI) was 63, malnutrition-inflammation score was 21 points, and laboratory tests showed an albumin of 2.1 g/dL, C-reactive protein of 0.22 mg/dL; these indicated malnutrition. He was diagnosed with PEW based [27] on the results of a biochemical examination, physical examination, and his low dietary intake. Invasion caused by inflammation of meningitis, insufficient nutritional intake, and complications owing to chronic renal failure were the main causes of malnutrition.

He was diagnosed with severe sarcopenia because of decreased muscle mass (calf circumference 28 cm), muscle strength (grip strength: right 15 kg, left 18 kg) , and physical function (walking was impossible) [28]. The causes of sarcopenia were considered to result from bed rest, invasion by meningitis, chronic renal failure, and low nutritional intake. Paralysis and decline of cognitive function were not observed. However, edema and pleural effusion were observed. He also received a diagnosis of possible sarcopenic dysphagia according to the relevant consensus diagnostic criteria because he presented with dysphagia and generalized sarcopenia. There was no obvious lesion suspected to be an organic disorder of the brain and because there was no history of paralysis and dementia (Mini Mental State Examination: 25 points), the cause of dysphagia was thought to be sarcopenia [29]. Functional Independence Measure (FIM) score was 58 points (motor domain score of 27, cognitive domain score of 31). Figure 1 shows the pathology-related figure of this case.

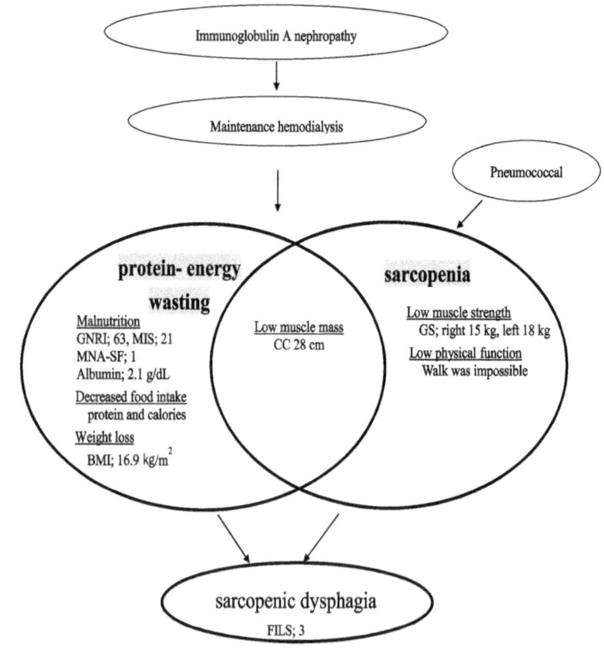

Fig. 1 Disease-related diagram of this case. Protein-energy wasting caused by dysphagia of sarcopenia, with meningitis, lack of activity, and sarcopenia due to low nutrition. Abbreviations: body mass index (BMI), calf circumference (CC), Food Intake Level Scale (FILS), Geriatric Nutritional Risk Index (GNRI), grip strength (GS), malnutrition-inflammation score (MIS), Mini Nutritional Assessment-Short Form (MNA-SF), protein-energy wasting (PEW)

Nutrition care management and outcome

He wished to resume oral intake and be discharged home despite having severe dysphagia. Therefore, a multi-disciplinary team approach—including doctors, nurses, physiotherapists, a speech-language-hearing therapist, and registered dietitians—was used to improve ADL, aid in the transition to oral intake of food, and accelerate discharge. The clinical course and intervention timeline are shown in Table 4.

The energy requirement was set to 1752 kcal/day as per the nutrition management plan during hospitalization. It was calculated using the Harris-Benedict equation [30], multiplied by the activity factor 1.2 and the stress factor 1.1, added to the daily energy accumulation (300 kcal/day), to improve muscle mass and strength. Protein requirement was set at 55.8 g of protein (1.2 g/kg dry weight). Similar to the previous hospital, 1200 kcal/day was administered from the nasogastric tube. The provided energy was gradually increased to 1500 kcal on day 2. On the 5th day, the provided nutrition reached 1800 kcal, 58.8 g of protein and 918 mL of water. After admission to our hospital, dry weight gradually decreased and reached 45.8 kg on the 15th day. Thereafter, dialysis treatment was continued without significant decrease in blood pressure.

Table 4 Trends in nutrition management and physical and mental functions

Hospital day		Admission	On day 7	On day 15	On day 29	On day 42	On day 64	On day 78	On day 92	Discharge On day 108
Nutrition management	Nutrition route	NG	NG and oral nutrition			Oral nutrition				
	Nutrition menu	Nutrient for renal failure	Nutrient for renal failure + Pureed	Nutrient for renal failure + Pureed	Pureed + ONS	Rice porridge and soft food + ONS	Diet for dialysis (soft and bite-sized)	Diet for dialysis (soft and bite-sized)	Diet for dialysis	Diet for dialysis
	Energy (kcal)	1200	1500 + 300	1500 + 300	1400 + 300	1400 + 300	1800	1800	2000	2000
	Protein (g)	42.0	53.2	53.2	66.7	66.7	60.0	60.0	65.0	65.0
Nutrition index	GNRI	63	–	–	70	–	75	–	77	79
	MNA-SF (point)	1	–	–	–	–	–	–	–	10
	nPCR (g/kg/day)	0.5	–	–	0.69	–	0.8	–	0.86	0.89
	%CGR	71	–	–	76	–	87	–	95	95
Biochemical examination	Albumin (g/dL)	2.1	–	2.3	2.6	2.9	2.9	2.9	3.0	3.1
	CRP (mg/dL)	0.22	–	–	0.30	–	0.24	–	0.20	0.26
	Potassium (mg/dL)	3.5	–	3.8	4.1	4.2	4.5	4.8	4.7	5.0
	Phosphorus (mg/dL)	3.3	–	3.6	4.2	4.0	4.5	4.9	4.8	5.1
	Sodium (mEq/L)	140	–	141	140	140	139	140	142	140
	Blood urea nitrogen (mg/dL)	41.6	–	42.8	43.9	49.8	57.5	62.5	62.2	70.5
	Creatinine (mg/dL)	7.38	–	7.41	7.51	8.30	8.45	8.55	9.22	9.50
	Cardiothoracic ratio (%)	56.8	–	–	51.5	–	50.5	–	51.5	–
Physical assessment	FIM (point)	58	–	–	–	–	82	–	115	–
	Grip strength; right (kg)	15	–	–	15	–	16	–	18	–
	Grip strength; left (kg)	18	–	–	17	–	18	–	20	–
	FILS	3	–	–	4	–	7	9	10	–
	Dry weight (kg)	46.5	46.0	45.8	–	46.0	46.5	–	47.0	47.5
	CC (cm)	28.0	–	–	28.2	28.4	–	–	28.8	29.1

Abbreviations: *CC* calf circumference, *CRP* C-reactive protein, *FIM* Functional Independence Measure, *FILS* Food Intake Level Scale, *GNRI* Geriatric Nutritional Risk Index, *MNA-SF* Mini Nutritional Assessment Short-Form, *NG* nasogastric tube, *nPCR* normalized protein catabolic rate, *ONS* oral nutritional supplements, *%CGR* % creatinine generation rate

On day 2, exercise training, physical activity training by physical therapist (PT), and swallowing training by the speech therapist (ST) began (PT: 20 min/day, ST: 20 min/day). On day 3, videoendoscopic examination (VE) of swallowing revealed disorders of bolus formation and transport. In addition, delayed swallowing reflex, a large amount of residuals in the epiglottic vallecula and pyriforms, and laryngeal penetration were also observed.

On day 7, ingestion of pudding (300 kcal) and thickened water began. On day 14, pureed food began to be offered only for one meal a day; from the 20th day, three meals were offered daily (1400 kcal + dietary supplement, 300 kcal). We continued physiotherapy, mainly focusing on lower limb muscular strength training and orthostatic exercises, and indirect swallowing training. The amount of enteral nutrition was modified based on physical activity and oral intake.

On day 42, the nasogastric tube was removed and rice porridge and soft food (combined with oral nutritional supplement) were started. VE on the 55th day showed no obvious larynx penetration and aspiration and improved throat clearance.

On day 81, in addition to PT—including walking training and stair ambulation—voluntary training was actively carried out. Therefore, we increased the provided energy to 2000 kcal and 65 g protein.

On day 108, he was discharged to go home, and he was able to walk outdoors. Dry weight increased to 47.5 kg, and the MNA-SF increased to 10 points, while GNRI was 79, indicating severe nutritional risk. The FIM score increased to 115 (+ 57) points (motor domain score of 81 [+ 54], cognitive domain score of 34 [+ 3]), and bilateral handgrip strength improved (right 18 [+ 3] kg, left 20 [+ 2] kg). His FILS level was 10, without developing pneumonia; sarcopenic dysphagia improved. He was no longer diagnosed with PEW because his dietary intake improved, although biochemical examination and physical examination did not show improvements. Walking ability improved, and handgrip strength showed a mild increase, although sarcopenia remains.

Ten months after discharge, he visits our hospital three times a week for maintenance dialysis.

Discussion

This case highlights two important issues with respect to nutritional intervention and management. Firstly, rehabilitation nutrition management aimed at increasing the dry weight, towards improving PEW in hemodialysis patients, may lead to improvement in physical function. Secondly, rehabilitation nutrition management may be useful in improving sarcopenic dysphagia in hemodialysis patients with PEW and sarcopenia.

Rehabilitation nutrition management aimed at increasing the dry weight in improving PEW in hemodialysis patients may lead to improvement in physical function. PEW is difficult to improve by nutritional supplementation alone because factors such as hyper catabolism accompanying dialysis, inflammation, loss of amino acids, insulin resistance, and endocrine abnormality may interfere with the treatment regimen [27]. Potential sources of sarcopenia, frailty, and protein-energy wasting in hemodialysis patients are shown in Fig. 2. The catabolism of protein and energy promotes not only fat loss but also protein loss, thus resulting in sarcopenia. Rehabilitation nutrition management evaluating sarcopenia is considered effective for improving physical functions. It is effective to raise awareness of sarcopenia, and early diagnosis and intervention are desired. Rehabilitation nutrition management improved physical function and facilitated the healing of pressure ulcers in a malnourished patient with type 2 diabetes. Based on this study, it may be useful to simultaneously perform nutritional support and rehabilitation for hemodialysis patients with PEW. We instituted nutrition control and rehabilitation by administering 38 kcal/dry weight/day for energy and 1.2 g/dry weight/day for protein [3]. By sharing

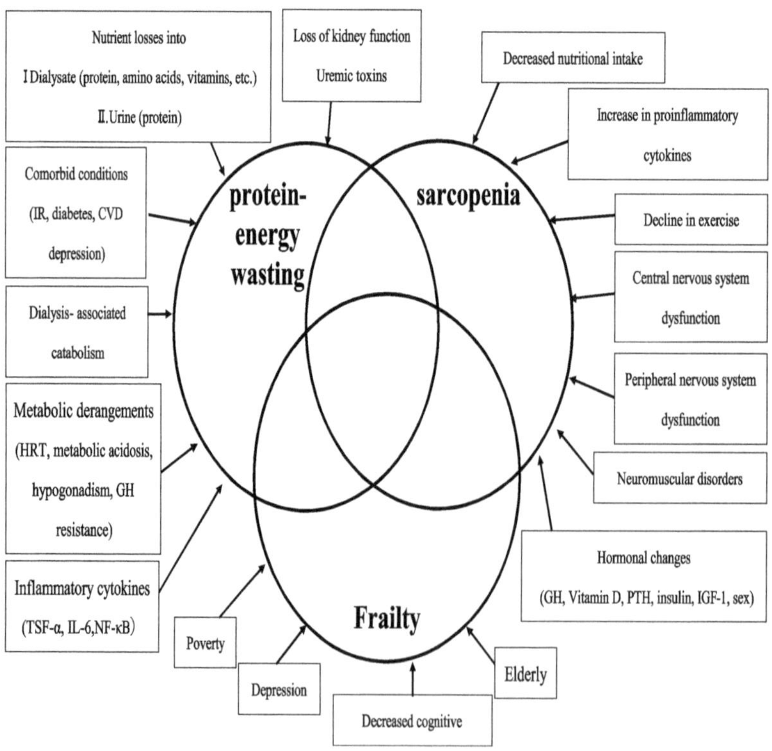

Fig. 2 Potential causes of sarcopenia, frailty, and protein-energy wasting in a hemodialysis patient. There are many factors in sarcopenia, frailty, and protein-energy wasting in hemodialysis patients, and these three factors often overlap. Abbreviations: cardiovascular disease (CVD), growth hormone (GH), hyperparathyroidism (HPT), insulin-like growth factor-1 (IGF-1), interleukin-6 (IL-6), insulin resistance (IR), nuclear factor-kappa B (NF-κB), parathyroid hormone (PTH), tumor necrosis factor-α (TSF-α)

information on momentum and swallowing function, we carried out nutrition management considering the energy requirement for functional improvement. This resulted in improvement in nutritional status and physical function, which resulted in the patient's ability to orally ingest food and to walk outdoors.

Rehabilitation nutrition management may be useful in improving sarcopenic dysphagia in hemodialysis patients with PEW and sarcopenia. There is a correlation between sarcopenia and swallowing dysphagia [31]. Sarcopenic dysphagia is caused by muscle mass reduction and muscle weakness of whole body and swallowing [3]. In this case, sarcopenia was found in the whole body due to increased bed rest, parenteral nutrition intake, nutritional deficiency, and infiltration by meningitis, despite oral ingestion before artificial respiration. The patient in this case had risk factors for sarcopenic dysphagia, such as decreased skeletal muscle index, low independence of ADL, and low BMI [32]. Skeletal muscle loss is related to swallowing function and that sarcopenia and reconstructed tongue may cause sarcopenic dysphagia. In this case, the swallowing function was improved mainly by resistance training, food training, and nutrition improvement, and so, it was considered to be affected by sarcopenic dysphagia. Improvement in swallowing function was observed by carrying out nutrition management aimed at dry weight increase in maintenance dialysis patients and mainly based on resistance training.

Conclusion

Rehabilitation nutrition management aimed at increasing the dry weight in improving PEW, and sarcopenia in maintenance hemodialysis patients may lead to improvement in physical function and sarcopenic dysphagia. Further investigations are necessary to verify the effect of rehabilitation nutrition approach on maintenance dialysis patients with PEW and sarcopenia.

Abbreviations

ADL: Activities of daily living; BMI: Body mass index; FILS: Food Intake Level Scale; FIM: Functional Independence Measure; GNRI: Geriatric Nutritional Risk Index; MNA-SF: Mini Nutritional Assessment Short Form; PEW: Protein-energy wasting; PT: Physical therapist; QOL: Quality of life; ST: Speech therapist; VE: Videoendoscopic examination

Acknowledgements

Not applicable.

Funding

The authors declare that there is no funding related to this manuscript.

Authors' contributions

All the authors have approved the manuscript and agree with submission to the esteemed journal. CU has participated in conception and design, acquisition of data, interpretation of data, drafting or revision of the manuscript, and approval of the final version of the manuscript. HW, KM, and SN have participated in conception and design, interpretation of data, drafting or revision of the manuscript, and approval of the final version of the manuscript.

Competing interests

The authors declare that they have no competing interests.

Author details

[1]Department of Nutrition, Sugiyama Hospital, 3-10 Yashirodai, Meito Ward, Nagoya, Aichi Prefecture 465-0092, Japan. [2]Department of Rehabilitation Medicine, Yokohama City University Medical Center, 4-57 Urafune-chou, Minami Ward, Yokohama, Kanagawa Prefecture 232-0024, Japan. [3]Palliative Care Center, Aichi Medical University, 1-1 Yazakokarimata, Nagakute, Aichi Prefecture 480-1195, Japan. [4]Department of Clinical Nutrition and Food Service, Nagasaki Rehabilitation Hospital, 4-11 Ginya-machi, Nagasaki, Nagasaki Prefecture 850-0854, Japan.

References

1. Sabatino A, Regolisti G, Karupaiah T, Sahathevan S, Sadu Singh BK, Khor BH, et al. Protein-energy wasting and nutritional supplementation in patients with end-stage renal disease on hemodialysis. Clin Nutr. 2017;36:663–71.
2. Carrero JJ, Stenvinkel P, Cuppari L, Ikizler TA, Kalantar-Zadeh K, Kaysen G, et al. Etiology of the protein-energy wasting syndrome in chronic kidney disease: a consensus statement from the International Society of Renal Nutrition and Metabolism (ISRNM). J Ren Nutr. 2013;23:77–90.
3. Wakabayashi H. Presbyphagia and sarcopenic dysphagia: association between aging, sarcopenia, and deglutition disorders. J Frailty Aging. 2014;3:97–103.
4. Fouque D, McKenzie J, de Mutsert R, Azar R, Teta D, Plauth M, et al. Use of a renal-specific oral supplement by haemodialysis patients with low protein intake does not increase the need for phosphate binders and may prevent a decline in nutritional status and quality of life. Nephrol Dial Transplant. 2008;23:2902–10.
5. Scott MK, Shah NA, Vilay AM, Thomas J III, Kraus MA, Mueller BA. Effects of peridialytic oral supplements on nutritional status and quality of life in chronic hemodialysis patients. J Ren Nutr. 2009;19:145–52.
6. Moretti HD, Johnson AM, Keeling-Hathaway TJ. Effects of protein supplementation in chronic hemodialysis and peritoneal dialysis patients. J Ren Nutr. 2009;19:298–303.
7. Malgorzewicz S, Rutkowski P, Jankowska M, Debska-Slizien A, Rutkowski B, Lysiak-Szydlowska W. Effects of renalspecific oral supplementation in malnourished hemodialysis patients. J Ren Nutr. 2011;21:347–53.
8. Magnard J, Deschamps T, Cornu C, Paris A, Hristea D. Effects of a six-month intradialytic physical ACTIvity program and adequate NUTritional support on protein-energy wasting, physical functioning and quality of life in chronic hemodialysis patients: ACTINUT study protocol for a randomised controlled trial. BMC Nephrol. 2013;14:259. https://doi.org/10.1186/1471-2369-14-259.
9. Ravel VA, Molnar MZ, Streja E, Kim JC, Victoroff A, Jing J, et al. Low protein nitrogen appearance as a surrogate of low dietary protein intake is associated with higher all-cause mortality in maintenance hemodialysis patients. J Nutr. 2013;14:1084–92.
10. Rattanasompattikul M, Molnar MZ, Lee ML, et al. Anti-Inflammatory and Anti-Oxidative Nutrition in Hypoalbuminemic Dialysis Patients (AIONID) study: results of the pilot-feasibility, double-blind, randomized, placebo-controlled trial. J Cachexia Sarcopenia Muscle. 2013;4:247–57.
11. Pasian C, Guebre-Egziabher F, Kalbacher E, Pommerol C, Fouque D. Nutritional care and clinical improvement in a renal ward: a pilot multimodal approach. Nephrol Ther. 2014;10:236–44.

12. Mpio I, Cleaud C, Arkouche W, Laville M. Results of therapeutics strategy of protein-energy wasting in chronic hemodialysis: a prospective study during 12 months. Nephrol Ther. 2015;11:97–103.
13. Hristea D, Deschamps T, Paris A, Lefrançois G, Collet V, Savoiu C, et al. Combining intra-dialytic exercise and nutritional supplementation in malnourished older haemodialysis patients: towards better quality of life and autonomy. Nephrology (Carlton). 2016;21:785–90.
14. Sohrabi Z, Eftekhari MH, Eskandari MH, Rezaianzadeh A, Sagheb MM. Intradialytic oral protein supplementation and nutritional and inflammation outcomes in hemodialysis: a randomized controlled trial. Am J Kidney Dis. 2016;68:122–30.
15. Martin-Alemañy G, Valdez-Ortiz R, Olvera-Soto G, Gomez-Guerrero I, Aguire-Esquivel G, Cantu-Quintanilla G, et al. The effects of resistance exercise and oral nutritional supplementation during hemodialysis on indicators of nutritional status and quality of life. Nephrol Dial Transplant. 2016;31:1712–20.
16. Jo IY, Kim WJ, Park HC, Choi HY, Lee JE, Lee SM. Effect of personalized nutritional counseling on the nutritional status of hemodialysis patients. Clin Nutr Res. 2017;6:285–95.
17. Hajira B, Manzoor M, Samiullah M, Chawla RK. Effect of dietary counselling on the nutritional status of end-stage renal disease patients. J Pak Med Assoc. 2017;67:1327–30.
18. Hosojima M, Shimada H, Obi Y, Kuwahara S, Kaseda R, Kabasawa H, et al. A randomized, double-blind, crossover pilot trial of Rice endosperm protein supplementation in maintenance hemodialysis patients. Sci Rep. 2017;7(1): 18003. https://doi.org/10.1038/s41598-017-18340-8.
19. Mamo Y, Esayas S. Fibrocalcific pancreatic diabetes in a young Ethiopian man. Ethiop Med J. 2003;41:69–75.
20. Kalantar-Zadeh K, Derose SF, Nicholas S, Benner D, Sharma K, Kovesdy CP. Burnt-out diabetes: impact of chronic kidney disease progression on the natural course of diabetes mellitus. J Ren Nutr. 2009;19:33–7.
21. Ikizler TA. A patient with CKD and poor nutritional status. Clin J Am Soc Nephrol. 2013;8:2174–82.
22. Wakabayashi H, Uwano R. Rehabilitation nutrition for possible sarcopenic dysphagia after lung cancer surgery: a case report. Am J Phys Med Rehabil. 2016;95:e84–9.
23. Maeda K, Akagi J. Treatment of sarcopenic dysphagia with rehabilitation and nutritional support: a comprehensive approach. J Acad Nutr Diet. 2016;116:573–7.
24. Hashida N, Shamoto H, Maeda K, Wakabayashi H, Suzuki M, Fujii T. Rehabilitation and nutritional support for sarcopenic dysphagia and tongue atrophy after glossectomy: a case report. Nutrition. 2017;35:128–31.
25. Wakabayashi H, Sakuma K. Rehabilitation nutrition for sarcopenia with disability: a combination of both rehabilitation and nutrition care management. J Cachexia Sarcopenia Muscle. 2014;5:269–77.
26. Kunieda K, Ohno T, Fujishima I, Hojo K, Morita T. Reliability and validity of a tool to measure the severity of dysphagia. The Food Intake LEVEL scale. J Pain Symptom Manag. 2013;46:201–6.
27. Fouque D, Kalantar-Zadeh K, Kopple J, Cano N, Chauveau P, Cuppari L, et al. A proposed nomenclature and diagnostic criteria for protein-energy wasting in acute and chronic kidney disease. Kidney Int. 2008;73:391–8.
28. Cruz-Jentoft AJ, Baeyens JP, Bauer JM, Boirie Y, Cederholm T, Landi F, et al. European working group on sarcopenia in older people. Sarcopenia: European consensus on definition and diagnosis report of the European working group on sarcopenia in older people. Age Ageing. 2010;39:412–23.
29. Mori T, Fujishima I, Wakabayashi H, Oshima F, Itoda M, Kunieda K, et al. Development, reliability, and validity of a diagnostic algorithm for sarcopenic dysphagia. JCSM Clinical Reports. https://doi.org/10.17987/jcsm-cr. v2i2.17.
30. Harris JA, Benedict FG. A biometric study of human basal metabolism. Proc Natl Acad Sci U S A. 1918;4:370–3.
31. Maeda K, Akagi J. Sarcopenia is an independent risk factor of dysphagia in hospitalized older people. Geriatr Gerontol Int. 2016;16:515–21.
32. Maeda K, Takaki M, Akagi J. Decreased skeletal muscle mass and risk factors of sarcopenic dysphagia: a prospective observational cohort study. J Gerontol A Biol Sci Med Sci. 2017;72:1290–4.

Sleep apnea syndrome caused lowering of cerebral oxygenation in a hemodialysis patient

Kiyonori Ito[1], Susumu Ookawara[1*], Mariko Fueki[2], Sojiro Imai[2], Takashi Hattori[2], Satoshi Kiryu[2], Yukari Sugai[3], Noriko Wada[3], Mitsutoshi Shindo[1], Yasushi Ohnishi[4], Noriaki Iino[5], Kaoru Tabei[4] and Yoshiyuki Morishita[1]

Abstract

Background: Sleep apnea syndrome (SAS) is a sleep disturbance, which is frequently comorbid in dialysis patients. SAS induces hypoxia, and therefore, systemic and cerebral oxygenation would be low. Near-infrared spectroscopy (NIRS) has recently been used to measure regional saturation of oxygen (rSO_2), as a marker of tissue oxygenation. Although cerebral rSO_2 was measured in patients in various clinical settings, few reports have previously shown the associations of changes in cerebral rSO_2 and systemic oxygenation using measurement of peripheral arterial oxygen saturation (SpO_2) in patients undergoing hemodialysis (HD) with SAS. We herein report a first HD case with SAS-induced reduction in cerebral oxygenation during sleep.

Case presentation: A 74-year-old woman underwent HD therapy for 1 month, because of advanced CKD caused by hypertension and obesity. In addition, she was diagnosed with obstructive sleep apnea with polysomnography about 4 years prior. Her apnea-hypopnea index (AHI) was 77.5 per hour, and therefore, continuous positive airway pressure (CPAP) was started. Thereafter, her AHI was improved to 3 to 6 per hour. However, she discontinued CPAP therapy at HD initiation. Since her oxygenation without CPAP would deteriorate, we evaluated her SpO_2 and cerebral rSO_2 by NIRS monitoring during sleep. We confirmed the deterioration in cerebral rSO_2 according to the SpO_2 decrease, and furthermore, the improvement in cerebral rSO_2 was apparently delayed even after the improvement in her SpO_2. The patient's cerebral oxygenation under CPAP therapy could not be evaluated because she refused to receive CPAP therapy after HD initiation. Therefore, as a comparison, we evaluated a 69-year-old male HD patient without SAS and found that in contrast to a patient with SAS, his SpO_2 and cerebral rSO_2 were maintained throughout sleep.

Conclusion: We observed deterioration in cerebral oxygenation during sleep in addition to a decrease in systemic oxygenation in a patient with SAS undergoing HD. Real-time cerebral NIRS monitoring during sleep might be a useful method for detection of SAS.

Keywords: Cerebral oxygenation, Sleep apnea syndrome, Hemodialysis, Regional saturation of oxygen (rSO2), Near-infrared spectroscopy (NIRS)

* Correspondence: su-ooka@hb.tp1.jp
[1]Division of Nephrology, First Department of Integrated Medicine, Saitama Medical Center, Jichi Medical University, 1-847 Amanuma-cho, Omiya-ku, Saitama 330-8503, Japan
Full list of author information is available at the end of the article

Background

Sleep apnea syndrome (SAS) is a sleep disturbance, which is frequently comorbid in dialysis patients [1, 2]. SAS induces hypoxia during apnea, and therefore, systemic and cerebral oxygenation would be low in these patients. However, few reports have examined regarding the changes in cerebral oxygenation during sleep in patients with SAS. Near-infrared spectroscopy (NIRS) has recently been used to measure regional saturation of oxygen (rSO_2), as a marker of tissue oxygenation. In particular, cerebral rSO_2 was measured in patients in various clinical settings, including hemodialysis (HD) patients [3–8]. It would be considered important to maintain cerebral rSO_2 levels because that low cerebral rSO_2 has been associated with cognitive impairment in patients with chronic kidney disease (CKD) [5, 8] and poor neurologic outcomes in post-cardiac arrest patients [7]. We aimed to examine the associations between changes in cerebral rSO_2 and those in systemic oxygenation using the measurement of peripheral arterial oxygen saturation (SpO_2%) in a patient undergoing HD with SAS.

Case presentation

A 74-year-old woman underwent HD therapy for 1 month, because of advanced CKD caused by hypertension and obesity. In addition, she was diagnosed with obstructive sleep apnea (OSA) with polysomnography about 4 years prior. Her apnea-hypopnea index (AHI) was 77.5 per hour and the arousal index was 76.1 per hour. Therefore, continuous positive airway pressure (CPAP) was started, and her AHI was improved to 3 to 6 per hour. However, she discontinued CPAP therapy at HD initiation. As systemic oxygenation would deteriorate without CPAP, we assessed her overnight SpO_2 using a pulse oximeter (PULSOX-Me300; TEIJIN PHARMA, Tokyo, Japan). Additionally, for the evaluation of cerebral oxygenation, we monitored cerebral rSO_2 using a regional saturation monitor (INVOS 5100c; Covidien Japan, Tokyo, Japan). Her vital sign and laboratory findings were as follows: blood pressure (BP) and pulse rate (PR) before evaluation; 127/71 mmHg, 76 beats/minute, BP and PR after evaluation; 121/59 mmHg, 80 beats/minute, hemoglobin (Hb): 9.5 g/dL, serum albumin (Alb); 2.7 g/dL, blood urea nitrogen (BUN): 48.2 mg/dL, serum creatinine (Cr): 4.13 mg/dL. Her physiological function examination findings were as follows: ejection fraction (EF): 60%, left ventricular systolic function was normal, mitral valve regurgitation was mild by echocardiography, and left and right carotid max intima-media thickness (IMT) were 1.1 and 1.1 mm, respectively by carotid ultrasonography. Cerebral rSO_2 level was evaluated as the rSO_2 ratio, which was defined as the ratio of rSO_2 at t (min) during sleep to the initial rSO_2 before bedtime [rSO_2 at t (min) during sleeping/initial rSO_2 before bedtime]. We confirmed the deterioration in cerebral rSO_2 according to the SpO_2 decrease in this HD patient with SAS. However, we could not directly comment on the influence of CPAP therapy on the improvement in systemic oxygenation because she refused to receive CPAP therapy after HD initiation. Therefore, as a comparison, changes in SpO_2 and cerebral rSO_2 were evaluated in a 69-year-old male HD patient without SAS. His vital sign and laboratory findings were as follows: BP and PR before evaluation 135/92 mmHg, 68 beats/minute, BP and PR after evaluation 148/100 mmHg, 61 beats/minute, Hb 11.1 g/dL, Alb 3.1 g/dL, BUN 55.7 mg/dL, and Cr 7.86 mg/dL. Results of his physiological function examination were as follows: EF: 71%, left ventricular systolic function was normal contraction, no valvular disease was noted by echocardiography, and left and right carotid IMT was 3.2 and 2.4 mm, respectively by carotid ultrasonography. Both patients provided informed consent before evaluation, and these examinations in each patient were performed on the day without HD therapy. The SpO_2 gradually decreased in patients with SAS from initiation to 3 h after sleep and then fell below 90%. According to the SpO_2 decrease during sleep, her cerebral rSO_2 simultaneously decreased; furthermore, the improvement in cerebral rSO_2 was apparently delayed even after the improvement in her SpO_2 (Fig. 1a). Her 3% Oxygen Desaturation Index was 19.0 times/hour by pulse oximetry. However, as shown in Fig. 1b, both his SpO_2 and cerebral rSO_2 ratio were maintained throughout sleep in the HD patient without SAS.

Discussion

We experienced a HD patient with SAS who showed a decrease in cerebral oxygenation in addition to a decrease in systemic oxygenation during sleep. In general, a decrease in systemic oxygenation would induce the deterioration of tissue oxygenation, including the brain. However, thus far, few reports have directly examined changes in cerebral oxygenation during sleep. Therefore, this case is a first report about nocturnal real-time monitoring of cerebral rSO_2 in a HD patient with SAS.

Sleep disorders, including SAS, are known as long-term complications in dialysis patients [1, 2]. Nocturnal hypoxia was associated with a poor prognosis for cardiovascular events [9], and patients with ischemic stroke have a high risk of obstructive sleep apnea, with lowest overnight SpO_2 values $< 80\%$ in more than half of observed patients [10]. Furthermore, in the clinical setting of HD therapy, cognitive impairment is common in patients undergoing HD and the pathogenesis of cognitive impairment would be associated with hemodynamic factors including changes in BP or anemia [11]. In particular, both intradialytic hypotension and anemia reportedly

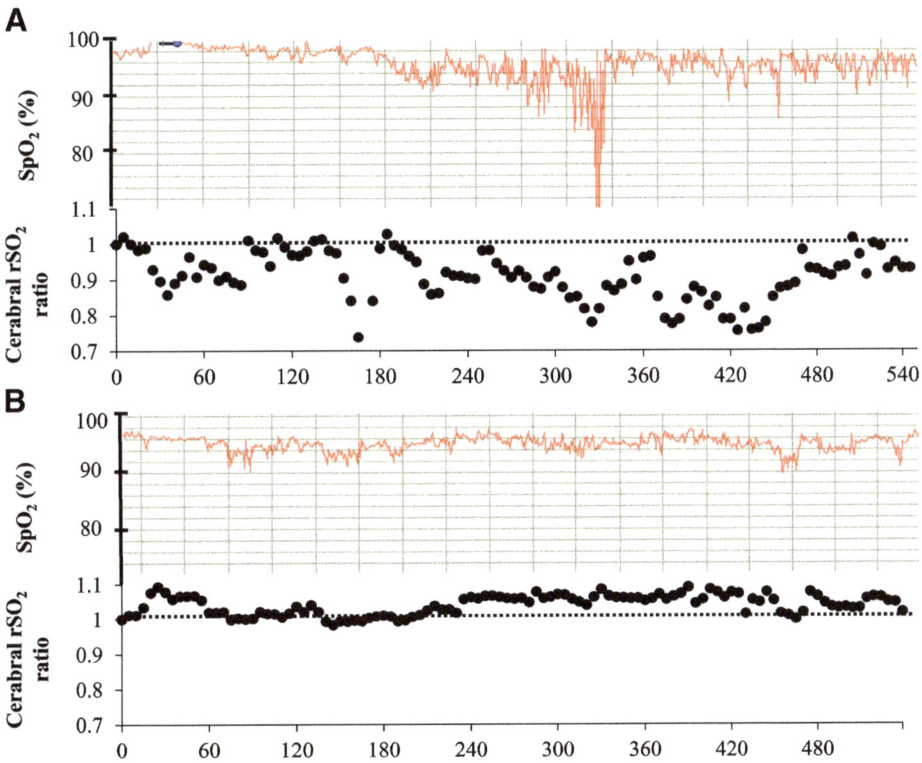

Fig. 1 Time course of SpO_2 and cerebral rSO_2 in a patient with obstructive SAS (**a**) and a patient without SAS (**b**). SpO_2 peripheral arterial oxygen saturation, rSO_2 regional saturation of oxygen, and SAS sleep apnea syndrome

induced the deterioration of cerebral oxygenation [12, 13]. In addition, the decrease in cerebral oxygen supply was associated with neuronal death, and hypoxia promoted the formation of amyloid ß peptide in experimental studies [14, 15]. Therefore, systemic oxygenation should be maintained to prevent worsening of cerebral oxygenation, which would be associated with the deterioration of cognitive function, in patients with SAS.

The measurement of cerebral rSO_2 by NIRS has recently been performed in various clinical settings, including cardiovascular surgery, pediatrics, and dialysis [3–8, 16–18]. We therefore, reviewed the literature for reports of cerebral rSO_2 values in dialysis patients (Table 1). Cerebral rSO_2 values in HD patients were lower than healthy control or non-dialysis patients [3, 8, 19–21] and were lower than peritoneal dialysis patients [22]. Therefore, the presence of renal dysfunction or dialysis therapeutic modality might influence the status of cerebral oxygenation. Furthermore, longer HD therapy itself might cause hypoxia of the brain because HD duration was negatively associated with cerebral rSO_2 [3, 19]. Regarding the association between cerebral rSO_2 and clinical parameters in maintenance HD patients, various factors, i.e., serum albumin, pH, Hb, and blood pressure, were related to cerebral rSO_2 [3, 13, 23]. Based on these previous reports, it would be important to maintain the nutritional status, and control Hb level and blood pressure in the clinical setting of HD therapy. On the other hand, it was also reported that there are little changes in cerebral rSO_2 during HD in spite of Hb increase induced by ultrafiltration in patients undergoing HD without intradialytic hypotension [6, 13, 20, 24]. However, thus far, there are few reports regarding the association between changes in systemic oxygenation and those in cerebral oxygenation in HD patients with or without SAS. Recently, evaluation of cerebral rSO_2 was reported to be useful for detection of SAS in addition to that using a pulse oximeter in children [18]. This report described that cerebral NIRS monitoring could detect SAS even in patients in whom SAS was ruled out with polysomnography, and AHI determined using cerebral rSO_2 had higher sensitivity for the detection of SAS compared with that using SpO_2 [18]. In HD patients with SAS, we noticed that a decrease in cerebral rSO_2 was observed more frequently than a decrease in SpO_2, and this result might be consistent with a previous report [18]. On the other hand, the HD patient without SAS in this study showed little changes in SpO_2 and cerebral rSO_2 during sleep. Therefore, in addition to the usefulness of polysomnography evaluation as a standard method for diagnosing SAS, cerebral rSO_2 measurement using NIRS might play an important role in the diagnosis of SAS in HD patients.

Table 1 Studies regarding cerebral oxygenation by near-infrared spectroscopy monitoring in dialysis patients

Authors	Year	Dialysis pattern	Number of patients	Main results about cerebral oxygenation	Reference
Prohovnik I, et al.	2007	HD	7	Cerebral rSO_2 in HD patients was lower than healthy control, and cerebral rSO_2 was negatively correlated with dialysis duration.	[19]
Papadopoulos G, et al.	2013	HD&PD	23 (HD), 9 (PD)	Cerebral rSO_2 in HD patients was lower than that in PD patients at preoperative condition.	[22]
Hoshino T, et al.	2014	HD	18	Cerebral rSO_2 in HD patients was lower than healthy control, and cerebral rSO_2 did not change during HD.	[20]
Ito K, et al.	2015	HD	54	Cerebral rSO_2 in HD patients was lower than healthy control, and cerebral rSO_2 was independently correlated with pH, dialysis duration, serum albumin, and diabetes mellitus.	[3]
Ito K, et al.	2017	HD	16	Cerebral rSO_2 in HD patients with severe anemia was lower than that in Hb well-controlled HD patients, and blood transfusion improved cerebral rSO_2.	[13]
MacEwen C, et al.	2017	HD	58	Cerebral rSO_2 was linearly dependent blood pressure below mean arterial pressure 60 mmHg.	[23]
Malik J, et al.	2017	HD	17	Cerebral rSO_2 was drop in the minimum value during the first 35 min, but cerebral rSO_2 did not change between before HD and after HD.	[24]
Ito K, et al.	2017	HD	108	Cerebral rSO_2 was correlated with aortic arch calcification by chest X-ray.	[4]
Matsukawa S, et al.	2017	HD	9	Cerebral rSO_2 in HD patients was lower than that in non-HD patients, although SpO_2 did not differ between HD and non-HD patients.	[21]
Kovarova L, et al.	2018	HD	39	Decreased cerebral rSO_2 was associated with cognitive impaired.	[5]
Ookawara S, et al.	2018	HD	44	Cerebral rSO_2 did not change during HD, and it was lower than liver rSO_2 from HD initiation to the end.	[6]

HD hemodialysis, *PD* peritoneal dialysis, *rSO_2* regional saturation of oxygen

Furthermore, the improvement in cerebral rSO_2 was apparently delayed even after the improvement in SpO_2 level (Fig. 1a). Although it is difficult to accurately state the mechanism of this phenomenon, we suspected two reasons regarding the difference between systemic and cerebral oxygenation improvement. First, NIRS monitoring was reported to have higher sensitivity for detecting SAS [18]. Therefore, the delay in cerebral oxygenation improvement might have the possibility to reflect the deep tissue oxygenation status, which was different from superficial arterial oxygenation status as shown in SpO_2 monitoring. Second, NIRS monitoring would mainly help observe venous oxygenation status (70–80%), against capillary (5%), or arterial blood (20–25%) [25]. On the other hand, SpO_2 monitoring could observe in the arterial blood oxygenation status. Brain cell would need the uptake of steady amount of oxygen into the cell according to the changes in oxygen supply in various conditions. In situations of decreased oxygen supply to brain such as severe anemia or hypoxic condition in SAS, cerebral rSO_2 would be low, which reflected the decrease of oxygen supply and the increase of oxygen extraction into the brain cell [13]. When hypoxic status in SAS transiently disappears during sleep, arterial oxygenation will be immediately improved, which lead to the SpO_2 increase. However, changes in oxygen extraction into brain cell might not be immediately normalized in response to the sudden increase of oxygen supply. As a result, there will be a lag time between the improvement in cerebral oxygenation and that of systemic oxygenation during sleep in this SAS patient. However, the mechanism of this phenomenon is yet not to be accurately clarified, and therefore, further studies are needed.

The use of CPAP improves systemic hypoxia in patients with SAS, and patients with OSA may have better outcomes under CPAP therapy through a decrease in the rate of recurrent myocardial infarction [26]. According to her prior medical records, the patient's AHI became relatively low under CPAP therapy compared to that without CPAP. Therefore, CPAP therapy would be effective in the prevention of systemic hypoxia during non-HD periods. Based on this result, cerebral oxygenation could be improved by CPAP therapy in patients with SAS in addition to the improvement of systemic oxygenation. However, further studies are needed to confirm the association between improvement in cerebral oxygenation and CPAP therapy in patients with SAS because we were unable to observe these associations in this study.

In conclusion, we observed cerebral oxygenation deterioration during sleep in addition to a decrease in systemic oxygenation in a patient undergoing HD with SAS. Furthermore, cerebral NIRS monitoring during sleep might be a useful method for the detection of SAS.

Acknowledgements
We thank the study participants and the clinical dialysis center staff in Minami-Uonuma City Hospital.

Funding
The authors declare that there is no funding related to this manuscript.

Authors' contributions
KI conceived and designed this study. KI, MF, SI, TH, SK, YS, NW, and MS performed this study. KI and OS analyzed the data. YO, NI, KT, and YM supervised the data collection and manuscript preparation. KI and OS drafted the manuscript. All authors read and approved the final manuscript.

Competing interests
The authors declared that they have no competing interests.

Author details
[1]Division of Nephrology, First Department of Integrated Medicine, Saitama Medical Center, Jichi Medical University, 1-847 Amanuma-cho, Omiya-ku, Saitama 330-8503, Japan. [2]Department of Clinical Engineering, Minami-Uonuma City Hospital, Niigata, Japan. [3]Department of Nursing, Minami-Uonuma City Hospital, Niigata, Japan. [4]Department of Internal Medicine, Minami-Uonuma City Hospital, Niigata, Japan. [5]Department of Nephrology, Uonuma Institute of Community Medicine, Niigata University Medical and Dental Hospital, Minami-Uonuma, Niigata, Japan.

References

1. Parker KP. Sleep disturbances in dialysis patients. Sleep Med Rev. 2003;7:131–43.
2. Forni Ogna V, Ogna A, Pruijm M, Bassi I, Zuercher E, Halabi G, et al. Prevalence and diagnostic approach to sleep apnea in hemodialysis patients: a population study. Biomed Res Int. 2015;2015:103686.
3. Ito K, Ookawara S, Ueda Y, Goto S, Miyazawa H, Yamada H, et al. Factors affecting cerebral oxygenation in hemodialysis patients: cerebral oxygenation associates with pH, hemodialysis duration, serum albumin concentration, and diabetes mellitus. PLoS One. 2015;10:e0117474.
4. Ito K, Ookawara S, Okochi T, Ueda Y, Kofuji M, Hayasaka H, et al. Deterioration of cerebral oxygenation by aortic arch calcification progression in patients undergoing hemodialysis: a cross-sectional study. Biomed Res Int. 2017;2017:2852514.
5. Kovarova L, Valerianova A, Kmentova T, Lachmanova J, Hladinova Z, Malik J. Low cerebral oxygenation is associated with cognitive impairment in chronic hemodialysis patients. Nephron. 2018;139:113–9.
6. Ookawara S, Ito K, Ueda Y, Miyazawa H, Hayasaka H, Kofuji M, et al. Differences in tissue oxygenation and changes in total hemoglobin signal strength in the brain, liver, and lower-limb muscle during hemodialysis. J Artif Organs. 2018;21:86–93.
7. Nishiyama K, Ito N, Orita T, Hayashida K, Arimoto H, Beppu S, et al. Regional cerebral oxygen saturation monitoring for predicting interventional outcomes in patients following out-of-hospital cardiac arrest of presumed cardiac cause: a prospective, observational, multicenter study. Resuscitation. 2015;96:135–41.
8. Miyazawa H, Ookawara S, Ito K, Ueda Y, Yanai K, Ishii H, et al. Association of cerebral oxygenation with estimated glomerular filtration rate and cognitive function in chronic kidney disease patients without dialysis therapy. PLoS One. 2018;13:e0199366.
9. Zoccali C, Mallamaci F, Tripepi G. Nocturnal hypoxemia predicts incident cardiovascular complications in dialysis patients. J Am Soc Nephrol. 2002;13:729–33.
10. Good DC, Henkle JQ, Gelber D, Welsh J, Verhulst S. Sleep-disordered breathing and poor functional outcome after stroke. Stroke. 1996;27:252–9.
11. Moeini M, Lu X, Avti PK, Damseh R, Belanger S, Picard F, et al. Compromised microvascular oxygen delivery increases brain tissue vulnerability with age. Sci Rep. 2018;8:8219.
12. Miyazawa H, Ookawara S, Tabei K. Aggravation of cerebral oxygenation due to intradialytic hypotension induced by blood volume reduction during hemodialysis: a case report. Ther Apher Dial. 2015;19:525–7.
13. Ito K, Ookawara S, Ueda Y, Miyazawa H, Kofuji M, Hayasaka H, et al. Changes in cerebral oxygenation associated with intradialytic blood transfusion in patients with severe anemia undergoing hemodialysis. Nephron Extra. 2017;7:42–51.
14. Peers C, Dallas ML, Boycott HE, Scragg JL, Pearson HA, Boyle JP. Hypoxia and neurodegeneration. Ann N Y Acad Sci. 2009;1177:169–77.
15. Peers C, Pearson HA, Boyle JP. Hypoxia and Alzheimer's disease. Essays Biochem. 2007;43:153–64.
16. Kobayashi K, Kitamura T, Kohira S, Torii S, Horai T, Hirata M, et al. Factors associated with a low initial cerebral oxygen saturation value in patients undergoing cardiac surgery. J Artif Organs. 2017;20:110–6.
17. Baik N, Urlesberger B, Schwaberger B, Avian A, Mileder L, Schmölzer GM, et al. Blood pressure during the immediate neonatal transition: is the mean arterial blood pressure relevant for the cerebral regional oxygenation? Neonatology. 2017;112:97–102.
18. Ullman N, Anas NG, Izaguirre E, Haugen W, Ortiz H, Arguello O, et al. Usefulness of cerebral NIRS in detecting the effects of pediatric sleep apnea. Pediatr Pulmonol. 2014;49:1036–42.
19. Prohovnik I, Post J, Uribarri J, Lee H, Sandu O, Langhoff E. Cerebrovascular effects of hemodialysis in chronic kidney disease. J Cereb Blood Flow Metab. 2007;27:1861–9.
20. Hoshino T, Ookawara S, Goto S, Miyazawa H, Ito K, Ueda Y, et al. Evaluation of cerebral oxygenation in patients undergoing long-term haemodialysis. Nephron Clin Pract. 2014;126:57–61.
21. Matsukawa S, Hamada M, Mizota T. Low preoperative regional cerebral oxygen saturation in hemodialysis patients. JA Clin Rep. 2017;3:13.
22. Papadopoulos G, Dounousi E, Papathanasiou A, Papathanakos G, Tzimas P. Cerebral oximetry values in dialyzed surgical patients: a comparison between hemodialysis and peritoneal dialysis. Ren Fail. 2013;35:855–9.
23. MacEwen C, Sutherland S, Daly J, Pugh C, Tarassenko L. Relationship between hypotension and cerebral ischemia during hemodialysis. J Am Soc Nephrol. 2017;28:2511–20.
24. Malik J, Kudlicka J, Lachmanova J, Valerianova A, Rocinova K, Bartkova M, et al. Tissue ischemia worsens during hemodialysis in end-stage renal disease patients. J Vasc Access. 2017;18:47–51.
25. Lemmers PMA, Toet MC, van Bel F. Impact of patent ductus arteriosus and subsequent therapy with indomethacin on cerebral oxygenation in preterm infants. Pediatrics. 2008;121:142–7.
26. Garcia-Rio F, Alonso-Fernández A, Armada E, Mediano O, Lores V, Rojo B, et al. CPAP effect on recurrent episodes in patients with sleep apnea and myocardial infarction. Int J Cardiol. 2013;168:1328–35.

Effects of electrical stimulation on muscle power and biochemical markers during hemodialysis in elderly patients

Misa Miura[1*], Aki Hirayama[1], Shigeru Oowada[2], Akihito Nishida[1], Chie Saito[3], Kunihiro Yamagata[3], Osamu Ito[4], Yo Hirayama[5] and Masahiro Kohzuki[6]

Abstract

Background: Decreased physical activity in hemodialysis (HD) patients causes various structural, metabolic, and functional abnormalities due to uremic changes in skeletal muscles. Electrical stimulation (ES) of the lower limbs was found to be effective in patients with cardiac insufficiency for exercise tolerance. This study compared the effects of ES and variable load ergometers on the lower limbs in HD patients.

Methods: We performed a prospective, double-center, open-label, randomized controlled trial. Eligible patients were aged over 65 years, had end-stage renal disease, and underwent maintenance HD. The primary endpoint was muscle power, and the secondary endpoints included changes in dialysis efficiency, serum phosphorus, and inflammatory markers. Thirty HD outpatients were randomly assigned to the following groups: exercise (EX), ES, or control (SED). In EX and ES groups, patients were instructed to exercise twice a week for 12 weeks, depending on their physical capabilities. The safety and efficacy of aerobic training and ES during HD were confirmed when a sudden decrease in blood pressure or any other side effects did not occur. A repeated measures analysis of variance was performed as the principal method to evaluate time (baseline vs. 12 weeks) and group (EX vs. ES vs. SED) comparisons for the experimental outcomes.

Results: The efficiency of HD significantly increased in the ES and EX groups ($p \leq 0.02$). Moreover, the ES group experienced a significant increase in muscle power ($p = 0.01$) and the weight bearing index ($p = 0.04$) and a significant decrease in serum phosphorus level ($p = 0.04$) and tumor necrosis factor-alpha (TNF-α) level ($p = 0.04$) from baseline to 12 weeks. Furthermore, there was a significant increase in serum TNF-α level ($p \leq 0.03$) over time in both the EX and SED groups.

Conclusion: The safety and efficacy of aerobic training and ES during HD were confirmed when a sudden decrease in blood pressure or any other side effects did not occur. Therefore, ES may improve the patient's condition, similar to lower limb exercises, and ES should be considered as an option for rehabilitation programs in HD patients.

Keywords: Elderly hemodialysis patients, Lower limb electrical stimulation, Aerobic exercise, Hemodialysis sessions

* Correspondence: m.miura@k.tsukuba-tech.ac.jp
[1]Faculty of Health Sciences, Tsukuba University of Technology, Kasuga 4-12-7, Tsukuba City, Ibaraki 305-8521, Japan
Full list of author information is available at the end of the article

Background

Chronic kidney disease (CKD) is a major contemporary health problem. The number of patients with CKD continues to increase globally, with a current estimate of 2.6 million CKD patients worldwide [1]. Patients with CKD are at a higher risk of various complications, such as high blood pressure and heart disease, in addition to the frequent occurrence of chronic inflammation, renal anemia, and sarcopenia [2]. While exercise is reported to improve chronic inflammation [3], recent reports have noted that electrical stimulation (ES) is effective not only in patients with moderate to severe heart failure [4], but also in hemodialysis (HD) patients [5]. ES and voluntary muscular contractions during cycle ergometer training are different ways of activating muscle fibers that influence a number of acute changes in the neuromuscular system [5]. ES activates type I muscle fibers, while anaerobic exercise activates type II muscle fibers. In addition, conventional training using cycle ergometers is a whole-body exercise, whereas ES is a static and localized body exercise. Therefore, ES might be effective for elderly patients undergoing HD who have disease complications.

Based on this perspective, achieving a higher training benefit in HD patients would be of great importance. However, effects of ES on physical function and indicators of biochemical changes in maintenance HD patients are unknown. Therefore, this study aimed to evaluate and compare the effects of ES on muscle strength, dialysis efficiency, and serum inflammatory markers, including cytokine factors in elderly patients undergoing maintenance HD.

Methods

Study design and participants

This study was a prospective, double-center, open-label, randomized controlled trial. Subjects included stable patients on maintenance HD who underwent outpatient HD treatments three times a week between February 2014 and March 2016 at two dialysis centers in Japan (Fig. 1). This study was approved by the Tohoku University Hospital Review Board (no. 2011-120-1) and the Tsukuba University of Technology Review Board (no. 05/02/2015). The study was also retrospectively registered on the UMIN Clinical Trials Registry (UMIN-CTR R 000032202).

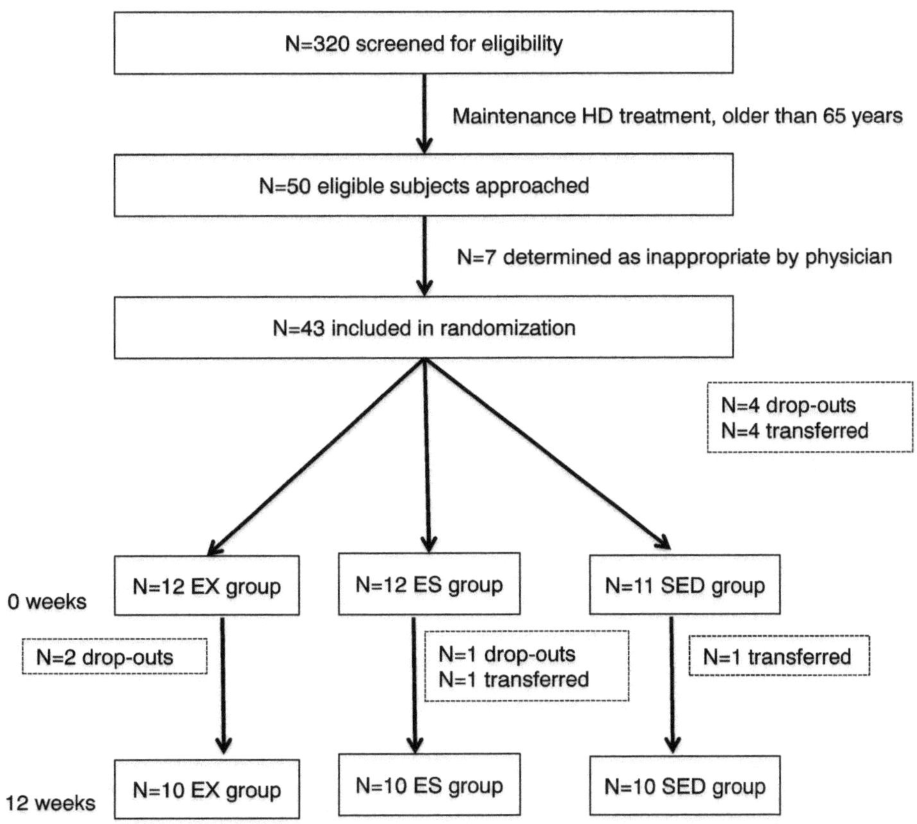

Fig. 1 Flow chart showing enrollment and grouping assignment of patients. Of 320 Japanese hemodialysis (HD) outpatients who were screened for eligibility, 50 consecutive patients who met the inclusion criteria were approached for study participation. Ultimately, 30 patients (23 men, 7 women) were included in this study. EX exercise, ES electrical stimulation, SED control

At the initiation of the present study, we identified 320 patients who were undergoing maintenance HD at both dialysis centers. The inclusion criteria were as follows: (1) patients who underwent dialysis treatment for at least 3 months and (2) age older than 65 years. The exclusion criteria were (1) acute coronary syndrome, particularly unstable angina and acute myocardial infarction; (2) systolic blood pressure ≥ 180 mmHg or diastolic blood pressure ≥ 110 mmHg; and (3) patients who were determined as inappropriate for the study by the attending physician. The first 50 eligible patients were consecutively approached to participate in this study; however, 7 patients were further excluded because a physician determined that they were inappropriate for this study. As a result, 43 patients were initially included. Of these 43 patients, 13 patients withdrew from participation due to poor physical conditions. Finally, 30 subjects (23 men and 7 women) were randomly assigned to one of three groups ($n = 10$ per group).

Randomization

Eligible patients were randomized to one of three groups described below. After the first evaluation, randomization was generated using online software (www.random.org). The three groups included a group that exercised on a variable load ergometer (EX group), a group that underwent low-frequency ES of the lower limbs (ES group), and a group that underwent standard HD treatment without exercise (SED). The median age of the subjects was 71.5 ± 1.6 years, and their mean time on dialysis was 10.7 ± 1.9 years. All subjects were minimally active and exercised less than once per week before the intervention. After patient selection, the sequence of numbers was generated by researchers who were blinded to the study. Prior to the start of the intervention program, the sequence of numbers was only disclosed to the expert nurse or the physical therapist who was responsible for applying the respective treatment (ES, EX, or SED) to ensure concealment of the allocation sequence and to keep patients blinded to the type of intervention.

Using the G*power statistics software (version 3.1; Heinrich-Heine-University, Düsseldorf, Germany), sample size calculation was performed based on a 5% alpha error and 80% power for a magnitude of effect of 1.181. To calculate the sample size, a mean between group difference of 3.9 ± 0.2 kgf for muscle power of the quadriceps femoris (MPQ) was used, as reported by Banerjee et al. [6]. According to the calculation performed, a sample of 10 subjects was required in each group.

Data collection

Physical parameters included baseline demographic characteristics, hand grip strength, leg muscle force, and weight bearing index (WBI) conversion. Biochemical parameters included dialysis efficiency, serum blood urea nitrogen (BUN), phosphorus, high-density lipoprotein cholesterol (HDL-C), low-density lipoprotein cholesterol/HDL-C (LDL-C/HDL-C), renal anemia indicators (ferritin [Fer] and transferrin saturation [TSAT]), nutritional status indicator (albumin), and inflammation markers (C-reactive protein [CRP], interleukin-6 [IL-6], and tumor necrosis factor-alpha [TNF-α]). At baseline and 12 weeks after the intervention, these parameters were collected before the HD session and under the same conditions; all procedures were carried out using the same protocol at both dialysis centers.

Hand grip strength

At baseline and 12 weeks after the intervention, hand grip strength was measured before the HD session and under the same conditions by the expert nurse and physical therapists who were not informed about the study details. Hand grip strength was measured using the Smedley Hand Dynamometer (OG Giken, Okayama, Japan). Measurements were completed using the arm opposite to the arm in which vascular access was installed before the HD session. All measurements were performed with the patient in a seated position, the shoulder in adduction and in a neutral position, the elbow in 90° flexion, and the forearm in a neutral position. The test was conducted three times with the subject exerting maximum force to ensure reliability, and the mean value of these three trials was recorded [7].

Maximum isometric knee extensor muscle power of the quadriceps femoris (MPQ) and WBI conversion

At baseline and 12 weeks after the intervention, physical conditions were measured before the HD session and under the same conditions. Maximum isometric knee extensor MPQ was measured using a handheld dynamometer (IsoforceGT-300; OG Wellness Technologies Co., Ltd., Okayama, Japan) by the expert nurse and physical therapists who were not informed about the study details. MPQ was measured from an initial seated position squarely with the hip and the knee joints at a 90° angle. The test was measured twice on each leg, and the maximum value was used. The WBI was calculated as WBI = MPQ/body weight [8].

Laboratory examination

At baseline and 12 weeks after the intervention, blood samples were collected after at least 12 h of fasting, and before the HD session, from an antecubital vein via venipuncture. Dialysis efficiency (represented using Kt/V) was calculated from body weight and BUN levels before and after dialysis using the Daugirdas formula [9] as follows. Single-pool Kt/V was calculated monthly using urea kinetic modeling equations derived from the following equation: (post: pre-dialysis plasma BUN ratio to estimate k. T/v and npcr: mathematical modeling) (second-generation logarithmic estimates of single-pool variable volume kt/v: an analysis of error). $Kt/V = -\ln(R - 0.008 \times t) + [(4-3.5 \times R) \times UF/W]$, where R is the ratio of post-dialysis to pre-dialysis serum BUN concentration, t is the duration of hemodialysis in hours, UF is the amount of ultrafiltration (in l) during the hemodialysis session, and W is the post-dialysis weight (in kg) [10]. Serum BUN, phosphorus, HDL-C, LDL-C/HDL-C, Fer, TSAT, albumin, CRP, IL-6, and TNF-α were analyzed at SRL Co., Ltd., Tokyo, Japan.

Conventional aerobic training (exercise with variable load ergometers)

Subjects exercised for 1 h or less during the first half of the HD session twice a week for 12 consecutive weeks using a cycle ergometer (TE2-70; Showa Denki Co., Ltd., Osaka, Japan). Exercise duration was determined based on an exercise intensity relative to levels 11–13 on the Borg Rating of Perceived Exertion (RPE) scale. RPE was recorded, and time limits were set depending on the subject's physical conditions. The exercise was performed at an intensity where the subject's heart rate did not exceed 30 bpm above resting heart rate.

Low-frequency ES

A low-frequency ES device (Espurge, Ito Co., Ltd., Tokyo, Japan) was used. Electrodes were attached to the bilateral quadriceps femoris and triceps surae muscles. ES was applied at 10 Hz below the subject's pain threshold and was turned on and off in 20-s cycles. Subjects underwent ES for 1 h or less during the first half of the HD session twice a week for 12 consecutive weeks [4, 5]. ES was applied such that the subject's heart rate did not exceed 30 bpm above resting heart rate.

Statistical analysis

Estimates of arithmetic mean and standard error were used as standard summary statistics while obtaining primary data. Prior to parametric data processing, we verified sample distribution normality (Shapiro-Wilk's test) and variance homogeneity. Two-way repeated measures analysis of variance was performed as the principal method to evaluate the outcomes of the experimental groups (ES, EX, and SED as independent, effect components) and sampling at different time points (as a dependent, pairwise component). A post hoc test was completed for variables with a significant difference depending on their parameters (Tukey-Kramer or Scheffé procedures). Greenhouse-Geisser correction was applied as Mauchly's test of sphericity was not met. SPSS 22.0 for Windows (IBM Corp., Armonk, NY, USA) was used for all analyses, and a value of $p < 0.05$ was considered statistically significant.

Results

Table 1 displays the subjects' baseline characteristics. There were no significant differences among the three groups at baseline in terms of age, male/female ratio, HD duration, body mass index, and diabetic nephropathy ratio (Table 1).

Physical parameters at baseline and 12 weeks after the intervention are presented in Table 2. With the exception of hand grip strength, there were no significant differences among the groups at baseline. After the 12-week intervention, the EX group showed a significant improvement in hand grip strength (from 19.7 ± 0.7 to 21.9 ± 0.8 kg; $p = 0.02$). In contrast, MPQ (from 13.1 ± 0.1 to 15.7 ± 1.6 kgf; $p = 0.01$) and WBI (from 0.2 ± 0.1 to 0.3 ± 0.1 kgf/kg; $p = 0.04$) significantly increased in the ES group only.

Biochemical parameters at baseline and 12 weeks after the intervention are presented in Table 3. Dialysis efficiency (evaluated via Kt/V) significantly improved in both the ES (from 1.3 ± 0.0 to 1.5 ± 0.0; $p = 0.01$) and EX groups (from 1.3 ± 0.0 to 1.5 ± 0.0; $p = 0.02$), but not in the SED group. Phosphorus level significantly decreased (from 6.0 ± 0.0 to 4.7 ± 0.1 mg/dl; $p = 0.04$) in the ES group. HDL-C level significantly decreased in the both the EX and ES groups; however, LDL-C/HDL-C level did not significantly change in these groups. Regarding immunological factors, in the EX group, serum CRP level significantly decreased (from 0.7 ± 0.1 to 0.4 ± 0.1 mg/dl; $p = 0.04$), while serum TNF-α level significantly increased (from 6.5 ± 1.0 to 7.0 ± 0.3 pg/ml; $p = 0.03$). Similarly, serum TNF-α level increased (from 6.2 ± 0.5 to 9.3 ± 0.8 pg/ml; $p = 0.02$) in the SED group, with no change detected in serum CRP after the 12-week intervention. Conversely, although serum CRP did not change, serum TNF-α level significantly decreased (from 6.7 ± 0.3 to 4.5 ± 0.1 pg/ml; $p = 0.04$) in the ES group.

Table 1 Patient baseline characteristics separated by experimental groups

Parameter	ES ($n = 10$)	EX ($n = 10$)	SED ($n = 10$)	p value*
Age (years)	68.6 ± 1.4	72.1 ± 0.7	69.9 ± 0.9	0.78
Male/female	7/3	8/2	8/2	0.85
Duration of HD (months)	126.0 ± 8.4	111.6 ± 4.8	123.6 ± 3.6	0.10
BMI (kg/m^2)	22.0 ± 0.9	22.0 ± 0.6	22.0 ± 0.7	0.99
Diabetic nephropathy	60.0%	70%	60%	0.89

Categorical data are presented as absolute number and percentage and continuous variables are presented as mean ± standard error
ES electrical stimulation of the leg extensors was applied to the patients during hemodialysis, *EX* the exercise-training group performed ergometer-training exercise during hemodialysis, *SED* the control group consisted of patients without exercise, *HD* hemodialysis, *BMI* body mass index
*Group comparisons were analyzed via the Kruskal-Wallis test and one-way analysis of variance for continuous parameters

Table 2 Changes in physical parameters in the ES ($n = 10$), EX ($n = 10$), and SED ($n = 10$) groups

Parameter	Mean ± SE		Time* (p value)	Repeated measures ANOVA† (p value)
	Baseline	12 weeks		
Hand grip (kg)				
ES	17.0 ± 0.7	18.8 ± 0.8	0.14	Group 0.01
EX	19.7 ± 0.7	21.9 ± 0.8	0.02	Time 0.04
SED	27.9 ± 0.7	26.1 ± 0.8	0.22	Interaction 0.41
Group‡ (p value)	0.01	0.44		
MPQ (kgf)				
ES	13.1 ± 0.1	15.7 ± 1.6	0.01	Group 0.53
EX	9.2 ± 0.3	10.0 ± 0.4	0.24	Time 0.04
SED	9.3 ± 0.2	9.1 ± 0.2	0.43	Interaction 0.78
Group‡ (p value)	0.30	0.01		
WBI (kgf/kg)				
ES	0.2 ± 0.1	0.3 ± 0.1	0.04	Group 0.69
EX	0.2 ± 0.0	0.2 ± 0.1	0.11	Time 0.02
SED	0.2 ± 0.0	0.2 ± 0.0	0.33	Interaction 0.73
Group‡ (p value)	0.32	0.51		

ES electrical stimulation, *EX* exercise, *SED* control, *SE* standard error, *ANOVA* analysis of variance, *MPQ* muscular power of the quadriceps, *WBI* weight bearing index
*Time-related differences within each group analyzed via post hoc test was completed for variables with a significant difference depending on their parameters (Tukey-Kramer or Scheffé procedures). Greenhouse-Geisser correction was applied as Mauchly's test of sphericity was not met pairwise
†Main effects (time and group) and interaction effect (time by group) analyzed via two-way repeated measures ANOVA
‡Group comparisons within each time point analyzed via post hoc test

There were no significant changes in other parameters and in group differences.

Discussion

To our knowledge, the present study was the first to investigate the effect of ES of skeletal muscles and aerobic training on physical function and biochemical parameters in elderly patients with CKD. Our major finding was that MPQ, WBI, Kt/V, serum phosphorus, and TNF-α level significantly changed from baseline to 12 weeks after the intervention in the ES group; however, there were no significant differences among the three groups at baseline for any parameters, except for hand grip strength. Additionally, in the EX and ES groups, HDL-C level significantly decreased from baseline to 12 weeks after the intervention, but no change was observed for LDL-C/HDL-C level. Therefore, these results support our hypothesis that training twice per week for 12 weeks during HD sessions in elderly patients with ESRD improves physical function and biochemical markers without any adverse effects.

However, the indicators of muscle power for the lower limbs (MPQ and WBI) significantly changed in the ES group only. The major difference between exercising on a cycle ergometer and lower leg ES is that the former is an endurance exercise of the lower limbs [11], whereas the latter induces muscle contraction without local articular exercise [4]. Both cycle exercise and lower limb ES involve muscle contraction. During cycle exercises, the appropriate number of motor units is recruited according to the exercise intensity, whereas ES may activate all motor units simultaneously [12]. That is, the major difference may be the possibility of ES to recruit the same number of motor units as high intensity exercises even at a low intensity. In the present study, the EX and ES groups conducted aerobic exercises at the same intensity (RPE 11–13). A preliminary experiment of expired gas measurement in two healthy individuals who underwent cycle ergometer exercise and lower leg ES revealed that the exercise was at or below an anaerobic threshold level for both tests. Therefore, the following reasons explain the lack of changes in muscle power in the EX group. Meanwhile, hand grip strength significantly improved in both the ES and EX groups. Several studies reported that improvement of muscle power in the lower limbs correlated with that in the upper limbs [13–15], which was similar with the results of the current study.

First, the exercise completed in this study was an endurance training of whole-body exercise [16], which may have improved endurance but was likely not enough to improve power in the EX group. The present study showed that in the ES group, MPQ increased while HDL-C significantly decreased with no changes in the other parameters. Although there is evidence that physical activity is beneficial in the general population, more work is required to determine the overall effects of exercise on physical activity in elderly patients with ESRD. Second, the exercise was performed at an RPE of 11–13 in the EX group, which may not have been high enough to reinforce muscle strength [17]. However, changes were observed in the ES and SED groups, as well as significant changes in inflammation markers CRP and TNF-α after the 12-week intervention. In addition, Kt/V significantly increased after the intervention in the ES and EX groups, whereas serum phosphorus and serum TNF-α levels significantly decreased in the ES group only. According to previous studies [4, 5, 18], ES of the legs was equally effective as exercise, but its effects were dependent on localized increases in muscular strength [19]. The present results also demonstrate that WBI increased because the leg muscles were strengthened. The reason for this finding is that ES only affects local function. Several investigators have examined the effects of repeated ES on muscle strength and reported increased

Table 3 Changes in biochemical parameters in the ES ($n = 10$), EX ($n = 10$), and SED ($n = 10$) groups

Parameter	Mean ± SE		Time* (p value)	Repeated measures ANOVA† (p value)
	Baseline	12 weeks		
Kt/V				
ES	1.3 ± 0.0	1.5 ± 0.0	0.01	Group 0.04
EX	1.3 ± 0.0	1.5 ± 0.0	0.02	Time 0.01
SED	1.3 ± 0.0	1.3 ± 0.0	0.47	Interaction 0.65
Group‡ (p value)	0.23	0.04		
BUN (mg/dl)				
ES	6.7 ± 0.3	5.5 ± 0.1	0.35	Group 0.93
EX	5.5 ± 0.1	5.0 ± 0.3	0.58	Time 0.49
SED	6.2 ± 0.5	6.3 ± 0.8	0.33	Interaction 0.95
Group‡ (p value)	0.977	0.908		
Phosphorus (mg/dl)				
ES	6.0 ± 0.0	4.7 ± 0.1	0.04	Group 0.04
EX	5.3 ± 0.1	5.1 ± 0.1	0.52	Time 0.04
SED	4.7 ± 0.1	5.4 ± 0.1	0.50	Interaction 0.43
Group‡ (p value)	0.39	0.59		
Potassium (mEq/l)				
ES	5.3 ± 0.1	5.0 ± 0.0	0.08	Group 0.93
EX	4.8 ± 0.1	4.6 ± 0.2	0.88	Time 0.74
SED	4.7 ± 0.1	4.8 ± 0.1	0.96	Interaction 0.63
Group‡ (p value)	0.55	0.59		
Alb (g/dl)				
ES	3.6 ± 0.0	3.5 ± 0.0	0.58	Group 0.72
EX	3.4 ± 0.1	3.5 ± 0.0	0.55	Time 0.95
SED	3.6 ± 0.0	3.6 ± 0.0	0.80	Interaction 0.07
Group‡ (p value)	0.69	0.91		
Hb (g/dl)				
ES	10.4 ± 0.1	10.3 ± 0.1	0.91	Group 0.21
EX	10.8 ± 0.1	10.3 ± 0.1	0.41	Time 0.49
SED	11.0 ± 0.1	11.0 ± 0.1	0.91	Interaction 0.77
Group‡ (p value)	0.766	0.309		
Fer (ng/ml)				
ES	118.9 ± 11.9	181.4 ± 15.9	0.24	Group 0.10
EX	133.7 ± 11.9	179.3 ± 17.4	0.11	Time 0.07
SED	84.5 ± 3.8	91.1 ± 6.1	0.79	Interaction 0.43
Group‡ (p value)	0.43	0.20		
TSAT (%)				
ES	22.6 ± 0.5	24.7 ± 0.8	0.48	Group 0.09
EX	21.9 ± 0.5	24.8 ± 0.6	0.50	Time 0.07
SED	23.5 ± 0.9	26.5 ± 1.0	0.53	Interaction 0.43
Group‡ (p value)	0.90	0.89		
HDL-C (mg/dl)				
ES	50.6 ± 1.1	47.9 ± 0.7	0.03	Group 0.16
EX	43.2 ± 0.8	45.1 ± 1.2	0.03	Time 0.04
SED	43.2 ± 1.3	43.4 ± 1.1	0.13	Interaction 0.69
Group‡ (p value)	0.27	0.47		
LDL-C/HDL-C				
ES	1.8 ± 0.1	1.9 ± 0.1	0.39	Group 0.52
EX	2.0 ± 0.1	2.0 ± 0.1	0.58	Time 0.22
SED	2.1 ± 0.0	2.2 ± 0.1	0.37	Interaction 0.87
Group‡ (p value)	0.51	0.79		
CRP (mg/dl)				
ES	0.4 ± 0.1	0.3 ± 0.1	0.47	Group 0.41
EX	0.7 ± 0.1	0.4 ± 0.1	0.04	Time 0.04
SED	0.2 ± 0.0	0.2 ± 0.0	0.70	Interaction 0.75
Group‡ (p value)	0.46	0.80		
IL-6 (pg/mL)				
ES	6.7 ± 0.2	6.9 ± 0.5	0.89	Group 0.61
EX	4.4 ± 0.2	4.6 ± 0.2	0.48	Time 0.25
SED	5.4 ± 0.3	6.5 ± 0.4	0.14	Interaction 0.93
Group‡ (p value)	0.38	0.55		
TNF-α (pg/ml)				
ES	6.7 ± 0.3	4.5 ± 0.1	0.04	Group 0.23
EX	6.5 ± 1.0	7.0 ± 0.3	0.04	Time 0.04
SED	6.2 ± 0.5	9.3 ± 0.8	0.03	Interaction 0.32
Group‡ (p value)	0.40	0.03		

ES electrical stimulation, *EX* exercise, *SED* control, *SE* standard error, *ANOVA* analysis of variance, *MPQ* muscular power of the quadriceps, *WBI* weight bearing index, *ES* electrical stimulation, *EX* exercise, *SED* control, *SE* standard error, *ANOVA* analysis of variance, *Kt/V* hemodialysis efficiency, *BUN* blood urea nitrogen, *Alb* albumin, *Hb* hemoglobin, *Fer* ferritin, *TSAT* transferrin saturation, *HDL-C* high-density lipoprotein cholesterol, *LDL-C* low-density lipoprotein cholesterol, *CRP* C-reactive protein, IL6 interleukin-6, *TNF-α* tumor necrosis factor-alpha

*Time-related differences within each group analyzed via post hoc test was completed for variables with a significant difference depending on their parameters (Tukey-Kramer or Scheffé procedures). Greenhouse-Geisser correction was applied as Mauchly's test of sphericity was not met pairwise

†Main effects (time and group) and interaction effect (time by group) analyzed via two-way repeated measures ANOVA

‡Group comparisons within each time point analyzed via post hoc test

strength of the skeletal muscles, improved muscle contraction in patients after knee surgery, and decreased atrophy. These findings indicate that ES might prevent and ameliorate disuse atrophy due to immobilization without requiring excessive effort.

However, there were no changes in anemia- and cholesterol-related factors from baseline to the end of the intervention. The exercise intensity and limited intervention duration (12 weeks) may not have been sufficient to induce changes in these factors. Problems specific to ES include the potential for local skin burns or irritation, electrode sensitivity, autonomic dysreflexia, surface burns, and skin inflammation. Previous studies reported that exercise training could be performed during HD sessions without any adverse effects. Likewise, our subjects did not experience any adverse effects, such as a sudden drop in blood pressure or cardiovascular disease.

On the other hand, previous studies reported that exercise improves inflammation; however, in the current study, serum CRP level significantly decreased after the intervention in the EX group and serum TNF-α level significantly increased. This elucidates that CRP is an indicator of systemic inflammation, whereas TNF-α can fluctuate with exercise and cause changes in psychological or physiological conditions, in addition to inflammation [20]. Therefore, it is reasonable that the CRP and TNF-α levels diverged in the present study.

In addition, serum phosphorus level decreased in the ES group only. We believe that this was an effect of muscle contraction on phosphorus metabolism, as explained in previous research [21]. The onset of poor physical condition was associated with bone metabolism, and the emergence of sarcopenia was accompanied by increased levels of inflammatory factors TNF-α and IL-6 [22].

Furthermore, subjects in both the EX and ES groups were able to safely undergo the intervention without shunt trouble, sudden drop in blood pressure, or the need for fluid replacement. Previous studies also reported that intra-dialytic exercise prolongs vital prognosis without adverse events [23]. Likewise, ES has also been safely conducted in previous studies without causing skin problems or new-onset heart failure [4, 24]. Therefore, ES of the lower limbs has beneficial effects on muscle power, systemic inflammation, and the prevention of falls in elderly patients undergoing HD.

Some limitations of our study should be considered. First, the study involved a relatively small sample size, and the study period was too short to determine long-term effects of exercise. Future examinations on efficacy should include a larger sample size and include a selection of resistance training adapted for Asian patients of advanced age.

Conclusion

ES of the legs and cycle exercise can be safely performed during dialysis. A comparison of ES and EX suggested that ES was more effective in improving muscle power of the lower limbs and TNF-α; therefore, ES might be effective for elderly patients with disease complications requiring HD.

Abbreviations

BUN: Blood urea nitrogen; CKD: Chronic kidney disease; CRP: C-reactive protein; ES: Electrical stimulation; ESRD: End-stage renal disease; EX: Exercise; Fer: Ferritin; HD: Hemodialysis; HDL-C: High-density lipoprotein cholesterol; IL-6: Interleukin-6; LDL-C: Low-density lipoprotein cholesterol; MPQ: Muscle power of the quadriceps femoris; RPE: Rating of perceived exertion; SED: Control; TNF-α: Tumor necrosis factor-alpha; TSAT: Transferrin saturation; WBI: Weight bearing index

Acknowledgements

The authors would like to thank PT. Sugiura and Nrs. Nose for the technical assistance with the evaluation.

Funding

This work was supported by the 2016 Renal Failure Pathological Research Grant of the Kidney Foundation in Japan.

Authors' contributions

MM contributed to the study design, study procedure implementation, data collection, and manuscript writing. All other authors contributed to the study design, data analysis, and manuscript writing. All authors read and approved the final manuscript.

Competing interests

The authors declare that they have no competing interests.

Author details

[1]Faculty of Health Sciences, Tsukuba University of Technology, Kasuga 4-12-7, Tsukuba City, Ibaraki 305-8521, Japan. [2]Asao Clinic, 1-8-10 Manpukuji, Asaoku, Kawasaki City, Kanagawa 215-0004, Japan. [3]Department of Nephrology, Faculty of Medicine, University of Tsukuba, 2-1-1 Amakubo, Tsukuba City, Ibaraki 305-8576, Japan. [4]Department of Internal Medicine and Rehabilitation, Faculty of Medicine, Tohoku Medical and Pharmaceutical University, Komatushima 4-4-1, Aobaku, Sendai City, Miyagi 981-0905, Japan. [5]Hirayama Hospital, Hanamigawa1494–3, Hanamigawaku, Chiba City, Chiba 262-0046, Japan. [6]Department of Internal Medicine and Rehabilitation Science, Tohoku University School of Medicine, 1-1 Seiryoumachi, Aobaku, Sendai City, Miyagi 980-8574, Japan.

References

1. Bello AK, Levin A, Tonelli M, Okpechi IG, Feehally J, Harris D, et al. Assessment of global kidney health care status. JAMA. 2017;317(18):1864–81.
2. Collister D, Ferguson T, Komenda P, Tangri N. The patterns, risk factors, and prediction of progression in chronic kidney disease: a narrative review. Semin Nephrol. 2016;36(4):273–82.
3. Johansen KL. Exercise in the end-stage renal disease population. J Am Soc Nephrol. 2007;18(6):1845–54.
4. Dobsák P, Nováková M, Fiser B, Siegelová J, Balcárková P, Spinarová L, et al. Electrical stimulation of skeletal muscles. An alternative to aerobic exercise training in patients with chronic heart failure? Int Heart J. 2006;47(3):441–53.

5. Dobsak P, Homolka P, Svojanovsky J, Reichertova A, Soucek M, Novakova M, et al. Intra-dialytic electrostimulation of leg extensors may improve exercise tolerance and quality of life in hemodialyzed patients. Artif Organs. 2012; 36(1):71–8. https://doi.org/10.1111/j.1525-1594.2011.01302.x
6. Banerjee P, Caulfield B, Crowe L, Clark AL. Prolonged electrical muscle stimulation exercise improves strength, peak VO2, and exercise capacity in patients with stable chronic heart failure. J Card Fail. 2009;15(4):319–26.
7. Wardlaw JM, Chappell FM, Stevenson M, De Nigris E, Thomas S, Gillard J, et al. Accurate, practical and cost-effective assessment of carotid stenosis in the UK. Health Technol Assess. 2006;10(30):1–182. iii-iv, ix-x
8. Muraki S, Akune T, Teraguchi M, Kagotani R, Asai Y, Yoshida M, et al. Quadriceps muscle strength, radiographic knee osteoarthritis and knee pain: the ROAD study. BMC Musculoskelet Disord. 2015;16:305.
9. Goldstein SL, Sorof JM, Brewer ED. Evaluation and prediction of urea rebound and equilibrated Kt/V in the pediatric hemodialysis population. Am J Kidney Dis. 1999;34(1):49–54.
10. Lertdumrongluk P, Streja E, Rhee CM, Park J, Arah OA, Brunelli SM, et al. Dose of hemodialysis and survival: a marginal structural model analysis. Am J Nephrol. 2014;39(5):383–91.
11. Elkington TJ, Cassar S, Nelson AR, Levinger I. Psychological responses to acute aerobic, resistance, or combined exercise in healthy and overweight individuals: a systematic review. Clin Med Insights Cardiol. 2017;11: 1179546817701725.
12. Doucet BM, Lam A, Griffin L. Neuromuscular electrical stimulation for skeletal muscle function. Yale J Biol Med. 2012;85(2):201–15.
13. Melo FCM, de Lima KKF, Silveira A, de Azevedo KPM, Dos Santos IK, de Medeiros HJ, et al. Physical training and upper limb strength of people with paraplegia: a systematic review. J Sport Rehabil. 2018;24:1–20. https://doi.org/10.1123/jsr.2017-0062
14. Baker J, Brown E, Hill G, Phillips G, Williams R, Davies B. Handgrip contribution to lactate production and leg power during high-intensity exercise. Med Sci Sports Exerc. 2002;34(6):1037–40.
15. Harvey S, Rissel C, Pijnappels M. Associations between bicycling and fall related physical performance in older adults. J Aging Phys Act. 2018;26(3): 514–19. https://doi.org/10.1123/japa.2017-0243
16. Hansen JS, Zhao X, Irmler M, Liu X, Hoene M, Scheler M, et al. Type 2 diabetes alters metabolic and transcriptional signatures of glucose and amino acid metabolism during exercise and recovery. Diabetologia. 2015; 58(8):1845–54.
17. Borde R, Hortobagyi T, Granacher U. Dose-response relationships of resistance training in healthy old adults: a systematic review and meta-analysis. Sports Med. 2015;45(12):1693–720.
18. Bruggemann AK, Mello CL, Dal Pont T, Hizume Kunzler D, Martins DF, Bobinski F, et al. Effects of neuromuscular electrical stimulation during hemodialysis on peripheral muscle strength and exercise capacity: a randomized clinical trial. Arch Phys Med Rehabil. 2017;98(5):822–31. e821
19. Dobsak P, Homolka P, Svojanovsky J, Reichertova A, Soucek M, Novakova M, et al. Intra-dialytic electrostimulation of leg extensors may improve exercise tolerance and quality of life in hemodialyzed patients. Artif Organs. 2012; 36(1):71–8.
20. Ramseyer VD, Garvin JL. Tumor necrosis factor-alpha: regulation of renal function and blood pressure. Am J Physiol Renal Physiol. 2013;304(10):F1231–42.
21. Friedman MA, Bailey AM, Rondon MJ, McNerny EM, Sahar ND, Kohn DH. Calcium- and phosphorus-supplemented diet increases bone mass after short-term exercise and increases bone mass and structural strength after long-term exercise in adult mice. PLoS One. 2016;11(3):e0151995.
22. Bian AL, Hu HY, Rong YD, Wang J, Wang JX, Zhou XZ. A study on relationship between elderly sarcopenia and inflammatory factors IL-6 and TNF-alpha. Eur J Med Res. 2017;22(1):25.
23. Chung YC, Yeh ML, Liu YM. Effects of intradialytic exercise on the physical function, depression and quality of life for haemodialysis patients: a systematic review and meta-analysis of randomised controlled trials. J Clin Nurs. 2017;26(13–14):1801–13.
24. Graham-Brown MP, March DS, Churchward DR, Young HM, Dungey M, Lloyd S, et al. Design and methods of CYCLE-HD: improving cardiovascular health in patients with end stage renal disease using a structured programme of exercise: a randomised control trial. BMC Nephrol. 2016;17(1):69.

Bacterial meningitis and multiple abscess formation in the iliopsoas, erector spinae, and vastus lateralis muscle in a maintenance hemodialysis patient treated with continuous epidural anesthesia for herpes zoster-related pain control

Shunsuke Yamada[1], Narihito Tatsumoto[1], Noriko Nakamura[1], Kosuke Masutani[1], Toshiro Maeda[2], Takanari Kitazono[1] and Kazuhiko Tsuruya[1,3*]

Abstract

Background: Infection is the second leading cause of mortality in patients who undergo maintenance hemodialysis. In this population, impairment in both cellular and humoral immunity contributes to the increased incidence of infection and infection-related hospitalization. However, these artificial devices occasionally enhance the risk of deep organ infection including muscle abscess, frequently leading to disability and mortality in hemodialysis patients.

Case presentation: A 54-year-old male undergoing maintenance hemodialysis was hospitalized because of the acute onset pain in the back and bilateral legs and declining consciousness which started at 7 days after the treatment of herpes zoster-related neuralgia with continuous epidural anesthesia. Physical examination revealed purulent discharge from the insertion site of the catheter. Serum biochemical tests showed increased inflammatory response and malnutrition. Magnetic resonance imaging revealed meningitis and multiple abscesses in the iliopsoas, erector spinae, gluteus medius, and vastus lateralis muscles, where conventional antibiotic treatment often fails to cure. *Staphylococcus aureus* was detected in the cerebrospinal fluid. Combination of intravenous antibiotics treatment and aggressive open surgical drainage of the muscle abscesses finally cured meningitis and multiple deep muscle abscesses in this patient.

Conclusions: Treatment with sensitive antibiotics and timely open surgical drainage is necessary to cure catheter-related meningitis and secondary deep muscle abscesses in hemodialysis patients. Our case also suggests that epidural anesthesia may not be a good therapeutic option for herpes zoster because patients with herpes zoster are immunologically more compromised during and shortly after reactivation of varicella zoster virus.

Keywords: Abscess, Epidural catheter, Erector spinae muscle, Hemodialysis, Iliopsoas muscle, Vastus lateralis muscle

* Correspondence: tsuruya@intmed2.med.kyushu-u.ac.jp
[1]Department of Medicine and Clinical Science, Graduate School of Medical Sciences, Kyushu University, 3-1-1 Maidashi, Higashi-ku, Fukuoka 812-8582, Japan
[3]Department of Integrated Therapy for Chronic Kidney Disease, Graduate School of Medical Sciences, Kyushu University, 3-1-1 Maidashi, Higashi-ku, Fukuoka 812-8582, Japan
Full list of author information is available at the end of the article

Background

Infection is the second leading cause of mortality, accounting for 18–25% of deaths in patients who undergo hemodialysis [1, 2]. Impairment in both cellular and humoral immunity contributes to the increased incidence of infection and infection-related hospitalization in hemodialysis patients [3–5]. Besides, dialysis patients have greater opportunities to receive various types of artificial medical devices for treatment and examination, catheterization for angiography and intravascular placement of catheters, and artificial grafts for dialysis access. These artificial devices greatly enhance the risk of deep organ infection including muscle abscess, frequently leading to disability and mortality in hemodialysis patients [6–10].

Herpes zoster is a self-limited dermatomal rash related to reactivation of the varicella zoster virus (VZV) in the dorsal root ganglion [11]. A recent population-based cohort study showed that hemodialysis patients are at 2.3 times higher risk of herpes zoster compared with the general population [12]. Standard treatment for herpes zoster and its related neuralgia includes anti-viral drugs (aciclovir, valaciclovir, famciclovir) and analgesics such as narcotics, topical lidocaine treatment, anticonvulsants, and nerve blocking [13–15]. Since anti-viral drugs are metabolized and secreted via the kidney, the dose should be reduced in dialysis patients. When patients with herpes zoster suffer from severe pain, epidural anesthesia is occasionally applied. However, when patients are suffering from active herpes zoster, they are immunologically more compromised than when they are not affected by that disease and put at an increased risk of infection. Here, we have a clinically important question whether epidural anesthesia is a safe treatment option for the pain control in hemodialysis patients with active herpes zoster.

We herein report the case of a patient undergoing maintenance hemodialysis who developed acute bacterial meningitis and multiple deep muscle abscesses related to epidural anesthesia during pain control for herpes zoster.

Case presentation

A 54-year-old male was hospitalized for the diagnosis and treatment for fever, backache, bilateral leg pain, and declining consciousness. He had been on maintenance hemodialysis due to endstage kidney disease with unknown etiology since he was 29 years old. At ages 46 and 49, he received surgeries for carpal tunnel syndrome secondary to dialysis-related amyloidosis. He received also total parathyroidectomy with auto-transplantation in the right forearm for the treatment of secondary hyperparathyroidism at age 47. He neither had a history of diabetes mellitus and immune deficiency nor received immunosuppressants. He had been on maintenance dialysis with the use of his arteriovenous fistula as a vascular access.

Three weeks prior to the admission, he developed herpes zoster in the left inguinal and groin area (L1–L2) and in the left waist area (L1–L2) and was treated with reduced dose of valacyclovir (250 mg/day). Because herpes zoster-related neuralgia was so severe and non-steroidal anti-inflammatory drugs were ineffective, he requested a more effective pain control and was then treated with continuous epidural anesthesia for the relief of severe pain. Seven days after starting continuous epidural anesthesia, epidural catheter was removed. At the time of catheter removal, purulent discharge was observed at the insertion site of epidural catheter. Although levofloxacin was initiated thereafter, he rapidly developed backache and bilateral leg pain and declining consciousness on the next day of catheter removal and was transferred to our hospital.

On admission, consciousness level was II-10 in the Japan Coma Scale. His height was 170 cm, his body weight was 62 kg, and his body mass index was 21.5 kg/m^2. Blood pressure was 156/84 mmHg in supine position. Heart rate was 104 bpm. Body temperature was 38.4 °C. A summary of blood test is shown in Table 1 including blood hemoglobin level of 106 g/L, white blood cell count of 28,600/μL (neutrophil 89.5%), platelet count of 8.7×10^4/μL, serum albumin level of 29 g/L, and C-reactive protein level of 215 nmol/L. These results suggested mild level of anemia and malnutrition, elevated inflammatory response, and the presence of bacterial infection.

Plain computed tomography did not show any mass lesion in the head. Because bacterial meningitis was highly suspected, cerebrospinal fluid was collected by lumbar puncture. The findings of the cerebrospinal fluid showed increased cell count with higher neutrophil dominance, increased levels of protein and lactate dehydrogenase, and decreased levels of glucose, indicating bacterial infection (Table 2).

Magnetic resonance imaging was performed for further evaluation. In the T2-weighted imaging, round high-intensity lesion at the L4/L5 level, indicative of epidural abscess, was observed (Fig. 1a). Also, round high-intensity lesions in the left iliopsoas muscle and in the bilateral erector spinae muscles were detected (Fig. 1b). Finally, he was diagnosed with bacterial meningitis and multiple abscesses in the iliopsoas and erector spinae muscles, which were probably triggered by the indwelling catheter for continuous epidural anesthesia.

Treatment with immunoglobulin (5 g/day for 3 days), antibiotics (vancomycin, 2 g/week; ampicillin 1 g/day; ceftriaxone, 2 g/day), and phenytoin were initiated on the first hospital day. On the fifth hospital day, blood

Table 1 Laboratory data on admission

Complete blood count	Value	Unit	*Serum biochemistries (continued)*	Value	Unit	*Immunology*	Value	Unit
Hemoglobin	106	g/L	Sodium	139	mmol/L	HBs antigen	−	
Hematocrit	32.8	%	Potassium	5.8	mmol/L	HBs antibody	−	
White blood cell	28.6	10^9/L	Chloride	99	mmol/L	HCV antibody	+	
Neutrophils	89.5	%	Lactate dehydrogenase	412	U/L	HTLV-1 antibody	+	
Platelet count	87	10^9/L	Amylase	246	U/L	TPHA test	−	
Serum biochemistries			Creatinine kinase	443	U/L	*Coagulation*		
Total protein	62	g/L	Calcium	2.33	mmol/L	Fibrinogen	15.6	μmol/L
Albumin	29	g/L	Phosphate	1.94	mmol/L	FDP	16.5	mg/L
Blood urea nitrogen	39.3	mmol/L	Magnesium	1.2	mmol/L	D-dimer	4.9	μg/mL
Creatinine	875	μmol/L	Iron	3.0	μmol/L	PT-INR	1.34	
Uric acid	595	μmol/L	Total cholesterol	2.87	mmol/L	APTT	36.7	s
Total bilirubin	5.1	μmol/L	Triglyceride	1.79	mmol/L	APTT-control	35.7	s
Direct bilirubin	1.7	μmol/L	HDL-cholesterol	0.36	mmol/L	Blood gas analysis		
Alanine aminotransferase	27	U/L	Glucose	4.2	mmol/L	pH	7.42	
Aspartate aminotransferase	14	U/L	C-reactive protein	215	nmol/L	pO_2	73.3	mmHg
Alkaline phosphatase	586	U/L				pCO_2	45.1	mmHg
Gamma-glutamyl transferase	186	U/L				HCO_3^-	28.4	mmol/L

APTT activated partial thrombin time, *HBs* hepatitis B surface, *FDP* fibrin/fibrinogen degradation product, *HCV* hepatitis C virus, *HDL* high-density lipoprotein, *HTLV-1* human T cell leukemia/lymphoma virus-1, *PT-INR* internationalized prothorombin time, *TPHA* Treponema pallidum hemagglutinin

culture turned out to be negative. However, culture result of cerebrospinal fluid disclosed *Staphylococcus aureus*. The *Staphylococcus aureus* was sensitive to cefazolin, gentamycin, amikacin, erythromycin, clindamycin, minocycline, vancomycin, teikoplanin, levofloxacin, and sulfamethoxazole/trimethoprim but resistant to ampicillin. Accordingly, ampicillin was discontinued and clindamycin was added instead. However, high fever lasted and serum inflammatory markers did not decrease. Hence, minocycline and sulfamethoxazole were added on after consulting our infection team. On the 14th hospital day, cell count and lactated dehydrogenase level in the cerebrospinal fluid decreased compared to the initial evaluation. His consciousness returned to almost normal.

Table 2 Findings of cerebrospinal fluid on admission

	Values
Cell count	14,330/3
Monocyte, %	20
Segmented, %	80
Total protein, mg/dL	345
Lactate dehydrogenase, U/L	788
Glucose, mg/dL	2
Sodium, mmol/L	140
Potassium, mmol/L	4.9
Chloride, mmol/L	108

Analysis of the cerebrospinal fluid obtained on the first hospital day is shown

However, fever lasted and serum levels of C-reactive protein remained high. At this point, echocardiography did not show any evidence of infective endocarditis, but gallium scintigraphy showed a strong accumulation around the left hip joint. Magnetic resonance imaging performed on the 19th hospital day showed bursitis around the femoral head and pyomyositis in the left gluteus minimus and medius muscles, large abscess in the left vastus lateralis muscle, which was probably spread from the abscess in the left iliopsoas muscle (Fig. 2). Although intravenous antibiotic administration (meropenem 1 g/day and vancomycin 2 g/week) was continued, multiple abscesses did not shrink. In addition, repeated culture of blood and cerebrospinal fluid did not detect any bacteria. Accordingly, surgical open drainage was performed on the 48th hospital day, followed by a drastic shrink of abscess in the vastus lateralis muscle and a decrease in serum inflammatory markers. Meropenem (1 g/day) was continued even after abscess disappeared. During the hospitalization, he also developed disuse atrophy and needed rehabilitation because of the long-term bedridden condition. On the 108th hospital day, he was finally transferred to another hospital for rehabilitation and maintenance hemodialysis. At 1 year after his discharge, he had completely recovered from multiple deep muscle abscesses and was on maintenance hemodialysis without relapse. Clinical course during the hospitalization is summarized in Fig. 3.

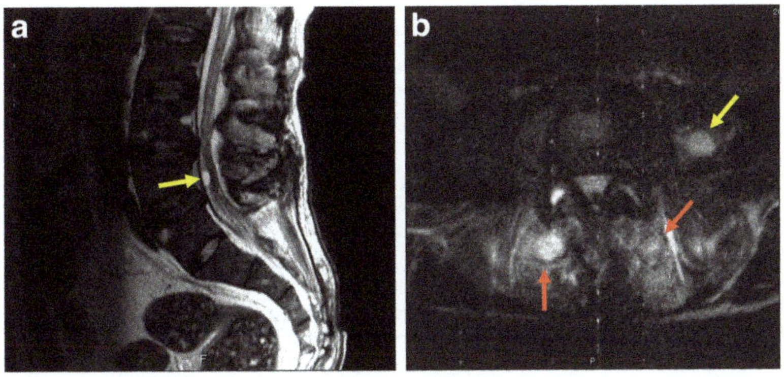

Fig. 1 Magnetic resonance imaging of the sagittal and cross-sectional spine. **a** Epidural abscess (yellow arrow) shown as a rounded high-intensity lesion at the L4/L5 level. **b** Abscess in the left iliopsoas muscle (yellow arrow, round high-intensity lesion) and bilateral erector spinae muscles (red arrows, round high-intensity lesions). L lumbar

Discussion

Herpes zoster is a process of reactivation of VZV which remains dormant in the sensory ganglia of the cranial nerve or the dorsal root ganglia after a previous varicella infection [16, 17]. Epidural anesthesia, occasionally used for pain control caused by various disorders in the general population, is also effective in hemodialysis patients. However, when patients are being affected by herpes zoster, it is unclear whether epidural anesthesia for pain control is a safe treatment, especially in hemodialysis patients. Generally, patients with active herpes zoster are immunologically being more compromised than when they are not affected by reactivation of VZV. As for hemodialysis patients, they are immunologically compromised because of their impaired immunity by uremic milieu. Besides, artificial devices such as catheter increase the risk of infection. Considering these medical conditions, epidural anesthesia may not be a good therapeutic option for the control of herpes zoster-related pain in hemodialysis patients with active herpes zoster, potentially causing severe infection as in the present case. Hence, further studies are necessary to determine

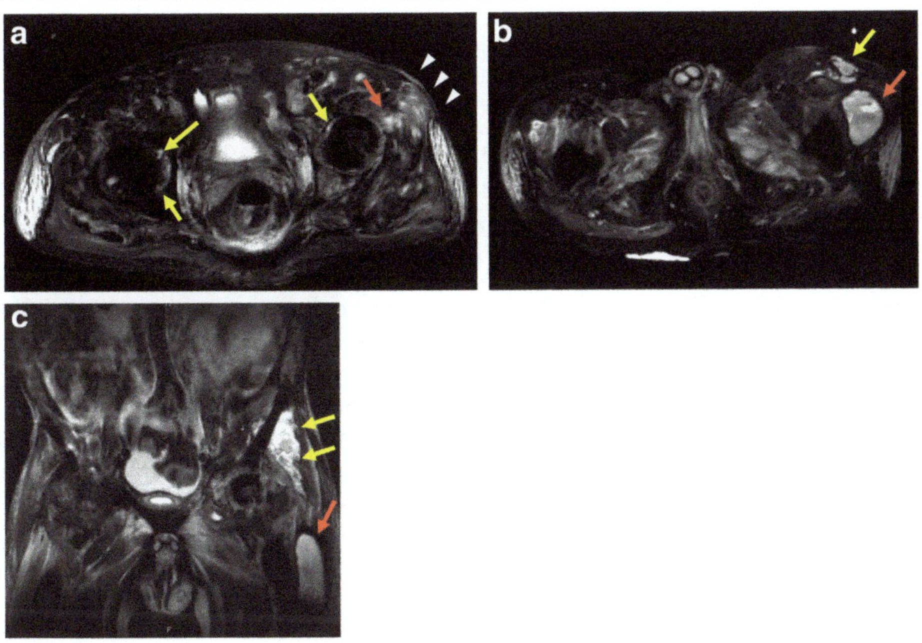

Fig. 2 Magnetic resonance imaging of the abdomen. **a** Bursitis around hip joints (yellow arrows) and pyomyositis in the left gluteus minimus (red arrow) and gluteus medius muscle (white arrow heads). **b** Abscess in the left gluteus medius (yellow arrow) and vastus lateralis muscle (red arrow) (cross-section). **c** Abscess in the left gluteus minimus and medius muscles (yellow arrow) and vastus lateralis muscle (red arrow) (coronal section)

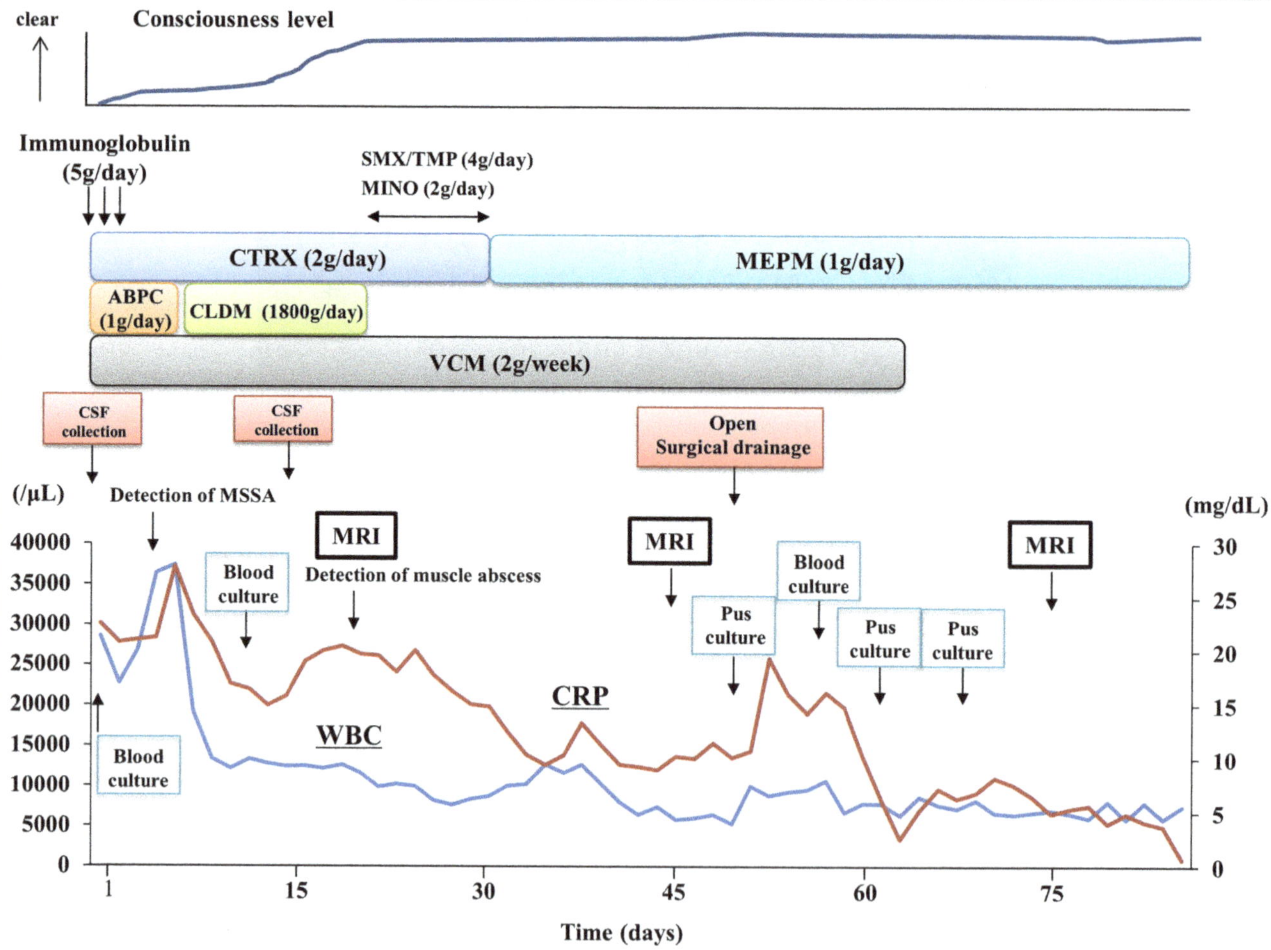

Fig. 3 Clinical course after hospitalization. ABPC ampicillin, CLDM clindamycin, CSF cerebrospinal fluid, CRP C-reactive protein, CTRX ceftriaxone, IMP/CS imipenem/cilastatin, MEPM meropenem, MINO minocycline, MRI magnetic resonance imaging, MSSA methicillin-sensitive *Staphylococcus aureus* SMX sulfamethoxazole, TMP trimethoprim, VCM vancomycin, WBC white blood cell

whether the risk for epidural catheter-related infection in hemodialysis patients with active herpes zoster is higher than those without active herpes zoster.

Psoas muscle abscess is a rare but lethal complication that is occasionally seen in hemodialysis patients [8–10, 18–28]. Triad of the classical psoas muscle abscess consists of fever, pain, and limp [29]. Psoas muscle abscess is generally classified into primary and secondary form, depending on the presence or absence of the underlying disease. Primary psoas abscess is caused by bloodstream-mediated infection from a distant site by bacteremia or sepsis. Secondary psoas abscess is usually related to direct spreading or expansion from the adjacent organs and often caused by inflammation and neoplasm of the intrapelvic organs such as inflammatory bowel diseases [23]. Risk factors of psoas muscle abscess include diabetes mellitus, intravenous drug use, immunosuppressive drugs, and human-immunodeficiency-virus infection [29]. Diagnosis often requires imaging such as computed tomography and magnetic resonance imaging and occasionally positron emission tomography. As for the causative bacteria, *Staphylococcus aureus* is the major pathogen detected in those reported cases. Notably, increasing number of cases is now caused by methicillin-resistant *Staphylococcus aureus*. Treatment involves intravenous administration of sensitive antibiotic agents for at least several weeks and interventions such as needle aspiration or open surgical drainage and debridement of the affected muscles [21]. A previous report showed that the prognosis of secondary psoas abscess is worse than primary psoas abscess, and unless open surgical drainage is performed, its prognosis is unacceptable [30].

Table 3 summarized the previous 22 reports including our case on psoas muscle abscess in hemodialysis patients [8–10, 19–28]. The age of the patients ranged from 45 to 78 years. Both male and female patients were affected. Primary infection sites included catheters for vascular access, enterocolitis, and discitis. The causative pathogens included *Staphylococcus aureus* and enteric bacteria, depending on the primary source of infection.

Table 3 Review of the literature on psoas muscle abscess in patients undergoing hemodialysis

Authors	Age (years)	Sex	Cause of ESKD	Dialysis Hx (years)	Treatment		Bacteria	Primary source of infection	Outcome
					Antibiotics	Surgical drainage			
The present case	54	M	CGN	26	Yes	Yes	SA	Epidural catheter	Remission
Peddi S et al. [8]	45	M	Unknown	0	Yes	No	MRSA	Internal jugular vein catheter for VA	Remission
Sato M et al. [9]	57	M	PCKD	14	Yes	Yes	*Bacteroides fragilis*	Diverticulitis	Remission
Sato M et al. [9]	58	M	PCKD	18	Yes	Yes	MSSA	Catheter for VA	Remission
Sato M et al. [9]	59	M	DMN	15	Yes	Yes	Enterococcus faecalis	Renal hematoma infection	Remission
Sato M et al. [9]	61	M	DMN	27	Yes	Yes	*Streptococcus agalactiae*	Enterocolitis	Remission
Sato M et al. [9]	67	M	DMN	2	Yes	Yes	MRSA	Discitis	Remission
Sato M et al. [9]	69	M	CGN	11	Yes	No	Streptococcus species	Endocarditis	Remission
Sato M et al. [9]	70	F	CGN	19	Yes	Yes	MSSA	Discitis	Remission
Sato M et al. [9]	78	M	CGN	5	Yes	Yes	MRSA	AVF infection	Death
Alif Adlan MT et al. [19]	53	F	Unknown	0.1	Yes	Yes	MSSA	Internal jugular vein catheter for VA	Remission
Hsiao PJ et al. [20]	47	F	Unknown	3	Yes	No	MRSA	Internal jugular vein catheter for VA	Remission
Kim JW et al. [21]	53	F	DMN	0.5	Yes	Yes	Unknown	Acupuncture	Remission
Lin CJ et al. [22]	66	M	DMN	0	Yes	Yes	MSSA	Femoral vein catheter for VA	Remission
Dovas S et al. [23]	66	F	CP	11	Yes	Yes	Bacteroides fragilis	Unknown	Remission
Chuang FR et al. [24]	55	M	CGN	0.1	Yes	Yes	Proteus vulgaris	Unknown	Death
Papoulidou et al. [25]	72	Unknown	Unknown	0.3	Yes	No	SA	Subclavian vein catheter for VA	Remission
Kato A et al. [26]	69	M	CGN	24	Yes	Yes	Bacteroides fragilis	Enterocolitis	Death
Kikuchi S et al. [27]	53	F	DMN	0.1	Yes	No	MRSA	Femoral vein catheter for VA	Remission
Kikuchi S et al. [27]	64	M	CGN	0.1	Yes	No	MRSA	Femoral vein catheter for VA	Remission
Tillman BF et al. [28]	48	M	TIN	2	Yes	Yes	MSSA	Discitis	Remission
Tillman BF et al. [28]	66	M	HTN	1	Yes	Yes	MSSA	AVF infection	Remission

Brackets indicate reference number cited in the main manuscript

AVF arteriovenous fistula, *CGN* chronic glomerulonephritis, *CP* chronic pyelonephritis, *DMN* diabetic nephropathy, *ESKD* endstage kidney disease, *F* female, *HTN* hypertensive nephrosclerosis, *Hx* history, *M* male, *MRSA* methicillin-resistant *Staphylococcus aureus*, *MSSA* methicillin-sensitive *Staphylococcus aureus*, *PCKD* polycystic kidney disease, *SA Staphylococcus aureus* (sensitivity to antibiotics is unknown), *TIN* tubulointerstitial nephritis, *VA* vascular access

All the catheter-related psoas muscle abscesses were caused by methicillin-sensitive or resistant *Staphylococcus aureus*. Most cases are treated with combination of intravenous antibiotics treatment and surgical drainage, leading to remission of psoas muscle abscess. As for psoas muscle abscess secondary to catheter-related infection, all previous cases were related to catheter used for vascular access and catheters inserted into the jugular, subclavian, or femoral veins for temporal or permanent use [7, 8, 19, 20, 22, 25, 27]. In this regard, our case is the first to report psoas muscle abscess caused by epidural catheter used for continuous epidural anesthesia.

Bacterial infection in the erector spinae muscle is not so common. *Staphylococcus aureus* occasionally causes abscess in the erector spinae muscle, named tropical myositis, which is restricted in the tropical regions [31, 32]. However, this disease entity is somewhat different from erector spinae muscle abscess caused by bacteremia. To our knowledge, abscess in the erector spinae muscle has not been reported in dialysis population. In the present case, *Staphylococcus aureus* was the causative pathogen and successfully treated by sensitive antibiotics. Our case indicates that abscess in the erector spinae muscle can be the possible cause of back pain in a particular medical condition. As for the route of abscess in the erector spinae muscle, two potential pathways were presumed. One was via bloodstream-mediated dissemination and should be prevented by controlling the primary infection promptly. Another was via the route made by lumbar punctures for continuous epidural anesthesia. Because lumbar puncture through para-median pathway penetrates erector spinae muscles, multiple punctures could cause infection of that muscle. In this regard, it may be said that epidural anesthesia may sometimes cause spinae muscle abscess especially in hemodialysis patients because epidural puncture is relatively difficult to do on dialysis patients and sometimes needs multiple punctures via the para-median pathway.

Abscess in the vastus lateralis muscles caused by non-tuberculous bacteria has rarely been reported both in the general population and hemodialysis patients. Since muscle abscess without trauma is usually caused by contamination of the bacteria into the bloodstream, it is reasonable to think that the site of abscess may be stochastic and there may be no common site of muscle abscess. Or blood supply to muscle may be more diverse depending on the location of the muscle, since the psoas muscle is known to have a huge blood supply compared to other muscles. This may be one of the reasons why cases of psoas muscle abscess have been the most. The mechanisms underlying bacterial lodging to muscle may be more complicated. Hence, further studies are necessary to determine why some muscles are prone to develop abscess and others are not under bacteremia or sepsis.

Drainage at an appropriate timing is critical in the management of deep muscle abscess including psoas muscle abscess. Open surgical drainage and percutaneous drainage are the two common modalities for abscess drainage. However, a previous study showed that open surgical drainage reduced total hospital days compared with needle aspiration, especially when abscess is larger [33]. As shown in Table 3, most of the remission cases experienced drainage as well as administration of sensitive antibiotics. In our case, open surgical drainage was performed at 29 days after psoas muscle abscess was detected by imaging. In our case, delayed surgical drainage might be responsible for the delayed remission of our case. One of the important messages of our case was that open surgical drainage without delay is necessary when abscess is larger and administration of sensitive antibiotics for 5–7 days is ineffective [26]. The importance of open surgical drainage is probably explained by the fact that delivery rate of antibiotic to the abscess site is lower than that of other infection sites [34].

As for the route of infection, primary deep muscle infection including iliopsoas muscle abscess is usually mediated by the bloodstream, namely secondary to bacteremia and/or sepsis [10, 18, 28]. However, judging from the distribution and progression of the multiple abscesses in the left-sided muscles, we cannot deny the possibility that abscess in the left iliopsoas muscle expanded into abscess in the left gluteus muscle and vastus lateralis muscle. As for dialysis population, vascular access is often the primary source of infection, even when vascular access infection looks absent [35]. In our case, considering that the epidural space is not directly connected to the iliopsoas muscle and erector spinae muscles and the muscle abscesses distributed bilaterally in our case, it is plausible to think that dissemination of *Staphylococcus aureus* in the epidural space via the bloodstream was ascribed to the multiple deep muscle abscesses. These results indicate that early control of bacterial meningitis with appropriate antibiotics is critically important to prevent secondary bacteremia and distant organ infection such as muscle abscess that can lead to life-threatening conditions.

Finally, it would be interesting and educational to discuss the best approach to this case. When purulent discharge from the insertion site of epidural catheter is noted, the catheter should be removed and purulent discharge and blood should be cultured to detect the causative organism. Repeat blood cultures until the causative pathogen is detected. Until the causative bacteria are identified, empiric therapy should be started with broad-spectrum antibiotics covering *Staphylococcus aureus* and Gram-positive bacteria, since these bacteria are the two major pathogens for epidural catheter-related infection. According to the guideline for bacterial meningitis in Japan, carbapenem and third-generation cephalosporins such as ceftriaxone are recommended because these drugs show a good penetration to the central nervous system [36, 37]. In recent years, the incidence of psoas abscess caused by methicillin-resistant *Staphylococcus aureus* is increasing. Hence, vancomycin should be included. Once the causative bacteria is detected and its susceptibility to antibiotics is determined, unneeded antibiotics should be discontinued and sensitive antibiotics should be continued for at least 4–6 weeks. If patients complicate bacteremia/septicemia/sepsis and distant organ infection is suspected as in the present case; imaging such as computed tomography and magnetic resonance imaging should be immediately performed to identify the location of the distant organ infection, then consider if there is a need for surgical intervention. Echocardiography should also be performed since dialysis population often are at increased risk for infective endocarditis. When the presence of intravascular infection or bloodstream-associated infection is suspected, continue treatment with sensitive antibiotics for weeks after blood culture becomes negative.

Conclusions

We presented here the case of a male patient receiving maintenance hemodialysis, whose bacterial meningitis and multiple abscess in the deep muscles were related to the indwelling epidural catheter and were successfully treated with antibiotics treatment and open surgical drainage. Our case confirms that treatment with sensitive antibiotics and open surgical drainage at an appropriate time is necessary to secondary deep muscle abscess in hemodialysis patients. Furthermore, our case suggests that epidural anesthesia may not be a good therapeutic option for the control of herpes zoster-related pain because patients with active herpes zoster is immunologically more compromised during and shortly after reactivation of VZV than when they are not affected by herpes zoster, especially in hemodialysis patients, who are already immunologically more compromised than the general population.

Authors' contributions

SY mainly drafted the manuscript. SY, NT, and NN performed acquisition of data and interpretation of data. KM, TM, and TK revised the manuscript. KT is responsible for the final version of the manuscript. All authors read and approved the final manuscript.

Competing interests

The authors declare that they have no competing interests.

Author details

[1]Department of Medicine and Clinical Science, Graduate School of Medical Sciences, Kyushu University, 3-1-1 Maidashi, Higashi-ku, Fukuoka 812-8582, Japan. [2]Division of Nephrology, Maeda Hospital, 2742-1 Tachibana-cho, Imari, Saga 848-0027, Japan. [3]Department of Integrated Therapy for Chronic Kidney Disease, Graduate School of Medical Sciences, Kyushu University, 3-1-1 Maidashi, Higashi-ku, Fukuoka 812-8582, Japan.

References

1. Renal Data System US. USRDS 2010 annual data report: atlas of chronic kidney disease and end-stage renal disease in the United States. Bethesda, MD: National Institute of Diabetes and Digestive and Kidney Diseases, National Institutes of Health; 2010.
2. Nakai S, Iseki K, Itami N, et al. Overview of regular dialysis treatment in Japan (as of 31 December 2009). Ther Apher Dial. 2012;16:11–53.
3. Chonchol M. Neutrophil dysfunction and infection risk in end-stage renal disease. Semin Dial. 2006;19:291–6.
4. Eleftheriadis T, Antoniadi G, Liakopoulos V, Kartsios C, Stefanidis I. Disturbances of acquired immunity in hemodialysis patients. Semin Dial. 2007;20:440–51.
5. Dalrymple LS, Mu Y, Nguyen DV, et al. Risk factors for infection-related hospitalization in in-center hemodialysis. Clin J Am Soc Nephrol. 2015;10: 2170–80.
6. Kanaa M, Wright MJ, Akbani H, et al. Cathasept line lock and microbial colonization of tunneled hemodialysis catheters: a multicenter randomized controlled trial. Am J Kidney Dis. 2015;66:1015–23.
7. Johns TS, Mokrzycki MH. Optimal approach for the diagnosis of hemodialysis catheter-related bacteremia. Clin J Am Soc Nephrol 2016 in press.
8. Peddi S, Ram R, Boreddy VD, et al. Multiple metastatic infections in a hemodialysis patient with untunneled internal jugular catheter. Hemodial Int. 2014;18:192–4.
9. Sato M, Iwasa Y, Otsubo S, et al. Psoas abscess in hemodialysis patients. Int Urol Nephrol. 2010;42:1113–6.
10. Okada A, Hangai M, Oda T. Bacteremia with an iliopsoas abscess and osteomyelitis of the femoral head caused by enterococcus avium in a patient with end-stage kidney disease. Intern Med. 2015;54:669–74.
11. Steiner I, Kennedy PG, Pachner AR. The neurotropic herpes viruses: herpes simplex and varicella-zoster. Lancet Neurol. 2007;6:1015–28.
12. Kuo CC, Lee CT, Lee IM, Ho SC, Yang CY. Risk of herpes zoster in patients treated with long-term hemodialysis: a matched cohort study. Am J Kidney Dis. 2012;59:428–33.
13. Sampathkumar P, Drage LA, Martin DP. Herpes zoster (shingles) and postherpetic neuralgia. Mayo Clin Proc. 2009;84:274–80.
14. Cook TM, Counsell D, Wildsmith JA; Royal College of Anaesthetists third National Audit Project. Major complications of central neuraxial block: report on the third National Audit Project of the Royal College of Anaesthetists. Br J Anaesth 2009;102:179–190.
15. Reynolds F. Neurological infections after neuraxial anesthesia. Anesthesiol Clin. 2008;26:23–52.
16. Gershon AA, Breuer J, Cohen JI, et al. Varicella zoster virus infection. Nat Rev Dis Primers. 2015;1:15016.
17. Gershon AA, Gershon MD, Breuer J, et al. Advances in the understanding of the pathogenesis and epidemiology of herpes zoster. J Clin Virol. 2010; 48(Suppl 1):S2–7.
18. Shields D, Robinson P, Crowley TP. Iliopsoas abscess—a review and update on the literature. Int J Surg. 2012;10:466–9.
19. Alif Adlan MT, Wan Mohd Rasis WA, Mohd Ramadhan MD. Fever with intradialytic pelvic pain: a case of iliopsoas abscess complicated with methicillin-sensitive staphylococcus aureus bacteraemia in an end stage renal failure patient. Med J Malaysia. 2016;71:72–3.
20. Hsiao PJ, Tsai MH, Leu JG, Fang YW. Iliopsoas abscess as a complication of tunneled jugular vein catheterization in a hemodialysis patient. Hemodial Int. 2015;19:330–2.
21. Kim JW, Kim YS. Psoas abscess formation after acupuncture in a hemodialysis patient. Hemodial Int. 2010;14:343–4.
22. Lin CJ, Lin HC, Wu CJ, Chen HH, Chen YC. Psoas muscle abscess as a complication of femoral vein catheterization in a hemodialysis patient. South Med J. 2008;101:566–7.

23. Dovas S, Liakopoulos V, Simopoulou T, et al. Psoas abscess in a dialysis patient with dialysis-related amyloidosis. Int Urol Nephrol. 2008;40:543–6.
24. Chuang FR, Lee CH, Chen JB, et al. Extra-renal abscess in chronic hemodialysis patients. Ren Fail. 2002;24:511–21.
25. Papoulidou F, Giannopoulos G, Pliakogiannis T, et al. Septic myositis in a chronic dialysis patient. Clin Nephrol. 2001;56:175–7.
26. Kato A, Takahashi T, Watanabe T, Furuhashi M, Maruyama Y, Hishida A. Psoas abscess with osteomyelitis in a patient undergoing long-term hemodialysis. Am J Nephrol. 2001;21:410–2.
27. Kikuchi S, Muro K, Yoh K, et al. Two cases of psoas abscess with discitis by methicillin-resistant Staphylococcus aureus as a complication of femoral-vein catheterization for haemodialysis. Nephrol Dial Transplant. 1999;14: 1279–81.
28. Tillman BF, Gibson RL, Stone WJ. Psoas abscess in chronic dialysis patients. J Urol. 1987;137:489–90.
29. Mallick IH, Thoufeeq MH, Rajendran TP. Iliopsoas abscesses. Postgrad Med J. 2004;80:459–62.
30. Ricci MA, Rose FB, Meyer KK. Pyogenic psoas abscess: worldwide variations in etiology. World J Surg. 1986;10:834–43.
31. Marshman LA, Bhatia CK, Krishna M, Friesem T. Primary erector spinae pyomyositis causing an epidural abscess: case report and literature review. Spine J. 2008;8:548–51.
32. Zheng YC, Chen CC, Wei KC, et al. Tropical pyomyositis of erector spinae complicated with spinal epidural abscess. Clin Neurol Neurosurg. 2015;128:84–9.
33. Santaella RO, Fishman EK, Lipsett PA. Primary vs secondary iliopsoas abscess. Presentation, microbiology, and treatment. Arch Surg. 1995;130:1309–13.
34. Obata A, Kaneto H, Kamei S, et al. Case of iliopsoas abscess that was markedly recovered after percutaneous and surgical drainage in a patient with poorly controlled type 2 diabetes. J Diabetes Investig. 2016;7:440–1.
35. Camins BC. Prevention and treatment of hemodialysis-related bloodstream infections. Semin Dial. 2013;26:476–81.
36. Ishikawa H, Kamei S. Revised Japanese guidelines for the clinical management of bacterial meningitis. Rinsho Shinkeigaku. 2014;54:1021–3.
37. Japanese Society of Chemotherapy Committee on guidelines for treatment of anaerobic infections; Japanese Association for Anaerobic Infection Research. Chapter 3-5. Appendix: pharmacokinetics of antimicrobial agents indicated for anaerobic infections. J Infect Chemother. 2011;17(Suppl 1):176–9.

Questionnaire survey on nutritional supplement therapy and exercise training at hemodialysis facilities in Japan

Satoko Sakurai[1], Norio Hanafusa[2*], Hideki Kato[1], Shinji Iizaka[3], Ryoko Murayama[4] and Masaomi Nangaku[1]

Abstract

Background: Nutritional therapy and exercise training (ET) are important interventions for hemodialysis patients. We investigated the status of nutritional therapy and ET provided at hemodialysis facilities across Japan.

Method: This was a cross-sectional study. The facilities investigated were 3993 facility member institutions of the Japanese Society for Dialysis Therapy in August 2015. Data was collected on the facility type, number of staff (doctors, nurses, and medic al engineers), presence of staff (clinical dietitians, pharmacists, and physical therapists), proportion of elderly patients (age ≥ 65 years), patients with albumin ≤ 3.5 g/dL, and types of oral nutritional supplements (ONS), intradialytic parenteral nutrition (IDPN), and ET in the facility. We summarized data on facilities and patient characteristics and calculated the proportion of the nutrition that were ONS, IDPN, and exercise interventions provided. We used multiple logistic analyses to examine the facility characteristics associated with the provision of nutritional support and ET.

Results: We obtained responses from 1048 facilities (response rate 26.2%) and 88,492 patients (27.6%). Patients aged ≥ 65 years accounted for 63.4% of all investigated patients. Patients with Alb ≤ 3.5 g/dL accounted for 37.6% of all investigated patients. Meals during hemodialysis sessions were provided at 601 facilities (64%), ONS were used at 382 facilities (40%), and IDPN was administered at 471 facilities (46%). Exercise during hemodialysis sessions was provided at 190 facilities (20%). These trends did not change after adjustment of response rates by affiliations of facility type and region. At the patient level, only a limited number of patients were provided with ONS, IDPN, and ET, 2.1, 2.7, and 3.0%, respectively. ONS and IDPN were less likely to be offered in hospitals than in clinics without beds (odds ratio (OR) 0.21; 95% confidence interval (CI) 0.09–0.45) (OR 0.37; 95% CI 0.17–0.82). ET was also less likely to be offered in hospitals (OR 0.20; 95% CI 0.08–0.49).

Conclusions: Nutritional support therapy is provided in a considerable number of hemodialysis facilities, ET is increasing but offered by fewer facilities compared to other countries, while a limited number of patients were provided with ET.

Keywords: Hemodialysis, Questionnaire, Nutritional therapy, Exercise training, National survey

Background

The aging population features prominently among hemodialysis patients and is influencing the epidemiological characteristics of this patient group. The average age of incident patients and prevalent patients is more than 65 years, and the increase in the dialysis population is currently due to an increase in patients aged 70 years or more [1]. Protein energy wasting (PEW), frailty, and sarcopenia are often found in patients with advanced chronic kidney disease and end-stage kidney disease [2, 3]. These conditions are reportedly associated with each other. Moreover, they are related to higher mortality and morbidity [4–6], especially among elderly individuals in whom physical functions and nutritional status have deteriorated. Older patients are more vulnerable than younger populations to further decline in these parameters [2, 7–9].

In the dialysis population, the two primary options to maintain and even improve nutritional condition and

* Correspondence: hanafusa@twmu.ac.jp
[2]Department of Blood Purification, Kidney Center Tokyo Women's Medical University, 8-1 Kawada-cho, Shinjuku-ku, Tokyo 162-8666, Japan
Full list of author information is available at the end of the article

physical function are nutritional therapy and exercise training (ET), provided either within or outside the dialysis facilities. For nutritional therapy, oral nutritional supplements (ONS) given during hemodialysis can be associated with better survival of dialysis patients [10–13]. In fact, some dialysis facilities offer meals during the sessions [14]. In the USA, dialysis facilities used to restrict eating during hemodialysis, but in recent years, they have been shifting toward allowing patients to eat meals [15]. Many studies and meta-analyses have shown that ET improves physical function, muscular strength, and functional capacity [16–18], although the details of how, when, and to whom ET should be given during hemodialysis sessions remain unclear.

The needs for nutritional therapy and ET in dialysis facilities are expected to continue to increase, as are the numbers of patients requiring such treatment. However, it is not clear how many facilities are offering nutritional therapy and ET, how many patients are receiving them, or what the detailed characteristics of these facilities are. Such information is fundamental and indispensable for the development of strategic plans for managing older dialysis patients.

This study sought to clarify the current status of nutritional therapy and ET interventions provided at hemodialysis facilities in Japan, in order to identify appropriate intervention points and approaches for initiatives at facilities in the future.

Methods

Study design

This was a cross-sectional study conducted using a nationwide questionnaire.

Study population

The study was conducted in member institutions of the Japanese Society for Dialysis Therapy (JSDT). In total, 3993 facilities were registered as member institutions of JSDT as of August 2015. The survey collected data on the facilities and patients receiving maintenance hemodialysis in these facilities during August 2015.

Study protocol

The questionnaire consisted of two parts. The first part contained questions regarding the facility itself, and the second part focused on the nutritional support and ET available at the facility (Additional file 1: Item S1). Questionnaires were sent to each facility by postal mail. We asked that completed questionnaires be returned by fax by the end of October 2015. We also requested that the conditions of dialysis treatments should not be changed while answering this questionnaire.

Data collection

The collected data included the following:

1. Facility details

Type: facility types were classified by their affiliation and size. The classification used by the JSDT annual survey for affiliations of facilities, i.e., national university hospital, private university hospital, national hospital, county municipalities hospital, hospital affiliated to the Japan Community Healthcare Organization, hospital affiliated to Japan Agricultural Cooperatives, other public hospital, private general hospital, private hospital, and private clinic. On the other hand, the original classification of four types according to their sizes were also investigated, i.e. clinic, clinic with beds, hospital (< 200 beds), and hospital (≥ 200 beds). The survey of medical facilities by Ministry of Health Labor and Welfare Japan determines the size of hospitals by the numbers of beds in the facility. The hospitals with 200 or more beds are considered large ones [19].

Region: prefecture and municipality in Japan.

Number of staff: number each of doctors, nurses, and clinical engineers.

Presence/absence of pharmacist, clinical dietitian, and physical therapist providing care for patients on dialysis.

Background of treated patients as a whole: number of patients aged ≥ 65 years, number of patients with albumin ≤ 3.5 g/dL. We used these cut-off values for the reasons as follows. Regarding the age, the elderly persons were defined as having a chronological age of 65 years in many countries including Japan at the time of this survey [20], about albumin level, the European Society for Clinical Nutrition and Metabolism (ESPEN) guideline described serum albumin < 3.5 g/dL as the criteria for severe undernutrition for which nutritional therapy is indicated [21].

2. Intervention provided at hemodialysis facilities: meals, ONS, intradialytic parenteral nutrition (IDPN), and ET

Statistical analyses

Results are summarized as means and standard deviations for data showing a normal distribution, and as medians and interquartile ranges (IQR) for data not showing a normal distribution. Detailed data are shown as numbers and percentages.

The following were excluded from analyses as outliers: facilities where the percentage of aged (≥ 65 years) or albumin ≤ 3.5 g/dL patients exceeded 100%.

Because the response rates, that is the proportion of facility that answered the question, differed by facility type and region, proportions of provision adjusted by affiliations of facility type and region were calculated as an average of the stratum-specific proportions weighted by their own proportion in the population. We used the JSDT classification for facility type adjustment and six districts (Hokkaido and Tohoku, Kanto, Chubu and Tokai, Kansai, Chugoku and Shikoku, and Kyusyu and Okinawa) for region adjustment. Differences between unadjusted and adjusted proportions of interventions provided were compared by a chi-square test.

Multiple logistic analyses were used to explore the factors associated with nutritional support and ET offered by the facility. Dependent variables included the provision of meals, ONS, IDPN, and ET at each facility. The facility-related factors investigated were as follows: facility type (original four types); region (six regions); number of staff (numbers of doctors, nurses, and clinical engineers) presented as quartiles; presence of staff (clinical dietitians, pharmacists, and physical therapists); proportion of elderly patients (age ≥ 65 years); and proportion of patients with albumin ≤ 3.5 g/dL. Reference data were set as follows: size of facility type; clinic without beds, region; Kanto, number of staff; the first quartile values, and presence/absence of staff; absence. We also performed a sensitivity analysis in which per-100-patient staffing level was used instead of actual number of staff as the covariate. In addition, we performed inverse probability of censoring weighted analysis of affiliations of facility type and region specifically for those facilities that provided responses to all items, excluding facilities with logically erroneous data for sensitivity analyses to remove the effect of response rate.

First, we performed multivariate analysis with region and affiliations of facility type as independent variables and actual response rates of these 60 facility groups. Accordingly, regression of facility group against response rate was determined to calculate the response probability of each facility group. Subsequently, a response probability for each facility was assigned based on region and affiliations of facility type. Then, we performed multivariate analysis to investigate factors affecting each therapy, with the reciprocal of the response probability included as the weight for each facility. The proportion of interventions provided was compared between hemodialysis facility groups with response probabilities dichotomized by the median, using the chi-square test to investigate the effects of the provision of interventions on the response probabilities.

We considered $p < 0.05$ statistically significant. All analyses were carried out using JMP Pro 11.0 (SAS Institute, NC, USA).

Ethical issues

The facility name was not specified in the questionnaire. No data that could identify individual patients were collected. Return of the completed questionnaire was deemed as facility consent to participate. This study was conducted in compliance with the Declaration of Helsinki.

Results

In total, 1048 facilities responded to the questionnaire (response rate 26.2%). Regarding facility characteristics, 41.3% of facilities were classed as a "clinic without bed" and 31.9% of facilities were located in the Kanto region (Table 1). The median number of total staff was 18 per facility (Table 2). In almost half of the facilities, pharmacists and physical therapists were working, irrespective of affiliation to the dialysis center, while clinical dietitians were working in 713 facilities (69.6%) (Table 3).

For patient characteristics, data were available regarding 88,492 patients (response rate 27.6%), of which only 9.6% were hospitalized; the remaining 90.4% were outpatients. Elderly patients were predominant, with 63.4% of the patients aged ≥ 65 years. The patients with serum albumin ≤ 3.5 g/dL accounted for 37.6% of all investigated patients. The median number of patients per facility was 70 (IQR 42–110) (Table 4).

Nutritional and exercise interventions provided

Meals during hemodialysis sessions were provided at 601 facilities (63.9%), ONS were used at 382 facilities (39.8%), and IDPN was performed at 471 facilities (45.8%). ET during hemodialysis sessions was provided at 190 facilities (20.2%). These trends did not change after adjustment by facility type and region. In contrast, the actual patient numbers were lower; that is, the proportions of patients who were offered ONS, IDPN, and ET were 2.1, 2.7, and 3.0%, respectively, of the total patients (Table 5) The proportions of the interventions provided in the facility were not associated with the probabilities of response rates for this survey (Additional file 2: Table S2). This fact indicated that the interest in providing these interventions or the interest in responding to this survey might not affect the actual provision of these therapies.

Table 1 Characteristics of facilities

		Number of facilities (%)
Total facilities		1048
Facility type	Clinic	430 (41.3)
	Clinic with beds	120 (11.5)
	Hospital (< 200 beds)	212 (20.4)
	Hospital (≥ 200 beds)	279 (26.8)
	Unanswered	7
Region	Hokkaido, Tohoku	132 (12.8)
	Kanto	328 (31.9)
	Chubu, Tokai	163 (15.9)
	Kansai	169 (16.5)
	Chugoku, Shikoku	101 (9.8)
	Kyushu, Okinawa	135 (13.1)
	Unanswered	20

Table 2 Number of each type of medical staff per facility and per number of patients and per facility

		Number of staff per facility, median (IQR)	Number of staff per number of 10 patients and facility, median (IQR)
Total staff		18 (12–26)	2.5 (1.9–3.5)
Disciplines	Doctor (full-time)	1 (1–3)	0.2 (0.1–0.5)
	Doctor (part-time)	1 (0–4)	0.2 (0–0.5)
	Nurse (full-time)	7 (4–11)	1.1 (0.8–1.6)
	Nurse (part-time)	1 (0–2)	0.1 (0–0.3)
	Clinical engineer (full-time)	4 (1–6)	0.5 (0.3–0.8)
	Clinical engineer (part-time)	0 (0–0)	0 (0–0)

Polymeric formula was the type of ONS most frequently used (56.1%) followed by amino acid formula (31.1%) and formula for kidney failure patients (19.8%) (Fig. 1). Figure 2 indicates the proportions of patients receiving various components of IDPN. More than half of the patients (59.2%) received amino acids only. Most of the patients receiving IDPN (91.3%) were given amino acids in some form; the proportion for glucose or lipids in some form was smaller (29.6 and 17.5%, respectively) (Fig. 2).

The types of ET offered by the facilities were diverse, including resistance training (RT) and aerobic training (AT), with each intervention type accounting for almost one-third of ET. Most patients (81.8%) performed ET three times per week (Fig. 3).

Regarding exercise duration, almost half (50.2%) of the patients performed ET for 15–29 min (Fig. 4). More than half of the facilities that did not offer ET at the time of the study (61.1%) were considering implementation of ET in the future.

Characteristic factors in facilities associated with each therapy

ONS were less likely to be offered in hospitals than in clinics without beds ($p < 0.01$). To our surprise, the presence of a clinical dietitian was not associated with the use of ONS ($p = 0.59$). For IDPN, a similar relationship was observed; the therapy was less likely to be used in large hospitals than in clinics ($p = 0.01$). The presence of pharmacists was not associated with the use of IDPN, similar to the finding for clinical dietitians for ONS ($p = 0.73$). ET was also less likely to be offered in hospitals ($p < 0.01$) and more likely in clinics with beds ($p = 0.03$). The presence of physical therapists was positively associated with the implementation of ET ($p < 0.01$).

Table 3 Facilities with and without relevant staff

	Number of facilities (%)		
	Pharmacist	Clinical dietitian	Physical therapist
With staff working in HD	276 (26.9)	495 (48.3)	200 (19.6)
With staff not working in HD	272 (26.5)	218 (21.3)	314 (30.8)
Without staff	478 (46.6)	312 (30.4)	506 (49.6)

HD hemodialysis

Table 4 Patient characteristics: breakdown of total patients and number of patients per facility

	Number of patients (%)	Number of patients per facility, median (IQR)	Rate of patients per facility (%, mean ± SD)
Total patients	88,492	70 (42–110)	
Inpatients	8501 (9.6)	1 (0–9)	
Outpatients	79,991 (90.4)	64 (34–104)	
Patients aged ≥ 65 years (n = 86,361)	54,770 (63.4)	44 (26–69)	(64.3 ± 14.4)
Patients with albumin ≤3.5 g/dL (n = 86,136)	32,331 (37.6)	24 (11–41)	(37.6 ± 20.4)

IQR interquartile range, *SD* standard deviation

The facilities with higher proportion of the patients aged ≥ 65 years were more likely to use ONS and IDPN. The facilities with higher proportion of the patients with serum albumin ≤ 3.5 g/dL were more likely to use IDPN, but ONS showed no significant difference (Table 6). In the results of the sensitivity analysis, we analyzed the same factors weighted by the reciprocals of the response probabilities and obtained similar results as the original analyses. Moreover, the proportion of the patients with lower albumin levels was positively associated with the implementation of ONS (Table 7). Further sensitivity analysis was conducted using per-100-patient staffing level and indicated similar results, except that the number of doctors was negatively associated with the likelihood of implementation of IDPN and that the number of clinical engineers was no longer significant (Additional file 3: Table S3).

Discussion

This is the first nationwide survey concerning the types of nutritional therapy and ET for patients on hemodialysis in

Table 5 Facilities and patients providing nutritional therapy and exercise training

	Number of patients (%)	Number of facilities	Unadjusted proportion (%)	Adjusted proportion (%)	p value[a]
Meals		601	(61.1)	(63.9)	0.21
ONS	1873 (2.1)	382	(38.9)	(39.8)	0.68
IDPN	2425 (2.7)	471	(45.3)	(45.8)	0.37
Exercise	2682 (3.0)	190	(19.2)	(20.2)	0.57

ONS oral nutritional supplements, *IDPN* intradialytic parenteral nutrition
Proportion of provision was adjusted for facility type and region
[a]Unadjusted vs adjusted

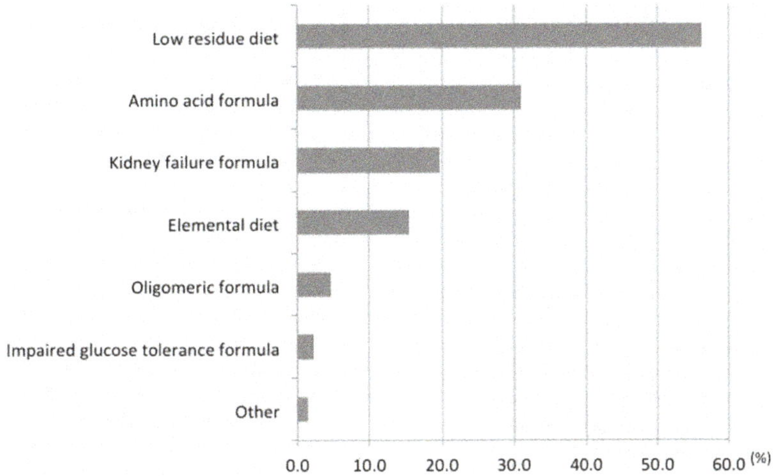

Fig. 1 Types of oral nutritional support. The low residue diet was most commonly used followed by amino acid formula and kidney failure formula. Oral nutritional supplements (ONS) were offered by 399 facilities; however, this answer included multiple answers so the proportion of each component was assessed among 523 answers

Japan. In this study, we adopted age and serum albumin as the patients' characteristics. The proportion of patients aged ≥ 65 years, which was 63.4% in this study, was almost identical to that of 61.8% found by JSDT for the entire Japanese dialysis population [1]. The prevalence of serum albumin < 3.5 g/dL was slightly greater at 37.5% in the present study than the 33.8% reported in a JSDT survey [22], a difference that may be due to the inclusion or exclusion of patients with serum albumin equal to 3.5 g/dL.

Approximately 40% of all facilities were administering ONS, predominantly the low residue diet that can be reimbursed by health insurance in Japan and has a well-balanced nutrient composition. About 50% of all facilities were offering IDPN. These results were independent of response probability. Although the typical composition of IDPN reported in the literature is a mixture of glucose, amino acids, and lipid emulsion [23], most facilities in the present study used only the amino acid formula for IDPN. This is possibly because the staff focused on the amino acids removed by the dialysis procedure [24]. Other reasons could be the higher costs of lipid emulsion compared with amino acid formula, as well as the time and labor required by medical staff to mix the components for IDPN preparations.

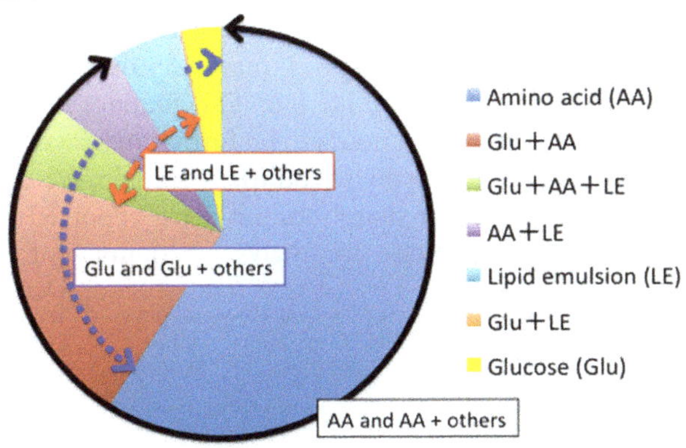

Fig. 2 Types of intradialytic parenteral nutrition. Proportion of each component and the mixtures used among the 2425 patients receiving intradialytic parenteral nutrition (IDPN) are shown. The amino acids formula alone was the most commonly used (59.0%). Including the combination of amino acids with glucose or lipid emulsion, 91.3% of patients received IDPN containing amino acids (black arc with arrows at both ends). On the other hand, 29.6% of the patients received IDPN containing glucose (blue scattered arc with arrows), and only 17.5% received IDPN containing lipids (red arc with arrows). Abbreviations: AA, amino acids; Glu, glucose; LE, lipid emulsion

ONS administration may be associated with better survival [12]. Although IDPN did not have an additive effect to ONS in malnourished dialyzed patients [25], IDPN works to facilitate protein anabolism in patients receiving long-term hemodialysis in the acute phase [26]. This is evidenced by significant concomitant increases in lean body mass and albumin synthesis in the liver [27]. Therefore, both ONS and IDPN can potentially ameliorate malnutrition. In the present study, the proportion of patients treated by nutritional therapy was as small as 2%, while the proportion of patients with serum albumin ≤ 3.5 g/dL was as high as 37.5%. Therefore, it is possible that patients who should have been treated by nutritional therapy did not receive it. However, hypoalbuminemia is not the sole indication for nutritional therapy, and this criterion could overestimate the actual proportion of patients needing nutritional therapy. Further clarification of the indications for nutritional therapy is required in actual clinical practice. A positive point to note, however, is that logistic analysis showed nutritional therapy is being administered to patients with low nutrition in some facilities in Japan.

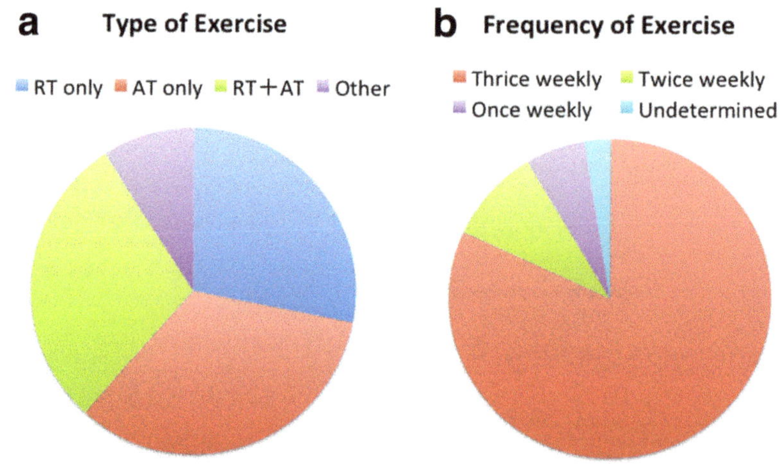

Fig. 3 Types and frequency of exercise training. Approximately 30% of patients underwent resistance training (RT) alone, aerobic training (AT) alone, or RT and AT (A). Further, 82% of patients exercised three times per week (B)

ET was enforced in about 20% of the facilities, and only 3% of all the patients were receiving ET. Patients on dialysis have extremely limited exercise capacity and poor physical functioning [28]. It has been reported that sedentary behavior in patients on hemodialysis is associated with an increased risk of death within 1 year even after adjusting for all covariates [29]. However, ET might increase aerobic capacity, muscle mass or strength, physical quality of life, and Kt/V [16, 30]. Additionally, ET during dialysis therapy is associated with few adverse events [16, 31, 32]. However, a study from the Dialysis Outcomes and Practice Patterns Study (DOPPS) showed that the percentage of units offering exercise programs was 14% in Japan from 2009 to 2011, while 27 and 37% of the facilities offered ET in Europe or Australia/New Zealand and in North America, respectively [33]. This difference between DOPPS and our study might indicate an increase in the facilities offering ET over the last few years, as the benefits of ET have become widely accepted.

ET performed on non-dialysis days is reportedly the most effective way of training, although difficulties in maintaining adherence have been demonstrated [34]. In the present study, a limited number of facilities (up to 20%) provided ET on hemodialysis days and only 9% provided ET on non-hemodialysis days. DOPPS showed that the proportion of facilities providing ET on dialysis and non-dialysis days was about 10% in japan from 2005 to 2006 [35]. After a decade, we found the facilities offering the exercise program on dialysis is increasing as discussed above, but the facilities offering ET on non-dialysis days have not increased. Recently it reported that two daily 10-min walking sessions during the off-dialysis days (every second day for patients on peritoneal dialysis) at a prescribed walking speed may improve physical performance and quality of life [36]. Our findings indicate that the awareness of ET needs to be further improved.

Each intervention type accounting for almost one-third of ET. Recently many studies have reported the evidences about exercise for dialysis patients. But the

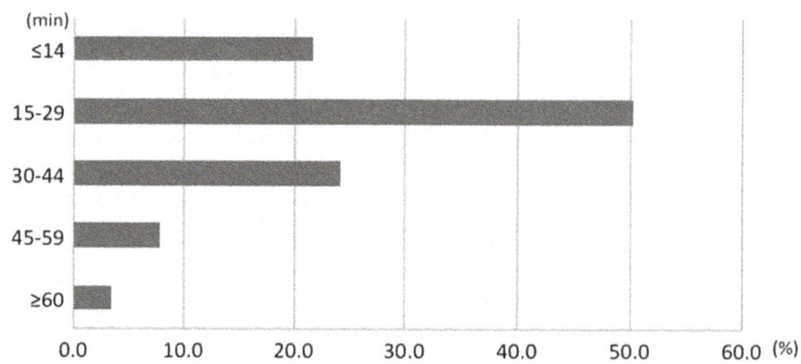

Fig. 4 Exercise duration. Half of the patients underwent exercise for 15–29 min during a single session

Table 6 Logistic regression analysis

Variable		ONS			IDPN			Exercise		
		OR	(95% CI)	*p* value	OR	(95% CI)	*p* value	OR	(95% CI)	*p* value
Clinic		1	reference		1	reference		1	reference	
Clinic with beds		0.66	0.38–1.11	0.12	1.15	0.68–1.96	0.60	0.50	0.28–0.95	0.03
Hospital (< 200 beds)		0.49	0.22–1.05	0.07	0.50	0.23–1.10	0.08	0.20	0.08–0.49	< 0.01
Hospital (≥ 200 beds)		0.21	0.09–0.45	< 0.001	0.37	0.17–0.82	0.01	0.08	0.03–0.20	< 0.001
Doctor	Q1	1	reference		1	reference		1	reference	
	Q2	0.95	0.59–1.53	0.83	0.76	0.48–1.21	0.25	0.85	0.46–1.63	0.62
	Q3	0.62	0.37–1.05	0.08	0.64	0.38–1.07	0.09	0.97	0.50–1.94	0.94
	Q4	0.85	0.50–1.45	0.55	0.86	0.51–1.45	0.56	1.39	0.71–2.79	0.34
Nurse	Q1	1	reference		1	reference		1	reference	
	Q2	1.21	0.81–1.84	0.36	0.83	0.55–1.24	0.36	1.00	0.56–1.79	1.00
	Q3	1.71	1.14–2.60	0.01	1.70	1.14–2.56	< 0.01	1.66	0.98–2.83	0.06
	Q4	1.64	1.03–2.60	0.04	1.71	1.08–2.70	0.02	1.58	0.90–2.81	0.11
Clinical engineer	Q1	1	reference		1	reference		1	reference	
	Q2	1.17	0.67–2.06	0.58	1.51	0.88–2.63	0.13	1.59	0.73–3.80	0.25
	Q3	1.92	1.09–3.44	0.03	2.65	1.51–4.71	< 0.001	1.95	0.88–4.72	0.10
	Q4	2.76	1.56–5.00	< 0.001	3.32	1.88–5.95	< 0.001	5.93	2.76–14.03	< 0.001
Presence of pharmacist (vs absence)		0.99	0.54–1.81	0.98	0.90	0.49–1.66	0.73	1.03	0.50–2.07	0.93
Presence of clinical dietitian (vs absence)		1.13	0.73–1.73	0.59	1.01	0.65–1.55	0.97	1.94	1.15–3.29	0.01
Presence of physical therapist (vs absence)		1.84	1.05–3.28	0.03	1.95	1.09–3.55	0.02	3.48	1.85–6.66	< 0.001
Regions	Hokkaido/Tohoku	0.79	0.44–1.27	0.29	1.58	0.95–2.64	0.08	2.85	1.48–5.46	< 0.01
	Kanto	1	reference		1	reference		1	reference	
	Chubu/Tokai	1.01	0.63–1.60	0.97	1.62	1.03–2.58	0.04	2.05	1.12–3.73	0.02
	Kansai	1.00	0.64–1.56	1.00	1.76	1.13–2.76	0.01	1.98	1.10–3.52	0.02
	Chugoku/Shikoku	0.90	0.51–1.57	0.71	1.51	0.87–2.63	0.15	2.03	0.97–4.16	0.06
	Kyushu/Okinawa	0.76	0.44–1.30	0.31	0.72	0.42–1.23	0.23	2.69	1.37–5.29	<0.01
Patients aged ≥ 65 years (per 10%)		1.14	1.01–1.28	0.03	1.16	1.03–1.30	0.01	1.07	0.93–1.25	0.35
Patients with albumin ≤ 3.5 g/dL (per 10%)		1.03	0.95–1.12	0.44	1.09	1.01–1.17	0.03	0.95	0.86–1.05	0.35

Abbreviations: *OR* odds ratio, *CI*, confidence interval

best way to offer ET in dialysis patients remains unclear. The current study demonstrated that the actual types of ET were diverse across the facility offering ET. Many investigations have employed ET as an intervention for at least 30 min, three times a week [16]. The duration of ET in Japanese facilities was found to be shorter in this study, possibly because the Japanese dialysis population investigated here was older than that in the reported clinical trials (aged 40–50 years) [16].

DOPPS reported an important finding: patients who exercise regularly showed better survival than those who do not (HR 0.73, 95% CI 0.69–0.78); moreover, patients who received treatment at a facility with a higher frequency of exercise also had better survival (HR per 10% increase in regularly exercising patients 0.92, 95% CI 0.89–0.94) [35]. These results demonstrate that the practice patterns implemented in a facility could affect the clinical outcomes of patients treated at that facility. So it is important for every dialysis facility to be aware of the usefulness and safety of ET in order to prevent PEW progression to further unfavorable outcomes. In fact, over half of the total facilities included in this survey intended to offer ET.

The present investigation into the background factors relating to the implementation of these therapies indicated that clinics tend to offer such therapies rather than hospitals. In general, clinics without beds manage larger numbers of chronic patients over longer terms, enabling them to provide these therapies more frequently than the other facility types. In contrast, we can consider that the patients in hospitals have different characteristics from those in clinics; they require the treatment for acute conditions because the hospitalized

Table 7 Logistic regression analysis with inverse probability of response rate weighting for facility type and region

Variable		ONS			IDPN			Exercise		
		OR	(95% CI)	*p* value	OR	(95% CI)	*p* value	OR	(95% CI)	*p* value
Clinic		1	reference		1	reference		1	reference	
Clinic with beds		0.68	0.52–0.88	< 0.01	1.18	0.96–1.54	0.22	0.56	0.41–0.78	< 0.001
Hospital (< 200 beds)		0.51	0.36–0.73	< 0.001	0.59	0.41–0.85	< 0.01	0.24	0.16–0.37	< 0.001
Hospital (≥ 200 beds)		0.22	0.15–0.33	< 0.001	0.43	029–0.64	< 0.001	0.10	0.06–0.16	< 0.001
Doctor	Q1	1	reference		1	reference		1	reference	
	Q2	0.94	0.74–1.18	0.56	0.89	0.71–1.12	0.33	0.88	0.65–1.20	0.41
	Q3	0.59	0.46–0.76	< 0.001	0.66	0.52–0.85	< 0.01	0.88	0.64–1.23	0.46
	Q4	0.85	0.66–1.09	0.20	0.84	0.65–1.08	0.18	1.64	1.19–2.30	< 0.01
Nurse	Q1	1	reference		1	reference		1	reference	
	Q2	1.07	0.87–1.30	0.52	0.89	0.73–1.08	0.23	1.14	0.87–1.51	0.34
	Q3	1.65	1.35–2.01	< 0.001	1.76	1.45–2.14	< 0.001	1.73	1.34–2.24	< 0.001
	Q4	1.62	1.30–2.01	< 0.001	1.69	1.35–2.10	< 0.001	1.70	1.30–2.24	< 0.01
Clinical engineer	Q1	1	reference		1	reference		1	reference	
	Q2	1.10	0.85–1.43	0.47	1.46	1.13–1.89	< 0.01	1.77	1.21–2.65	< 0.01
	Q3	1.84	1.41–2.42	< 0.001	2.74	2.10–3.60	< 0.001	1.93	1.30–2.93	< 0.01
	Q4	2.66	1.41–3.51	< 0.001	3.36	2.56–4.44	< 0.001	6.36	4.34–9.52	< 0.001
Presence of pharmacist (vs absence)		1.05	0.78–1.41	0.76	0.81	0.60–1.10	0.17	1.04	0.74–1.47	0.80
Presence of clinical dietitian (vs absence)		1.13	0.91–1.40	0.26	1.02	0.82–1.27	0.83	2.05	1.58–2.66	< 0.001
Presence of physical therapist (vs absence)		1.76	1.36–2.29	< 0.001	1.97	1.51–2.59	< 0.001	2.41	1.80–3.25	< 0.001
Regions	Hokkaido/Tohoku	0.69	0.54–1.27	< 0.01	1.60	1.24–2.07	< 0.001	2.86	2.06–3.96	< 0.001
	Kanto	1	reference		1	reference		1	reference	
	Chubu/Tokai	0.99	0.72–1.12	0.33	1.52	1.23–1.90	< 0.001	2.33	1.76–3.07	< 0.001
	Kansai	1.00	0.80–1.23	0.92	1.53	1.24–1.91	< 0.001	1.77	1.33–2.34	< 0.001
	Chugoku/Shikoku	0.71	0.55–0.92	< 0.01	1.35	1.05–1.75	0.02	2.40	1.72–3.33	< 0.001
	Kyushu/Okinawa	0.63	0.49–0.81	< 0.001	0.63	0.49–0.81	< 0.001	3.00	2.20–4.09	< 0.001
Patients aged ≥ 65 years (per 10%)		1.13	1.07–1.20	< 0.001	1.22	1.16–1.30	< 0.001	1.04	0.96–1.11	0.34
Patients with albumin ≤3.5 g/dL (per 10%)		1.04	1.00–1.08	0.03	1.09	1.06–1.14	<0.001	0.98	0.93–1.03	0.36

Abbreviations: *OR* odds ratio, *CI* confidence interval

patients in other nephrology department tend to have many comorbidities.

The results obtained from the analyses where staff number was standardized by patient number confirmed that IDPN is being predominantly offered in clinics without beds.

Interestingly, our results indicate that the number of staff—key elements of each facility—was positively correlated with the implementation of nutritional therapy or ET. In particular, the results obtained from the analyses standardized by facility type and region revealed stronger associations between these factors.

Curiously, the proportions of the older patients or the patients with lower albumin levels were positively associated with the implementation of ONS or IDPN. On the other hand, ET did not have such associations with the proportions of the patients with such background. This fact shows the medical director of the facility might have different criteria to implement ET from those for ONS and IDPN.

Surprisingly, the provision of ONS or IDPN was independent of the presence of dietitians or pharmacists in the facility. This might indicate these therapies might be readily available irrespective of the professionals available, although the involvement of dietitians or pharmacists might improve the quality or effectiveness of these therapies.

There are several limitations to this study. The first is that this observational study did not examine the data of individual patients. Therefore, we could not investigate the detailed relationship between patient characteristics and the interventions or clinical outcomes. However, the aim of the study was to investigate the overall status of these therapies in Japan, which has not been investigated previously. Second, the response rate for the questionnaire was not high 26% of all facilities. Although detailed patient characteristics were not investigated and we cannot eliminate the effects of differences in patients characteristics between responded and non-responded facilities, the proportions of older patients or the patients with albumin of 3.5 g/dl or less were not virtually different from the entire dialysis population in Japan. On the other hand, the response rate did differ across the facility types. However, adjustment by affiliations of facility type or region yielded no significant differences in the proportion of facilities offering these interventions.

Conclusions

Many hemodialysis facilities provided nutritional intervention and for ET are also increasing, while a limited number of patients provided ET. And the number of staff was positively correlated with the implementation of nutritional therapy or ET. We consider it important to assess the indications for nutritional therapies and ET for each patient appropriately and to provide patients with appropriate and detailed knowledge about such therapies for their proper and wider use. Moreover, the standardization of nutritional therapy and ET is needed in the future.

Abbreviations

95% CI: 95% confidence interval; AA: Amino acids; AT: Aerobic training; DOPPS: The Dialysis Outcomes and Practice Patterns Study; ESPEN: The European Society for Clinical Nutrition and Metabolism; Glu: Glucose; IDPN: Intradialytic parenteral nutrition; IQR: Interquartile ranges; JSDT: The Japanese Society for Dialysis Therapy; LE: Lipid emulsion; ONS: Oral nutritional supplements; OR: Odds ratio; PEW: Protein energy wasting; RT: Resistance training

Acknowledgements

We are grateful to all the staff who took time responding to the questionnaire. The abstract of this article was presented at the 17th International Congress on Nutrition and Metabolism in Renal Disease, Okinawa, in April 2016; the 61st Annual Meeting of the Japanese Society for Dialysis Therapy, Osaka, in June 2016; and the 4th the Japanese Society on Renal Nutrition and Metabolism, Kobe, in June 2016.

Funding

None to declare.

Authors' contributions

SS and NH designed the study, collected and analyzed the data, and wrote the draft version of the manuscript. SI and RM contributed to the questionnaire design. SI contributed to the data analysis. HK, RM, and MN reviewed and finalized the manuscript for intellectual content. All authors read and approved the final manuscript.

Competing interests

Satoko Sakurai: none. Norio Hanafusa: NH received research funding from Meiji Co., Ltd., a manufacturer of oral nutritional supplements and was also a former member of a division that is funded by Terumo Corporation. However, this study has no association with that funding and the relationship did not affect the interpretation of this study's results. Hideki Kato: none. Shinji Iizaka: none. Ryoko Murayama: RM is a member of a division that is funded by Terumo Corporation. However, this study has no association with that funding and the relationship did not affect the interpretation of this study's results. Masaomi Nangaku: MN served as consultancy or advisory boards of Akebia, Bayer, Kyowa Hakko Kirin, Daiichi Sankyo, Astellas, Taisho, Mitsubishi Tanabe, JT, speaker bureaus of Kyowa Hakko Kirin, Daiichi Sankyo, MSD, Astellas, AstraZeneca, Alexion, Mitsubishi Tanabe, JT, and Chugai. However, this study has no association with that funding and the relationship did not affect the interpretation of this study's results. This research did not receive any specific grant from funding agencies in the public, commercial, or not-for-profit sectors.

Author details

[1]Division of Nephrology and Endocrinology, The University of Tokyo Graduate School of Medicine, Tokyo, Japan. [2]Department of Blood Purification, Kidney Center Tokyo Women's Medical University, 8-1 Kawada-cho, Shinjuku-ku, Tokyo 162-8666, Japan. [3]School of Nutrition, College of Nursing and Nutrition, Shukutoku University, Chiba, Japan. [4]Department of Advanced Nursing Technology, The University of Tokyo Graduate School of Medicine, Tokyo, Japan.

References

1. Masakane I, Nakai S, Ogata S, et al. An overview of regular dialysis treatment in Japan (as of 31 December 2013). Ther Apher Dial. 2015;19:540–74.
2. Cruz-Jentoft AJ, Baeyens JP, Bauer JM, et al. Sarcopenia: European consensus on definition and diagnosis: report of the European working group on sarcopenia in older people. Age Ageing. 2010;39:412–23.
3. Fried LP, Tangen CM, Walston J, et al. Frailty in older adults: evidence for a phenotype. J Gerontol A Biol Sci Med Sci. 2001;56:M146–56.
4. Isoyama N, Qureshi AR, Avesani CM, et al. Comparative associations of muscle mass and muscle strength with mortality in dialysis patients. Clin J Am Soc Nephrol. 2014;9:1720–8.
5. Johansen KL, Chertow GM, Jin C, Kutner NG. Significance of frailty among dialysis patients. J Am Soc Nephrol. 2007;18:2960–7.
6. Kalantar-Zadeh K, Kilpatrick RD, Kuwae N, et al. Revisiting mortality predictability of serum albumin in the dialysis population: time dependency, longitudinal changes and population-attributable fraction. Nephrol Dial Transplant. 2005;20:1880–8.
7. Kim JC, Kalantar-Zadeh K, Kopple JD. Frailty and protein-energy wasting in elderly patients with end stage kidney disease. J Am Soc Nephrol. 2013;24:337–51.
8. Fouque D, Kalantar-Zadeh K, Kopple J, et al. A proposed nomenclature and diagnostic criteria for protein-energy wasting in acute and chronic kidney disease. Kidney Int. 2008;73:391–8.
9. Rockwood K, Stadnyk K, MacKnight C, McDowell I, Hebert R, Hogan DB. A brief clinical instrument to classify frailty in elderly people. Lancet. 1999;353:205–6.
10. Sohrabi Z, Eftekhari MH, Eskandari MH, Rezaianzadeh A, Sagheb MM. Intradialytic oral protein supplementation and nutritional and inflammation outcomes in hemodialysis: a randomized controlled trial. Am J Kidney Dis. 2016;68:122–30.
11. Weiner DE, Tighiouart H, Ladik V, Meyer KB, Zager PG, Johnson DS. Oral intradialytic nutritional supplement use and mortality in hemodialysis patients. Am J Kidney Dis. 2014;63:276–85.
12. Lacson E Jr, Wang W, Zebrowski B, Wingard R, Hakim RM. Outcomes associated with intradialytic oral nutritional supplements in patients undergoing maintenance hemodialysis: a quality improvement report. Am J Kidney Dis. 2012;60:591–600.
13. Caglar K, Fedje L, Dimmitt R, Hakim RM, Shyr Y, Ikizler TA. Therapeutic effects of oral nutritional supplementation during hemodialysis. Kidney Int. 2002;62:1054–9.
14. Kistler B, Benner D, Burgess M, Stasios M, Kalantar-Zadeh K, Wilund KR. To eat or not to eat-international experiences with eating during hemodialysis treatment. J Ren Nutr. 2014;24:349–52.

15. Benner D, Burgess M, Stasios M, et al. In-center nutrition practices of clinics within a large hemodialysis provider in the United States. Clin J Am Soc Nephrol. 2016;11:770–5.
16. Sheng K, Zhang P, Chen L, Cheng J, Wu C, Chen J. Intradialytic exercise in hemodialysis patients: a systematic review and meta-analysis. Am J Nephrol. 2014;40:478–90.
17. Heiwe S, Jacobson SH. Exercise training in adults with CKD: a systematic review and meta-analysis. Am J Kidney Dis. 2014;64:383–93.
18. Segura-Orti E. Exercise in haemodyalisis patients: a literature systematic review. Nefrologia. 2010;30:236–46.
19. Military of Health Labour and Welfare. Survey of Medical facilities 2013. [http://www.mhlw.go.jp/toukei/saikin/hw/iryosd/13/dl/1-1.pdf] Accessed 1 Sep 2017.
20. Ouchi Y, Rakugi H, Arai H, et al. Redefining the elderly as aged 75 years and older: proposal from the Joint Committee of Japan Gerontological Society and the Japan Geriatrics Society. Geriatr Gerontol Int. 2017;17:1045–7.
21. Cano NJ, Aparicio M, Brunori G, et al. ESPEN guidelines on parenteral nutrition: adult renal failure. Clin Nutr. 2009;28:401–14.
22. Japanese Society for Dialysis Therapy. An overview of regular dialysis treatment in Japan as of Dec.31 2015. [http://member.jsdt.or.jp/member/contents/cdrom/2015/pdf/chohyo/IMP04176.pdf] Accessed 1 Sep 2017.
23. Fouque D. Causes and interventions for malnutrition in patients undergoing maintenance dialysis. Blood Purif. 1997;15:112–20.
24. Ikizler TA, Flakoll PJ, Parker RA, Hakim RM. Amino acid and albumin losses during hemodialysis. Kidney Int. 1994;46:830–7.
25. Cano NJ, Fouque D, Roth H, et al. Intradialytic parenteral nutrition does not improve survival in malnourished hemodialysis patients: a 2-year multicenter, prospective, randomized study. J Am Soc Nephrol. 2007;18:2583–91.
26. Hiroshige K, Iwamoto M, Kabashima N, Mutoh Y, Yuu K, Ohtani A. Prolonged use of intradialysis parenteral nutrition in elderly malnourished chronic haemodialysis patients. Nephrol Dial Transplant. 1998;13:2081–7.
27. Pupim LB, Flakoll PJ, Ikizler TA. Nutritional supplementation acutely increases albumin fractional synthetic rate in chronic hemodialysis patients. J Am Soc Nephrol. 2004;15:1920–6.
28. Johansen KL. Physical functioning and exercise capacity in patients on dialysis. Adv Ren Replace Ther. 1999;6:141–8.
29. O'Hare AM, Tawney K, Bacchetti P, Johansen KL. Decreased survival among sedentary patients undergoing dialysis: results from the dialysis morbidity and mortality study wave 2. Am J Kidney Dis. 2003;41:447–54.
30. Ikizler TA. Exercise as an anabolic intervention in patients with end-stage renal disease. J Ren Nutr. 2011;21:52–6.
31. Smart N, Steele M. Exercise training in haemodialysis patients: a systematic review and meta-analysis. Nephrol (Carlton). 2011;16:626–32.
32. Cheema BS, Singh MA. Exercise training in patients receiving maintenance hemodialysis: a systematic review of clinical trials. Am J Nephrol. 2005;25:352–64.
33. Lopes AA, Lantz B, Morgenstern H, et al. Associations of self-reported physical activity types and levels with quality of life, depression symptoms, and mortality in hemodialysis patients: the DOPPS. Clin J Am Soc Nephrol. 2014;9:1702–12.
34. Konstantinidou E, Koukouvou G, Kouidi E, Deligiannis A, Tourkantonis A. Exercise training in patients with end-stage renal disease on hemodialysis: comparison of three rehabilitation programs. J Rehabil Med. 2002;34:40–5.
35. Tentori F, Elder SJ, Thumma J, et al. Physical exercise among participants in the dialysis outcomes and practice patterns study (DOPPS): correlates and associated outcomes. Nephrol Dial Transplant. 2010;25:3050–62.
36. Manfredini F, Mallamaci F, D'Arrigo G, et al. Exercise in patients on dialysis: a multicenter, randomized clinical trial. J Am Soc Nephrol. 2017;28:1259–68.

Permissions

All chapters in this book were first published in RRT, by BioMed Central; hereby published with permission under the Creative Commons Attribution License or equivalent. Every chapter published in this book has been scrutinized by our experts. Their significance has been extensively debated. The topics covered herein carry significant findings which will fuel the growth of the discipline. They may even be implemented as practical applications or may be referred to as a beginning point for another development.

The contributors of this book come from diverse backgrounds, making this book a truly international effort. This book will bring forth new frontiers with its revolutionizing research information and detailed analysis of the nascent developments around the world.

We would like to thank all the contributing authors for lending their expertise to make the book truly unique. They have played a crucial role in the development of this book. Without their invaluable contributions this book wouldn't have been possible. They have made vital efforts to compile up to date information on the varied aspects of this subject to make this book a valuable addition to the collection of many professionals and students.

This book was conceptualized with the vision of imparting up-to-date information and advanced data in this field. To ensure the same, a matchless editorial board was set up. Every individual on the board went through rigorous rounds of assessment to prove their worth. After which they invested a large part of their time researching and compiling the most relevant data for our readers.

The editorial board has been involved in producing this book since its inception. They have spent rigorous hours researching and exploring the diverse topics which have resulted in the successful publishing of this book. They have passed on their knowledge of decades through this book. To expedite this challenging task, the publisher supported the team at every step. A small team of assistant editors was also appointed to further simplify the editing procedure and attain best results for the readers.

Apart from the editorial board, the designing team has also invested a significant amount of their time in understanding the subject and creating the most relevant covers. They scrutinized every image to scout for the most suitable representation of the subject and create an appropriate cover for the book.

The publishing team has been an ardent support to the editorial, designing and production team. Their endless efforts to recruit the best for this project, has resulted in the accomplishment of this book. They are a veteran in the field of academics and their pool of knowledge is as vast as their experience in printing. Their expertise and guidance has proved useful at every step. Their uncompromising quality standards have made this book an exceptional effort. Their encouragement from time to time has been an inspiration for everyone.

The publisher and the editorial board hope that this book will prove to be a valuable piece of knowledge for researchers, students, practitioners and scholars across the globe.

List of Contributors

Taro Horino, Yoshiko Shimamura, Koji Ogata, Kosuke Inoue and Yoshio Terada
Department of Endocrinology, Metabolism and Nephrology, Kochi Medical School, Kohasu, Okoh-cho, Nankoku 783-8505, Kochi, Japan

Kazuo Kimura, Shigeru Otsubo and Kosaku Nitta
Department of Medicine, Kidney Center, Tokyo Women's Medical University, Tokyo, Japan

Takashi Akiba and Kazuo Kimura
Department of Nephrology, Sekikawa Hospital, Tokyo, Japan

Katsuya Kajimoto
Department of Cardiology, Sekikawa Hospital, Tokyo, Japan

Shigeru Otsubo
Department of Blood Purification, Tohto Sangenjaya Clinic, 2-13-2 Taishido, Setagaya-ku, Tokyo 154-0004, Japan

Shoichiro Daimon
Department of Nephrology, Daimon Clinic for Internal Medicine, Nephrology and Dialysis, Oshino 1-400, Nonoichi 921-8802, Japan

Ichiro Mizushima
Division of Rheumatology, Department of Internal Medicine, Kanazawa University Graduate School of Medicine, Kanazawa, Japan

Kentaro Wada
Division of Nephrology and Dialysis, Department of Internal Medicine, Nippon Kokan Fukuyama Hospital, 1844, Tsunoshita, Daimon-cho, Fukuyama, Hiroshima 721-0927, Japan

Haruhito A. Uchida
Department of Chronic Kidney Disease and Cardiovascular Disease, Okayama University Graduate School of Medicine, Dentistry and Pharmaceutical Sciences, Okayama, Japan

Yuko Wada
Division of Nephrology and Dialysis, Department of Internal Medicine, Central Hospital, Hiroshima, Japan

Yoshifumi Abe, Atsuhiko Matsunaga, Kei Yoneki, Manae Harada, Takaaki Watanabe and Kyo Shigeta
Department of Rehabilitation Sciences, Kitasato University Graduate School of Medical Sciences, 1-15-1 Kitasato, Sagamihara, Kanagawa 252-0373, Japan

Ryota Matsuzawa
Department of Rehabilitation, Kitasato University Hospital, Sagamihara, Kanagawa, Japan

Atsushi Yoshida and Kei Yoneki
Sagami Junkanki Clinic, Sagamihara, Kanagawa, Japan

Toshiki Kutsuna
Department of Rehabilitation, Kitasato University East Hospital, Sagamihara, Kanagawa, Japan

Masahiko Kimura
School of Allied Health Sciences, Kitasato University, Sagamihara, Kanagawa, Japan

Yasuo Takeuchi
School of Medicine, Kitasato University, Sagamihara, Kanagawa, Japan

Satoru Mitsuboshi, Hitoshi Yamada and Kazuhiko Nagai
Department of Pharmacy, Kaetsu Hospital, 1459-1 Higashikanazawa, Akiha-ku, Niigata-shi, Niigata 956-0814, Japan

Hideo Okajima
Department of Internal Medicine, Kaetsu Hospital, 1459-1 Higashikanazawa, Akiha-ku, Niigata-shi, Niigata 956-0814, Japan

Hirotoshi Kodama, Akihiro Fujinoki and Tatsuo Inoue
Division of Blood Purification Center, Kamifukuoka General Hospital, 931 Fukuoka, Fujimino, Saitama 356-0011, Japan

Akira Tsuji, Koujirou Ooshima and Kaori Ishizeki
Department of Blood Purification, National Defense Medical College Hospital, 3-2 Namiki, Tokorozawa, Saitama 359-8513, Japan

Takaaki Watanabe, Toshiki Kutsuna, Kei Yoneki, Manae Harada, Takahiro Shimoda and Atsuhiko Matsunaga
Department of Rehabilitation Sciences, Kitasato University Graduate School of Medical Sciences, 1-15-1 Kitasato, Sagamihara, Kanagawa 252-0373, Japan

Toshiki Kutsuna
Department of Physical Therapy, School of Health Sciences, Tokyo University of Technology, 5-23-22 Nishikamata, Ota-ku, Tokyo 144-8535, Japan

Yusuke Matsunaga
Department of Sleep Medicine, Kitasato University Graduate School of Medical Sciences, 1-15-1 Kitasato, Sagamihara, Kanagawa 252-0373, Japan

Norio Murayama
School of Allied Health Sciences, Kitasato University, 1-15-1 Kitasato, Sagamihara, Kanagawa 252-0373, Japan

Ryota Matsuzawa
Department of Rehabilitation, Kitasato University Hospital, 1-15-1 Kitasato, Sagamihara, Kanagawa 252-0375, Japan

Yasuo Takeuchi
Department of Nephrology in Internal Medicine, Kitasato University School of Medicine, 1-15-1 Kitasato, Sagamihara, Kanagawa 252-0373, Japan

Atsushi Yoshida
Department of Hemodialysis Center, Sagami Circulatory Organ Clinic, 4-21-15 Sonan, Sagamihara, Kanagawa 252-0312, Japan

Shoichiro Daimon
Department of Nephrology, Daimon Clinic for Internal Medicine, Nephrology and Dialysis, Oshino 1-400, Nonoichi, Ishikawa-pref 921-8802, Japan

Hiromi Nuka, Kinya Kitada, Yasunori Suzuki, Fae Kim and Mitsuhiro Kawano
Division of Rheumatology, Department of Internal Medicine, Kanazawa University Graduate School of Medicine, Kanazawa, Japan

Kenji Maeda and Toshiro Iida
Daiko Sunadabashi Clinic, Nagoya, Japan

Shigehito Yoshizaki
Daiko Sunadabashi Branch Clinic, Nagoya, Japan

Tomoyoshi Terada and Seiichi Era
Department of Physiology and Biophysics, Graduate School of Medicine, Gifu University, Gifu, Japan

Keiichiro Sakashita
Laboratory of Dialysis Medical Care and Technology, Nagoya, Japan

Hajime Arikawa
Department of Early Childhood Education, Chubu Gakuin College, Seki, Gifu, Japan

Takashi Shigematsu
Department of Nephrology, Wakayama Medical University, Wakayama 641-8509, Japan

Jun Minakuchi
Department of Nephrology and Blood Purification, Kawashima Hospital, Tokushima, Japan

Satoshi Funakoshi
Department of Nephrology and Blood Purification, Nagasaki Jin Hospital, Nagasaki, Japan

Junichiro Hashiguchi
Department of Blood Purification, Nagasaki Jin Clinic, Nagasaki, Japan

Hiroshi Yoshimoto
Division of Nephrology and Dialysis, Department of Medicine, Social Insurance Chuo General Hospital, Tokyo, Japan

Kyoko Ito
Department of Blood Purification, Heisei Hidaka Clinic, Takasaki, Japan

Takuya Ban and Tetsunosuke Kunitomo
Toray Medical Co., Ltd., Tokyo, Japan

Kentaro Wada
Division of Nephrology and Dialysis, Department of Internal Medicine, Nippon Kokan Fukuyama Hospital, 1844, Tsunoshita, Daimon-cho, Fukuyama City, Hiroshima 721-0927, Japan

Haruhito A. Uchida
Department of Chronic Kidney Disease and Cardiovascular Disease, Okayama University Graduate School of Medicine, Dentistry and Pharmaceutical Sciences, Okayama, Japan

Yuko Wada
Division of Nephrology and Dialysis, Department of Internal Medicine, Central Hospital, Hiroshima, Japan

Satoko Oyama, Chihiro Hirose, Kenichiro Hori, Katsuhiro Sugano, Jie Zhang and Kimio Tomita
The Chronic Kidney Disease Research Center, Tomei Atsugi Hospital, 232, Funako, Atsugi City, Kanagawa 243-8571, Japan

Miyuki Tamura
Pharmaceutical Research Laboratories, Sanwa Kagaku Kenkyusho Co., Ltd., Nagoya 461-8631, Japan

Kojiro Nagai, Sayo Ueda and Toshio Doi
Department of Nephrology, Institute of Biomedical Sciences, Tokushima University Graduate School, Tokushima, Japan

Kenji Tsuchida
Department of Dialysis Vascular Surgery, Tsuchida Dialysis Access Clinic, Osaka, Japan

Jun Minakuchi
Department of Kidney Disease (Dialysis & Transplantation), Kawashima Hospital, Tokushima, Japan

Kojiro Nagai
Tokushima University Graduate School, 3-18-15, Kuramoto-cho, Tokushima 770-8503, Japan

Kenji Tsuchida
Tsuchida Dialysis Access Clinic, 2-10-18, Fujiidera DH building 4F, Oka, Fujiidera City, Osaka 583-0027, Japan

Ayako Hasegawa, Fumiko Kojima, Mio Ueda and Yoshiko Tanaka
Department of Nephrology, Shinjuku Ishikawa Clinic, Tokyo, Japan

Kosaku Nitta
Department of Medicine, Kidney Center, Tokyo Women's Medical University, 8-1 Kawada-cho, Shinjuku-ku, Tokyo 162-8666, Japan

Shigeru Nakai, Kazunori Kawaguchi, Kazuyoshi Sakai and Nobuya Kitaguchi
Faculty of Clinical Engineering Technology, Fujita Health University School of Health Sciences, Dengakugakubo 1-98, Kutsukake-cho, Toyoake, Aichi 470-1192, Japan

Kenji Wakai
Department of Preventive Medicine, Nagoya University Graduate School of Medicine, Tsurumai-cho 65, Showa-ku, Nagoya, Aichi 466-8550, Japan

Eiichiro Kanda
Department of Nephrology, Tokyo Kyosai Hospital, Nakameguro 2-3-8, Meguro-ku, Tokyo 153-8934, Japan

Toshiyuki Mochizuki and Kenichi Morihisa
Physical Therapy Service, Ibuki Clinic, 1-37 Kofuku-cho, Kadoma, Osaka 571-0066, Japan

Yoshimi Matsuo
Graduate School of Health and Sports Sciences, Mukogawa Women's University, 6-46 Ikebiraki, Nishinomiya, Hyogo 663-8558, Japan

Mayumi Sasaki
Nursing Department, Ibuki Clinic, 1-37 Kofuku-cho, Kadoma, Osaka 571-0066, Japan

Sakuyoshi Tabata
Department of Internal Medicine, Ibuki Clinic, 1-37 Kofuku-cho, Kadoma, Osaka 571-0066, Japan

Toyofumi Fukuda and Ibuki Yajima
Department of Urology, Ibuki Clinic, 1-37 Kofuku-cho, Kadoma, Osaka 571-0066, Japan

Naoko Takahashi, Taku Yoshizawa, Aiko Okubo and Junko Kumagai
Akane-Foundation Omachi Tsuchiya Clinic, 2-8-35 Omachi Higashi, Asa Minami-ku, Hiroshima 731-0124, Japan

Hideki Kawanishi and Shinichiro Tsuchiya
Department of Artificial Organs, Akane-Foundation, Tsuchiya General Hospital, Hiroshima, Japan

Misaki Moriishi
Akane-Foundation Nakajima Tsuchiya Clinic, Hiroshima, Japan

Takao Masaki
Department of Nephrology, Hiroshima University Hospital, Hiroshima, Japan

Toshiya Ebata
Chitofuna Dermatology Clinic, Tokyo, Japan

Eri Amano, Taro Horino, Satoshi Inotani, Tatsuki Matsumoto, Kazu Hamada-Ode, Yoshiko Shimamura, Kosuke Inoue and Yoshio Terada
Department of Endocrinology, Metabolism and Nephrology, Kochi Medical School, Kochi University, Kohasu, Oko-cho, Nankoku, Kochi 783-8505, Japan

Osamu Ichii
Laboratory of Anatomy, Department of Biomedical Sciences, Graduate School of Veterinary Medicine, Hokkaido University, Kita 18, Nishi 9, Kita-Ku, Sapporo 060-0818, Japan

Masayuki Tanemoto
Division of Nephrology, Department of Internal Medicine, 418-1 Kamihayami, Kuki, Saitama 346-8530, Japan

Yu Ishimoto, Yukio Kosako, Yukio Okazaki and Masayuki Tanemoto
Dialysis Unit, Shin-Kuki General Hospital, 418-1 Kamihayami, Kuki, Saitama 346-8530, Japan

Yoshimitsu Takahashi and Takashi Oite
Department of Clinical Engineering and Medical Technology, Faculty Medical Technology, Niigata University of Health and Welfare, 1398 Shimami-cho, Kita-ku, Niigata 950-3198, Japan

Ichiei Narita and Suguru Yamamoto
Division of Clinical Nephrology and Rheumatology, Niigata University Graduate School of Medical and Dental Sciences, Niigata, Japan

Junichiro J. Kazama
Department of Nephrology and Hypertension, Fukushima Medical University, Fukushima 951-8520, Japan

Yoshitaka Shimizu, Tatsu Fujiura and Hidetaka Wakabayashi
Department of Rehabilitation Medicine, Yokohama City University Medical Center, 4-57 Urafune-chou, Minami ward, Yokohama City 232-0024, Japan

Kinuko Dote and Nobuyuki Takahashi
Department of Medicine, Kori Hospital, Kansai Medical University, 8-45 Korihondori-cho, Neyagawa City, Osaka 572-8551, Japan

Tomoko Niki
Department of Laboratory Medicine, Kori Hospital, Kansai Medical University, Neyagawa City, Osaka, Japan

Tomoya Ishiguro
Department of Neurointervention, Osaka City General Hospital, Osaka City, Osaka, Japan

Ichiro Shiojima
Department of Internal Medicine, Kansai Medical University, Hirakata City, Osaka, Japan

Yoshiaki Tanaka, Haruki Uojima, Naohisa Wada, Kousuke Kubota, Hisashi Hidaka, Takahide Nakazawa and Wasaburo Koizumi
Department of Gastroenterology, Internal Medicine, Kitasato University School of Medicine, Sagamihara, Kanagawa, Japan

Yasuo Takeuchi, Togo Aoyama and Takanori Masaki
Department of Nephrology, Internal Medicine, Kitasato University School of Medicine, Sagamihara, Kanagawa, Japan

Ji Hyun Sung, Makoto Kako and Haruki Uojima
Department of Gastroenterology, Shonan Kamakura General Hospital, Kamakura, Kanagawa, Japan

Shuzo Kobayashi and Takayasu Ohtake
Department of Kidney Disease and Transplant Center, Shonan Kamakura General Hospital, Kamakura, Kanagawa, Japan

Tomoaki Fujikawa
Department of Gastroenterology, Shonan Fujisawa Tokushukai Hospital, Fujisawa, Kanagawa, Japan

Yasuhiro Yamanouchi
Department of Kidney Disease, Shinfuji Hospital, Fuji, Shizuoka, Japan

Akitaka Shibuya
Department of Healthcare Administration, Kitasato University School of Medicine, Sagamihara, Kanagawa, Japan

Shun Minatoguchi, Atsushi Nomura, Takahiro Imaizumi, Hideaki Shimizu and Yoshiro Fujita
Department of Nephrology, Chubu Rosai Hospital, Nagoya, Japan

Takaya Ozeki, Takahiro Imaizumi and Shun Minatoguchi
Department of Nephrology, Nagoya University Graduate School of Medicine, 65 Tsurumai-cho, Showa-ku, Nagoya 466-8550, Japan

Sho Sasaki
Division of Nephrology and Hypertension, St. Marianna University School of Medicine Hospital, Kawasaki, Japan

Takaya Ozeki
Department of Nephrology, Toyohashi Municipal Hospital, Toyohashi, Japan

Daisuke Uchida
Department of Nephrology and Hypertension, Kawasaki Municipal Tama Hospital, Kawasaki, Japan

Hiroo Kawarazaki
Department of Nephrology, Inagi Municipal Hospital, Tokyo, Japan

Fumihiko Sasai
Department of Nephrology, Showa University Fujigaoka Hospital, Yokohama, Japan

Keigo Tomita
Department of Nephrology, Iizuka Hospital, Iizuka, Japan

Chiharu Uno
Department of Nutrition, Sugiyama Hospital, 3-10 Yashirodai, Meito Ward, Nagoya, Aichi Prefecture 465-0092, Japan

Hidetaka Wakabayashi
Department of Rehabilitation Medicine, Yokohama City University Medical Center, 4-57 Urafune-chou, Minami Ward, Yokohama, Kanagawa Prefecture 232-0024, Japan

Keisuke Maeda
Palliative Care Center, Aichi Medical University, 1-1 Yazakokarimata, Nagakute, Aichi Prefecture 480-1195, Japan

Shinta Nishioka
Department of Clinical Nutrition and Food Service, Nagasaki Rehabilitation Hospital, 4-11 Ginya-machi, Nagasaki, Nagasaki Prefecture 850-0854, Japan

Kiyonori Ito, Susumu Ookawara, Mitsutoshi Shindo and Yoshiyuki Morishita
Division of Nephrology, First Department of Integrated Medicine, Saitama Medical Center, Jichi Medical University, 1-847 Amanuma-cho, Omiya-ku, Saitama 330-8503, Japan

Satoshi Kiryu, Mariko Fueki, Sojiro Imai and Takashi Hattori
Department of Clinical Engineering, Minami-Uonuma City Hospital, Niigata, Japan

Yukari Sugai and Noriko Wada
Department of Nursing, Minami-Uonuma City Hospital, Niigata, Japan

Kaoru Tabei and Yasushi Ohnishi
Department of Internal Medicine, Minami-Uonuma City Hospital, Niigata, Japan

Noriaki Iino
Department of Nephrology, Uonuma Institute of Community Medicine, Niigata University Medical and Dental Hospital, Minami-Uonuma, Niigata, Japan

Misa Miura, Aki Hirayama and Akihito Nishida
Faculty of Health Sciences, Tsukuba University of Technology, Kasuga 4-12-7, Tsukuba City, Ibaraki 305-8521, Japan

Shigeru Oowada
Asao Clinic, 1-8-10 Manpukuji, Asaoku, Kawasaki City, Kanagawa 215-0004, Japan

Chie Saito and Kunihiro Yamagata
Department of Nephrology, Faculty of Medicine, University of Tsukuba, 2-1-1 Amakubo, Tsukuba City, Ibaraki 305-8576, Japan

Osamu Ito
Department of Internal Medicine and Rehabilitation, Faculty of Medicine, Tohoku Medical and Pharmaceutical University, Komatushima 4-4-1, Aobaku, Sendai City, Miyagi 981-0905, Japan

Yo Hirayama
Hirayama Hospital, Hanamigawa1494−3, Hanamigawaku, Chiba City, Chiba 262-0046, Japan

Masahiro Kohzuki
Department of Internal Medicine and Rehabilitation Science, Tohoku University School of Medicine, 1-1 Seiryoumachi, Aobaku, Sendai City, Miyagi 980-8574, Japan

Shunsuke Yamada, Narihito Tatsumoto, Noriko Nakamura and Kosuke Masutani Takanari Kitazono and Kazuhiko Tsuruya
Department of Medicine and Clinical Science, Graduate School of Medical Sciences, Kyushu University, 3-1-1 Maidashi, Higashi-ku, Fukuoka 812-8582, Japan

Toshiro Maeda
Division of Nephrology, Maeda Hospital, 2742-1 Tachibana-cho, Imari, Saga 848-0027, Japan

Kazuhiko Tsuruya
Department of Integrated Therapy for Chronic Kidney Disease, Graduate School of Medical Sciences, Kyushu University, 3-1-1 Maidashi, Higashi-ku, Fukuoka 812-8582, Japan

Satoko Sakurai, Hideki Kato and Masaomi Nangaku
Division of Nephrology and Endocrinology, The University of Tokyo Graduate School of Medicine, Tokyo, Japan

Norio Hanafusa
Department of Blood Purification, Kidney Center Tokyo Women's Medical University, 8-1 Kawada-cho, Shinjuku-ku, Tokyo 162-8666, Japan

Shinji Iizaka
School of Nutrition, College of Nursing and Nutrition, Shukutoku University, Chiba, Japan

Ryoko Murayama
Department of Advanced Nursing Technology, The University of Tokyo Graduate School of Medicine, Tokyo, Japan

Index

CPSIA information can be obtained
at www.ICGtesting.com
Printed in the USA
LVHW060856030122
707669LV00002B/194

9 781639 272754